COVID-19

The SARS-CoV-2 virus, and the associated COVID-19 pandemic, is perhaps the greatest threat to life, and lifestyles, the world has known in more than a century. The scholarship included here provides critical insights into the institutional responses, communal consequences, cultural adaptations, and social politics that lie at the heart of this pandemic. This volume maps out the ways in which the pandemic has impacted (most often disproportionately) societies, the successes and failures of means used to combat the virus, and the considerations and future possibilities – both positive and negative – that lie ahead. While the pandemic has brought humanity together in some noteworthy ways, it has also laid bare many of the systemic inequalities that lie at the foundation of our global society. This volume is a significant step toward better understanding these impacts.

The work presented here represents a remarkable diversity and quality of impassioned scholarship and is a timely and critical advance in knowledge related to the pandemic. This volume and its companion, *COVID-19: Volume I: Global Pandemic, Societal Responses, Ideological Solutions*, are the result of the collaboration of more than 50 of the leading social scientists from across five continents. The breadth and depth of the scholarship is matched only by the intellectual and global scope of the contributors themselves. The insights presented here have much to offer not just to an understanding of the ongoing world of COVID-19, but also to helping us (re-)build, and better shape, the world beyond.

J. Michael Ryan, PhD, is an assistant professor of sociology at Nazarbayev University, Kazakhstan. He has previously held academic positions in Portugal, Egypt, Ecuador, and the United States of America. Before returning to academia, Dr. Ryan worked as a research methodologist at the National Center for Health Statistics in Washington, DC. He is the editor of multiple volumes, including *Trans Lives in a Globalizing World: Rights, Identities, and Politics* (Routledge 2020), *Core Concepts in Sociology* (Wiley 2019), and *Gender in the Middle East and North Africa: Contemporary Issues and Challenges* (Lynne-Rienner 2020).

COVID-19

Volume II: Social Consequences and Cultural Adaptations

Edited by J. Michael Ryan

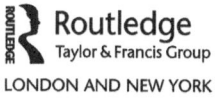

LONDON AND NEW YORK

First published 2021
by Routledge
2 Park Square, Milton Park, Abingdon, Oxon OX14 4RN

and by Routledge
52 Vanderbilt Avenue, New York, NY 10017

Routledge is an imprint of the Taylor & Francis Group, an informa business

British Library Cataloguing-in-Publication Data
A catalogue record for this book is available from the British Library

Library of Congress Cataloging-in-Publication Data
A catalog record for this book has been requested

ISBN: 978-0-367-69511-8 (hbk)
ISBN: 978-0-367-69512-5 (pbk)
ISBN: 978-1-003-14206-5 (ebk)

Typeset in Bembo
by Apex CoVantage, LLC

CONTENTS

FIGURES

TABLES

PREFACE

One of my principal concerns when bringing together these volumes has been that the scholarship contained within them might be out of date before they ever even come to print. Given the (un)usually lengthy times required to bring most academic work to ink, that is not an entirely uncommon concern, but given the rapidly changing pace of the current global situation, it is certainly one that has been amplified. I have attempted to mitigate that concern by allowing contributors opportunities to update up to the very last possible minute. More importantly, I have come to terms with the fact that no piece of printed scholarship, and even less so that dealing with contemporary public issues, can achieve such a goal. That said, I do not believe that a couple of out-of-date numbers or the absence of a few recently passed policies will greatly impact the sound academic scholarship presented in the chapters that follow. Instead, I believe the work here can serve as a foundational building block for the no-doubt litany of COVID-19 and pandemic related scholarship that is sure to be the focus of significant study and research for some time to come. These volumes are, in fact, quite cutting edge.

They were brought together with remarkable speed – from call to papers to final drafts in roughly four months. That is an incredibly tight time frame to bring together an academic volume, but particularly one containing the caliber of scholarship included here. To that end, I am eternally grateful to all of the contributors for their sound scholarly work, their careful attention to feedback and rapid responses, their general commitment to this project, and, more importantly, to doing their part to help us all better understand and combat this pandemic. I am also grateful to Routledge for their willingness to sponsor this project and for their flexibility and willingness to accelerate their end of the publication process in order to bring this important scholarship to light in time for it to (hopefully) make a difference. My editor, Rebecca Brennan, has been an especially enthusiastic supporter from the beginning, and credit is due to her as much as anyone for the ability to make these projects happen.

The world of COVID-19

The world ahead is uncertain. That is not new. What is new is that the contemporary cohort (and I do hope that remains singular) will be forever marked by the presence of the SARS-CoV-2 virus and the associated COVID-19 pandemic. The aim of this volume (in tandem with its companion volume) is to help map out the ways in which this pandemic has impacted (most often disproportionately) global society, the successes and failures of means used to combat the virus, and the considerations and future possibilities – both positive and negative – that lie ahead.

On an ethical level, my sincere hope is that the outstanding scholarship in these volumes will help individuals and societies, especially in a collective sense, to better understand the impact of COVID-19. While the medical understandings of the virus have taken center stage (and, to most degrees, rightfully so), there has been a general gap in understanding the social, cultural, economic, psychological, political, and other less-medical aspects. These volumes are an effort to help fill that gap.

On a professional level, my sincere hope is that these volumes will further demonstrate my commitment to public sociology and what I personally view as the purpose of social science – to better understand, inform, and improve society. I firmly believe that the academy has an obligation to provide research, insights, and understandings of the human condition, especially in times of crisis and rapid social change. These volumes are a response to that obligation.

On a personal level, I have been rewarded, indeed honored, by getting to work with some of the brightest, most highly motivated minds at work in the world today. Indeed, the contributions in these companion volumes are the result of a collaboration between more than 50 of the world's leading social scientists representing nearly a dozen countries from across five continents. They represent a truly global effort and the kinds of things communities can achieve when they work together. I have had the opportunity to engage in fascinating discussions with these scholars from across a wide range of disciplines and from around the world. I have been appreciative of that opportunity and look forward to future discussions with many of the brilliant minds and good-natured souls that I have met through this project well after the volumes are in print.

As a final note, I have been encouraged by the critical analyses, sharp insights, and timely scholarship presented in these volumes. Many present dark pictures of how the world was (not) prepared, reacted to, responded to, and administered the current pandemic, but it is only by walking through darkness that we can come to the light, and I personally feel a sense of optimism, though sometimes buried, in each and every one of these chapters. Rather than be solely depressed by the current situation, we should all find means to learn from it and inspiration to work together toward a brighter future. It has often been said that the only way to unite global humanity is to confront a common outside threat. Perhaps this is the one? The choice is ours. Let us make the right one.

With warmest wishes for better days ahead,

J. Michael Ryan
Nur-Sultan, Kazakhstan
August 2020

TIMELINE OF COVID-19

Timeline of COVID-19 Pandemic
J. Michael Ryan

The COVID-19 pandemic has impacted every country on the planet. As the most significant global pandemic to strike the human population in more than a century, it has wrought devastating effects on the vast majority of the world's population (though some, it should be noted, have profited quite generously from the global misery). With that in mind, it is difficult, nay, impossible, to construct a timeline that includes events considered significant to every individual, community, or country. The following timeline makes no such attempt. Instead, I have tried to include events that are either globally significant (e.g., announcements by the WHO) or at least representative of a global condition (e.g., lockdowns). I have also paid particular attention to events that are helpful in understanding the context of the various chapters presented in this volume. It should be noted that some of the dates listed might conflict with other reports, though usually by no more than a day in either direction. The reasons include differences in reporting (for example, there is no universal agreement on the number of cases reported in particular countries) and time zone differences (though I have made every attempt to list dates based on the point of origin of the event). Despite those considerations, this timeline does present the most comprehensive, global chronology of events yet compiled (or at least in publication) as of the time of writing.

Month	Date	Event
Nov	17, 2019	First unconfirmed case of COVID-19 traced back to Hubei province in China
Dec	31	The WHO reports that the People's Republic of China has alerted the organization to cases of pneumonia with an unknown cause in Wuhan City, Hubei Province.
Jan	1, 2020	Officials close the Huanan food market in Wuhan, suspected to be the source of the novel coronavirus
Jan	7	Chinese officials report that they have identified a new coronavirus
Jan	9	China reports the first confirmed case of a death related to the novel coronavirus
Jan	13	Thailand reports a case of novel coronavirus, the first reported outside of China
Jan	16	Japan reports a case of novel coronavirus, the second reported outside of China
Jan	20	The United States of America confirms its first case in Washington State
Jan	21	The WHO confirms human-to-human transmission of the virus
Jan	23	Wuhan is placed under quarantine
Jan	24	France reports three cases of novel coronavirus, the first reported in Europe
Jan	25	Australia, Canada, and Malaysia confirm their first cases
Jan	26	China becomes first country to close all schools and universities across the country
Jan	27	Germany, Cambodia, and Sri Lanka all confirm their first cases
Jan	27	The Bill & Melinda Gates Foundation commits their first $10 million USD to combat the virus
Jan	29	The United Arab Emirates report the first case in the Eastern Mediterranean region
Jan	30	India confirms its first case
Jan	30	WHO declares the COVID-19 outbreak a "public health emergency of international concern"
Jan	31	Russia, Spain, Sweden, Italy, and the UK all confirm their first cases
Feb	2	The first confirmed COVID-19 death outside of China is reported in the Philippines
Feb	3	China launches the first clinical trials into remdesivir for treating COVID-19
Feb	5	The Bill & Melinda Gates Foundation commits $100 million USD to combat the virus
Feb	6	The first death is reported in the USA
Feb	7	WHO announces a "severe global disruption" in the market for personal protective equipment
Feb	7	Li Wenliang, a doctor who initially tried to raise the alarm on COVID-19, dies – his death sparks a global outrage
Feb	8	WHO director-general Tedros Adhanom Ghebreyesus criticizes the levels of misinformation spreading around the virus, saying "we're not just battling the virus; we're also battling the trolls and conspiracy theorists that push misinformation and undermine the outbreak response"
Feb	8	Italy places the entire country under lockdown
Feb	9	The death toll for the novel coronavirus tops 800, now surpassing the death toll of SARS

Month	Date	Event
Feb	9	National University of Singapore announces that it will move all classes of 50 students or more online
Feb	10	The death toll for the novel coronavirus tops 900, now surpassing the death toll of MERS
Feb	10	The UK health department declares COVID-19 an "imminent threat"
Feb	11	WHO officially labels the novel coronavirus as COVID-19
Feb	11	The confirmed death toll tops 1,000
Feb	14	Egypt reports their first case, also the first in Africa
Feb	15	France reports the first death from COVID-19 outside of Asia
Feb	15	The UN's Food and Agricultural Organization raises alarms over record locust swarms threatening food supplies in Africa
Feb	19	Iran confirms its first case
Feb	21	Lebanon and Israel confirm their first cases
Feb	24	US biotech firm Moderna begins testing a potential vaccine
Feb	26	Brazil reports its first case, also the first in South America
Feb	26	For the first time there are more daily reported cases outside of China than inside of China
Feb	28	Mexico, Ireland, New Zealand, Nigeria, and Iceland all report their first cases
Feb	28	Stock markets worldwide report their largest single week decline in more than a decade
Mar	2	Portugal, Indonesia, Morocco, Saudi Arabia, and Senegal all report their first cases
Mar	3	Chile, Argentina, and Ukraine all report their first cases
Mar	4	Poland reports its first case
Mar	5	South Africa and Palestine report their first cases
Mar	6	Peru, Colombia, Slovakia, Cameroon, and Togo report their first cases
Mar	7	Confirmed global cases reach 100,000
Mar	8	Over 100 countries confirm cases of COVID-19
Mar	9	Poland joins a list of countries implementing a national ban on mass gatherings and nationwide closings of educational and cultural institutions
Mar	10	Harvard University announces it will suspend in-person classes and shift to online learning where possible
Mar	11	The WHO issues statement declaring COVID-19 a pandemic
Mar	11	Cuba, Honduras, and Turkey all confirm their first cases
Mar	12	A National Basketball Association (NBA) player tests positive for the virus and the league suspends play indefinitely. All other major US sports leagues quickly follow suit in the coming days.
Mar	12	Actor Tom Hanks and his wife Rita Wilson confirm they have tested positive for the virus
Mar	12	Broadway temporarily halts all shows
Mar	13	The USA declares COVID-19 a national emergency
Mar	13	Kazakhstan, Puerto Rico, and Kenya confirm their first cases
Mar	13	Sophie Trudeau, wife of Canadian prime minister Justin Trudeau, tests positive for the virus
Mar	14	Spain announces a nationwide lockdown
Mar	15	The European Union restricts exporting personal protective equipment outside of the EU

(*Continued*)

(Continued)

Month	Date	Event
Mar	15	The Union of European Football Associations (UEFA) postpones all Champions League and Europa League soccer matches indefinitely
Mar	16	Moderna becomes first company to kick off human trials of a potential vaccine
Mar	16	Walt Disney World temporarily closes due to the virus
Mar	17	The European Union bans most nonessential incoming travel
Mar	17	The University of Minnesota begins testing hydroxychloroquine, a well-known malaria treatment drug, in relation to COVID-19
Mar	17	The International Organization for Migration and the UN Refugee Agency temporarily suspend refugee resettlements
Mar	17	President Emmanuel Macron announces France will go into lockdown
Mar	18	Eurovision Song Contest, one of the world's most watched events, is cancelled for the first time in its 64-year history
Mar	18	Non-EU citizens are barred from entering the EU
Mar	19	California becomes the first state in the USA to issue a stay-at-home order
Mar	19	Wuhan reports no new daily cases for the first time since the pandemic began
Mar	19	The state of California announces lockdown measures
Mar	19	Netflix announces they will reduce their bandwidth in Europe for 30 days to help with crippling bandwidth overload as more people are home and streaming
Mar	20	Papua New Guinea, Cape Verde, and Madagascar report first confirmed cases
Mar	20	Cannes Film Festival is postponed for 2020
Mar	22	Opera legend Plácido Domingo tests positive for the virus
Mar	23	UN secretary-general António Guterres calls for a global ceasefire to help combat COVID-19
Mar	24	India announces nationwide lockdown
Mar	24	The Summer Olympics and Paralympics are officially postponed until July 2021
Mar	24	Ryanair, one of the largest carriers in Europe, announces that they will ground all flights until at least June
Mar	24	New Zealand introduces the bubble metaphor to help control the spread of the pandemic
Mar	25	74th Annual Tony Awards are postponed indefinitely
Mar	25	Etihad Airlines announces that they will be grounding all flights
Mar	25	Prince Charles tests positive for the virus
Mar	26	The USA becomes the country with the most reported confirmed infections
Mar	27	The United States Congress passes the CARES Act, the largest economic recovery package in history, providing for more than $2 trillion in COVID-19 relief
Mar	27	UK prime minister Boris Johnson tests positive for the virus
Mar	27	The International Monetary Fund (IMF) announces a global recession
Mar	28	Portugal announces that all foreigners will be treated as residents to ensure that they have treatment to healthcare and public services

Month	Date	Event
Mar	31	El Salvador announces their first COVID-related death
Apr	1	For the first time since WWII, the Wimbledon tennis tournament is cancelled
Apr	2	Confirmed global cases top 1 million
Apr	5	South Sudan reports its first confirmed case
Apr	7	Countries around the world have already pledged more than $4.5 trillion worth of emergency measure spending – Malta and Japan top the list in terms of spending as percentage of GDP, each over 20%
Apr	8	China lifts the lockdown on the city of Wuhan
Apr	10	Confirmed global death toll tops 100,000
Apr	10	Burning Man Festival cancelled for 2020
Apr	10	Pope Francis leads a Good Friday service in an empty St. Peter's Square
Apr	10	EU finance ministers agree to a 500-euro bailout for member countries who have been heavily impacted by the virus
Apr	15	The number of confirmed global cases passes 2 million
Apr	15	The first anti-shutdown protests in the USA are held in Lansing, Michigan. Trump praises the protestors, which helps to spur more such protests across the country.
Apr	15	The Bill & Melinda Gates Foundation increases funding to $250 million to combat the virus
Apr	16	The first reported case of COVID-19 is reported in Cox's Bazar, the world's largest refugee camp located in Bangladesh
Apr	16	Poland implements a nationwide face mask order
Apr	17	The "One World: Together at Home" concert, curated by Lady Gaga, takes place
Apr	20	NYC Gay Pride Parade, one of the world's largest, is cancelled for the first time in its 50-year history
Apr	20	US oil prices fell below zero for the first time in history
Apr	21	The number of confirmed global cases passes 2.5 million
Apr	21	Jeff Bezos, already the world's richest man, is reported to have made nearly $25 billion since the pandemic began, a number that would more than triple over the next three months amid crumbling economies and widespread unemployment
Apr	21	The World Food Programme announces that COVID-19 could double the number of people facing food crisis
Apr	21	The European Union issues aviation safety measures, including face mask requirements
Apr	22	The World Bank announces that global remittances could fall by almost 30% for 2020
Apr	22	The Papua New Guinea controller announces a new confirmed case in the Eastern Highlands Province, bringing the total confirmed number of cases in the country to eight
Apr	23	It is announced that newly popular web application Zoom has passed more than 300 million daily users
Apr	24	Trump suggests the possibility of injecting disinfectants to beat the virus
Apr	25	The global death toll passes 200,000
Apr	26	The city of Toronto announces that several hundred homeless people are being moved to hotels to help prevent the spread of the virus, a move becoming increasingly common in many countries

(Continued)

(Continued)

Month	Date	Event
Apr	27	The Los Angeles Lakers return their $4.6 million payroll protection bailout amid public outcry
Apr	28	The number of confirmed cases in the United States passes 1 million, the first country to reach that mark
Apr	28	As measles outbreaks appear in several countries, UNICEF issues statement warning about the negative impacts of children missing routine vaccinations
Apr	30	Russian prime minister Mikhail Mishustin tests positive for the virus
Apr	30	The Little League World Series (baseball) cancels its 2020 tournament
May	3	Italy reopens its borders to tourists
May	3	Clothing retailer J. Crew files for bankruptcy citing COVID-19 as a cause
May	5	Neil Ferguson, UK coronavirus advisor, resigns after violating the lockdown rules he helped to implement
May	5	Trump announces that the country's coronavirus task force will be phased out
May	8	The USA blocks a UN Security Resolution calling for a global ceasefire so that countries can focus on COVID-19 because they mention the WHO
May	8	United States Food and Drug Administration approves first at-home test for COVID-19 using saliva
May	8	US unemployment rate hits 14.7%, the highest levels since the Great Depression
May	9	South Korea sees a new outbreak of cases linked to nightclubs
May	10	The first case appears in Wuhan, China, in over a month
May	10	Avianca, the world's second oldest airline and one of the largest in Latin America, files for bankruptcy
May	14	The number of deaths globally passes 300,000
May	14	Pope Francis invites people of all faiths to pray together for an end to the virus
May	15	WHO announces links between COVID-19 and multisystem inflammatory syndrome in children and adolescents
May	15	A study finds that homelessness in the United States could increase by as much as 45%
May	18	United Nations secretary-general Antonio Guterres argues that the virus must be a "wake-up call" and that we must reshape our economies and societies to be fairer and more inclusive
May	19	A migrant worker in India is found dead after trying to walk home due to travel lockdowns; it will not be an isolated case
May	19	Cambridge University announces all classes to be online until summer 2021
May	20	Mount Everest becomes visible from Kathmandu for first time in decades amidst a radical drop in air pollution levels due to the lockdown
May	20	The Arab Coordination Group commits $10 billion to fight the virus
May	21	The number of confirmed cases globally passes 5 million
May	22	Confirmed cases on the African continent pass 100,000

Month	Date	Event
May	22	Executives at US biotech firm Moderna cash in over $30 million in stock as the company announces promising vaccine results
May	22	WHO announces that more than 80 million babies could be missing childhood vaccinations as a direct result of the pandemic
May	25	George Floyd, an African American man, is murdered by police in Minneapolis, setting off a wave of global protests against racial inequality
May	25	Brazilian president Jair Bolsonaro repeats his claim that COVID-19 is just a "little flu"
May	27	The death toll in the USA reaches 100,000
May	28	Tyson Food Plant in Iowa (USA) is shut down after an outbreak, launching a series of closures of meatpacking plants
May	28	Chinese president Xi Jinping, pledges $2 billion to help fight coronavirus during a meeting of the WHO
May	28	The Boston Marathon (which has earlier been postponed in April) is cancelled for 2020
May	29	Trump announces that the USA will be terminating their relationship with the WHO
May	29	Passengers on a flight to Lanzarote in Spain's Canary Islands are quarantined upon landing after a passenger received positive test results mid-flight
May	30	India announces an end to national lockdown
June	1	It is estimated that Elon Musk made more than $750 million in the last week alone
June	2	A new report finds that ethnic minorities in the UK are up to 50% more likely to die from COVID-19 than White people are
June	2	OECD announces an estimated 60% drop in international tourism during 2020 due to the virus
June	3	A new model suggests that stricter lockdowns are better for economies than longer-term more moderate ones
June	5	The WHO recommends that all people wear masks in public spaces
June	8	New Zealand is declared "virus free" after having no new reported cases for two weeks
June	8	The World Bank estimates the global economy could shrink by between 5% and 8% for 2020, and more than 90% of national global economies are expected to suffer
June	8	The World Bank estimates an additional 70 to 100 million could be pushed into extreme poverty (meaning living on less than $1.90 a day) as a direct result of the pandemic
June	8	Environmentalists raise the concern that there will soon be more masks than jellyfish in the Mediterranean due to improper waste disposal
June	10	Confirmed cases in the USA pass 2 million
June	15	France reopens borders with most EU and Schengen member countries
June	16	Peruvian president Martín Vizcarra refers to the virus as "the most serious crisis in our history"
June	16	It is announced that COVID related data in the United States will now be collected in part by a private technology firm rather than the CDC

(*Continued*)

(Continued)

Month	Date	Event
June	17	The WHO announces that further trials into hydroxychloroquine will be halted
June	17	President of Honduras, Juan Orlando Hernández, tests positive for the virus
June	18	President of Kazakhstan, Nursultan Nazarbayev, tests positive for the virus
June	19	The number of confirmed cases in Brazil reaches 1 million, the second country to hit that landmark
June	19	Confirmed global counts pass 250,000 new cases in a single day
June	21	Spain eases lockdown measures
June	21	Trump holds a political rally in Tulsa, OK, sparking political outrage for having a large gathering
June	21	Former Iraqi soccer star Ahmed Radhi dies from COVID-19
June	23	Tennis star Novak Djokovic tests positive for the virus
June	23	UNICEF predicts an additional 120 million children could be pushed into poverty in South Asia
June	24	South Africa announces launch of first vaccine trial in that country
June	25	The Centers for Disease Control and Prevention announce that the actual number of cases may be ten times higher than what is being counted
June	27	The New York Stock Exchange has returned to pre-COVID levels
June	28	Confirmed global cases reach 10 million
June	28	Confirmed global deaths reach 500,000
June	28	More than 100 influential world leaders issue a statement calling for any COVID-19 vaccine to be a global common good
June	29	Broadway announces they will remain closed through the end of 2020
June	29	WHO director-general says the pandemic is "not even close to being over"
July	1	Portugal begins welcoming tourists from 15 non-European countries for purposes of boosting their tourist industry
July	1	Tokyo Disney reopens to the public after having been closed for four months
July	2	Miami-Dade County issues a curfew to help curb the dramatic increase in cases there
July	3	The CDC announces an outbreak among college students who went on spring break vacations, one of many as a result of ignoring lockdown and safety measures
July	4	The Lleida province in northeastern Spain orders a new lockdown amidst a wave of new outbreaks there
July	5	Kazakhstan becomes the first country in the world to go back into full lockdown
July	6	Businesses in Washington State (USA) can no longer legally serve customers unless they are wearing a mask
July	6	A new report by the International AIDS Society suggests that efforts to combat COVID could cause more than 1 million extra deaths from other illnesses
July	6	Harvard University announces all fall 2020 instruction will be online

Month	Date	Event
July	7	Jair Bolsonaro, president of Brazil, tests positive for COVID-19
July	7	Serbia reintroduces lockdown measures after cases begin to spike
July	7	The European Commission predicts that the Eurozone economy will contract by more than 8% in 2020
July	8	Confirmed cases in the USA top 3 million
July	8	Brooks Brothers files for bankruptcy
July	8	Melbourne goes back into lockdown as cases there begin to surge again
July	8	Bolsonaro vetoes COVID-19-related protections for Brazil's Indigenous populations
July	9	Oxfam announces that more than 12,000 people could die a day from COVID-related hunger by the end of the year
July	10	WHO director-general says, "the greatest threat we now face is not the virus itself. Rather, it's the lack of leadership and solidarity at the global and national levels"
July	10	A bus driver in France who was beaten by passengers refusing to wear mandatory masks dies
July	11	Trump wears a mask in public for the first time since the pandemic began
July	12	Bollywood star Amitabh Bachchan tests positive for the virus
July	12	Massive protests erupt in Israel over the government's handling of the pandemic
July	13	Kazakhstan marks July 13th as a National Day of Mourning for COVID-19 victims
July	17	Confirmed cases in Brazil top 2 million
July	17	Confirmed cases in India top 1 million
July	20	Oxford announces promising results of a new vaccine trial; the UK has already ordered 100 million doses. There are already 24 vaccines in human trials around the world.
July	20	London witnesses another protest against the wearing of masks
July	20	The Dominican Republic declares a state of emergency amidst soaring number of cases
July	20	Venezuela returns to lockdown status as 20% of their total cases were reported in just the previous week
July	21	European Union leaders agree on a new 750 billion euro stimulus plan to help fund Europe's recovery from the virus
July	21	Trump announces that he will soon resume regular public briefings related to the virus, a practice he had discontinued since April, calling them "a waste of time"
July	21	Climate activist Greta Thunberg announces that she will donate 100,000 euros to combat the spread of COVID-19 in the Brazilian Amazon
July	21	The government of the Bahamas announces that they are banning travelers from the US and other countries where COVID-19 is surging
July	22	University of California Berkeley announces that all classes for the fall will be online
July	22	Confirmed global cases reach 15 million
July	22	A new study reports that as many as nearly one in four people in Delhi might have already contracted the virus

(Continued)

(Continued)

Month	Date	Event
July	22	Jeff Bezos, already the world's richest man, adds $13 billion to his wealth in a single day
July	23	Confirmed cases in the USA top 4 million
July	23	China announces $1 billion in loans to Latin America and the Caribbean for vaccine access
July	24	The Republican Party in the USA announces that their national convention will be cancelled
July	24	Uganda records its first coronavirus death; the country so far has just over 1,000 confirmed cases
July	24	Sao Paulo, Brazil, announces their legendary Carnival festivities will be postponed until at least May or June 2021
July	25	Emirates Airlines announces they will cover all medical expenses if a passenger catches COVID-19
July	25	Vietnam records its first locally transmitted case in 100 days
July	25	North Korea reports its first case, blaming it on a man reportedly returning from South Korea
July	26	India reports its single highest daily increase so far – nearly 50,000 cases
July	27	The first phase 3 vaccine trial begins in the USA
July	27	Tedros Adhanom Ghebreyesus, director-general of the WHO, says that coronavirus "has changed our world. It has brought people, communities and nations together, and driven them apart" and "it has shown what humans are capable of, both positively and negatively"
July	27	The Netherlands begins allowing "lovers" of citizens to enter the country recognizing that partner relationships are not always legal ones
July	27	Hong Kong makes it compulsory to wear masks in public
July	27	China reports its highest number of local COVID-19 infections since March
July	27	A Brazilian healthcare union representing more than 1 million workers files charges against President Bolsonaro of "crimes against humanity" for his response to the pandemic
July	27	Papua New Guinea confirms its first COVID-19-related death
July	28	A new report suggests that nearly 7 million more children could suffer from acute malnutrition as a direct result of the consequences of the pandemic
July	28	Bolivia declares a "state of public calamity" due to the financial impact of the virus
July	28	A new report from the UN World Tourism Organization states that the global tourism industry lost more than $320 billion between January and May
July	28	Colombia reports high daily increase in new cases since the beginning of the pandemic
July	29	Russia claims that they will approve the world's first COVID-19 vaccine and do so in less than two weeks
July	29	Hajj begins in Saudi Arabia with 1,000 pilgrims, rather than the usual 2 million

Month	Date	Event
July	30	The USA economy is reported to have shrunk at a 32.9% annual rate between April and June, the deepest decline since the government began keeping records in 1947. Meanwhile, Europe's economy shrank by 11.9%.
July	30	Amazon reports that sales have soared 40% in the three months ending June. Meanwhile, the number of people using Facebook, WhatsApp, and Instagram report a jump of 15%.
July	30	A new report suggests that just two weeks of physical distancing policies cut the spread of the virus by 65% globally
July	31	Vietnam records its first COVID-19 death
July	31	Hong Kong postpones Legislative Council elections
July	31	*The Lancet*, a leading medical journal, calls widespread false information related to the pandemic a threat to public health
Aug	1	A large demonstration takes place in Berlin to protest COVID-19 restrictions
Aug	2	Confirmed cases in South Africa top 500,000
Aug	2	Confirmed cases in the Philippines top 100,000, prompting President Rodrigo Duterte to reimpose stricter lockdowns on Manila
Aug	3	Retail legend Lord & Taylor files for bankruptcy
Aug	3	Mexico announces that school will begin with remote learning in the fall, a decision that impacts more than 30 million students
Aug	3	Portugal sees a 96% decline in overnight stays by foreigners in the month of June – tourism accounts for roughly 10% of Portugal's GDP; Spain also reports a 97.7% drop in tourism – tourism accounts for roughly 11% of Spain's GDP
Aug	4	Confirmed cases in Latin America and the Caribbean top 5 million
Aug	4	Virgin Atlantic files for bankruptcy
Aug	5	Kosovo prime minister Avdullah Hoti tests positive for the virus
Aug	5	The Indianapolis 500, one of the world's largest sporting events, says it will run without fans – before the pandemic expectations had been that more than 300,000 spectators would attend the event
Aug	5	Twitter temporarily restricts the Trump campaign's ability to tweet over false COVID-19 claims that children are "almost immune"; Facebook also took down similar posts
Aug	5	Kenya cancels the entire 2020–21 academic school year for students in pre-K through high school, a decision affecting more than 18 million students (colleges and universities will still hold classes, but will do so online until at least January 2021)
Aug	5	*Foreign Policy* magazine's COVID-19 Global Response Index ranks the USA 31st among 36 countries – New Zealand tops the list with the best response score
Aug	7	Confirmed cases in Africa top 1 million, more than half of those are located in South Africa
Aug	7	Confirmed cases in India pass 2 million – it took over six months to reach the first million, only 12 more days to reach 1.5 million, and only nine more days to reach 2 million
Aug	7	Italy extends COVID-19 safety measures through September
Aug	7	Ireland's prime minister Micheál Martin announces new regional lockdowns amidst rising number of cases in the country

(Continued)

(Continued)

Month	Date	Event
Aug	7	Howard University announces that classes will be entirely online for fall 2020
Aug	7	The US state of California tops more than 10,000 deaths related to COVID-19, more than in many individual countries, including more than twice as many as in China
Aug	9	Confirmed cases in Brazil top 3 million the same day that confirmed deaths top 100,000 in that country
Aug	9	Confirmed cases in the USA top 5 million – it took the country 99 days to reach 1 million cases, and only an additional 103 days to quintuple that number
Aug	10	Paris joins an increasingly long list of cities making masks compulsory at outdoor sites
Aug	10	Dr. Mike Ryan, executive director of the World Health Organization's Health Emergencies Programme, announces, "the virus is proving exceptionally difficult to stop"
Aug	10	Actor Antonio Banderas announces that he has tested positive for the virus
Aug	11	Employment in the UK fell by the biggest quarterly amount since 2009
Aug	11	Russia announces that they have approved the world's first COVID-19 vaccine, calling it Sputnik-V, and claims that some 20 countries have already requested more than a billion doses. As they have not released any scientific data related to the vaccine, many leading global health experts remain skeptical.
Aug	11	New Zealand records first locally transmitted cases in 102 days
Aug	11	The USA strikes a deal worth more than $1.5 billion to buy 100 million doses of COVID-19 vaccine from Moderna
Aug	12	Confirmed cases in Kazakhstan top 100,000
Aug	12	UK economic output shrank by more than 20% in the second quarter, the worst quarterly slump on record, and pushing that country into the deepest recession of any major global economy
Aug	12	Confirmed cases in the US state of Texas pass 500,000
Aug	12	It is announced that the Masters golf tournament will be held without spectators
Aug	12	Churchill Downs racetrack announces that the already delayed Kentucky Derby will be run with less than 15% of their regular attendance
Aug	12	A new report indicates that there was a 58% drop in the number of civilians killed or injured by explosives between April and July as compared to a year ago
Aug	12	Spain's Galicia region bans smoking in public places if physical distancing is not possible
Aug	12	A report by the WHO indicates that as many as 800 million children are not able to properly wash their hands at school
Aug	13	The WHO and IMF estimate that the global economy is losing more than $375 billion a month due to the pandemic. The cumulative loss is expected to top $12 trillion over two years.
Aug	13	Pharmaceutical company AstraZeneca signs an agreement with Mexico-based Slim Foundation to produce vaccine for the entirely of Latin America, minus Brazil

Month	Date	Event
Aug	13	A survey by the CDC found that more than 40% of respondents report struggling with additional mental health issues as a result of the pandemic
Aug	14	Columbia University becomes the latest to announce that all undergrad classes will be online
Aug	14	Confirmed cases in Peru and Mexico both top 500,000
Aug	15	California becomes first state in the USA to pass 600,000 cases
Aug	15	Mexico announces 30 days of national mourning to honor the country's COVID-19 victims
Aug	16	The confirmed death toll in India tops 50,000
Aug	16	New Zealand announces that their general election will be postponed for four weeks due to a renewed outbreak of the virus
Aug	16	Japan reports a 7.8% decline in GDP in the second quarter, the worst since modern recording started there in 1980
Aug	16	The number of confirmed cases in Bolivia tops 100,000 amidst protests over election postponement
Aug	17	Dr. Ashish Jha, director of the Harvard Global Health Institute, argues that the USA had the worst response to COVID-19 of any major country
Aug	17	COVID-19 is now the third leading cause of death in the USA, just behind heart disease and cancer but ahead of lung disease and diabetes
Aug	18	South Korea suspects in-person church services after an outbreak there is tied to a religious sect
Aug	18	The University of North Carolina Chapel Hill moves all classes to online after an outbreak among students. Many other universities are doing the same after significant outbreaks among students who have returned to campus.
Aug	18	Lebanon announces a renewed countrywide lockdown amidst a surge in confirmed cases
Aug	18	The Pan American Health Organization announces that despite having only 13% of the world's population, the Americas account for more than 64% of deaths related to COVID-19 globally
Aug	19	Apple becomes the first US corporation to top a net worth of more than $2 trillion. Their stock prices have doubled since March 2020.
Aug	19	The New York Police Department creates a special Asian Hate Crime Task Force in response to a marked increase in anti-Asian hate crimes during the pandemic
Aug	19	Confirmed cases in Colombia top 500,000
Aug	19	During a general audience, Pope Francis states, "On the one hand, it is imperative to find the cure for a small but terrible virus, which is bringing the whole world to its knees. On the other hand, we must cure a great virus, that of social injustice, inequality of opportunity, marginalization and lack of protection for the weakest."
Aug	20	Sweden records the highest death tally in 150 years in the first half of 2020
Aug	20	The Brazilian Congress overrules President Bolsonaro's veto and rules that masks are mandatory in indoor spaces. They also uphold the government's responsibilities to protect Indigenous peoples.

(*Continued*)

(Continued)

Month	Date	Event
Aug	20	The White House formally declares that teachers are essential workers, a move largely seen as a political attempt to resume and maintain in-person classes
Aug	21	WHO director-general states, "With more connectedness, the virus has a better chance of spreading . . . but at the same time, we also have technology to stop it, and the knowledge to stop it"
Aug	21	South Korea goes back into a stricter lockdown following a spike in cases
Aug	21	Paraguay announces social quarantine in the country's capital, Asunción, and its central region due to an increase in cases in that country
Aug	23	The FDA in the USA issues emergency use authorization for convalescent plasma for COVID-19 treatment
Aug	24	A 33-year-old man living in Hong Kong is the first person confirmed to have had COVID-19 twice; other confirmed cases of being infected twice follow in the days after
Aug	24	Olympic superstar Usain Bolt announces he has tested positive for COVID-19
Aug	24	Kentucky Fried Chicken suspends its famous "finger lickin' good" slogan due to coronavirus
Aug	25	Indian Institute of Technology Bombay uses avatars for virtual graduation ceremony
Aug	25	WHO announces that the pandemic is disrupting polio vaccination efforts in Africa
Aug	25	A survey from KPMG indicates that nearly 70% of large company CEO's plan to downsize their office space
Aug	26	Argentina's annual Tango World Championships begin virtually
Aug	27	Pew Research Center releases a report that shows the USA and UK ranking worst in terms of how their populations feel the government has handled the coronavirus; Denmark and Australia rank at the top of the list
Aug	28	Lord & Taylor, the first department store established in the USA, announces that it will be going out of business
Aug	28	Brazil's "paradise islands" reopen only to tourists who have already had COVID-19
Aug	29	Notting Hill Carnival begins in the UK, but only in virtual format
Aug	30	Nearly 40,000 people protest in the streets of Berlin against coronavirus restrictions
Aug	30	Global confirmed cases top 25 million with more than 840,000 confirmed deaths
Aug	31	Confirmed cases in the USA top 6 million with more than 180,000 confirmed deaths
Aug	31	An official report shows that the Indian economy shrank by 23.9% in the three months ending June, the fastest contraction on record for that country
Aug	31	The US Department of Health and Human Services offers a $250 million contract to a PR firm to "defeat despair and inspire hope" against the pandemic
Sept	1	Confirmed cases in Russia top 1 million cases with just over 17,000 confirmed deaths

Month	Date	Event
Sept	1	Zoom reports that their company's profits rose by nearly 3,300% compared to the same period one year ago
Sept	1	A recent survey by the World Economic Forum and Ipsos among 27 countries shows that 74% of adults would get a vaccine if available – the highest rate of support was 97% in China; the lowest rate of support was 54% in Russia
Sept	1	Spain reports that they had 75% tourists in July compared to a year ago
Sept	1	Brazil officially enters into recession with a 9.7% fall in GDP in the second quarter as compared to the first quarter
Sept	1	Elon Musk becomes the third richest person in the world. His personal wealth has increased more than $80 billion since the beginning of the pandemic.
Sept	2	Pope Francis holds his first public audience since March
Sept	2	Australia enters recession for the first time in nearly 30 years
Sept	2	The USA announces that they will not participate in an international effort to develop and distribute a vaccine because it is linked to the WHO
Sept	2	More than 570,000 healthcare workers across the Americas have been infected by the virus
Sept	2	The Moria refugee camps in Greece confirm their first case of COVID-19
Sept	3	Actor Dwayne "The Rock" Johnson announces that he and his family have tested positive for the virus
Sept	4	Confirmed cases in Brazil top 4 million with nearly 125,000 confirmed deaths
Sept	4	A recent WHO survey of 105 countries shows that 46% of those countries reported disruptions in malaria treatment and diagnosis
Sept	4	The WHO announces that COVID-19 deaths are likely undercounted at this time
Sept	4	WHO director-general Tedros Adhanom Ghebreyesus states, "the first priority must be to vaccinate some people in all countries, rather than all people in some countries," making the point that people, not countries, should be given priority when a vaccine becomes available
Sept	4	According to an article in *The Lancet*, Russia's COVID-19 vaccine generates an immune response
Sept	5	Confirmed cases in India top 4 million with nearly 70,000 confirmed deaths
Sept	7	Confirmed cases in Egypt top 100,000
Sept	7	Confirmed cases in Spain top 500,000, more than any other country in Western Europe
Sept	8	Nine of the leading vaccine makers announce a pledge to follow "high ethical standards" in vaccine development and release
Sept	8	Some World Cup–qualifying games are moved to 2021 because of the pandemic
Sept	9	Drug maker AstraZeneca pauses coronavirus vaccine trial after a volunteer comes down with an unexplained illness
Sept	9	A new report suggests that the USA undercounted coronavirus cases by as much as 90% and that there might have been over 6.4 million cases by as early as April 18

(*Continued*)

(Continued)

Month	Date	Event
Sept	12	Delhi's subway system reopens after having been closed for more than five months
Sept	13	Confirmed daily cases in France top 10,000 in a day, the highest count since the pandemic began
Sept	13	Confirmed daily cases globally reach 307,930, the highest 24-hour increase since the pandemic began
Sept	13	The Gates Foundation releases their annual Goalkeepers Report, which argues that the pandemic has set global progress back by "25 years in 25 weeks"
Sept	16	Confirmed cases in India top 5 million cases
Sept	16	A new analysis by UNICEF indicates that an additional 150 million children have been plunged into poverty as a result of the pandemic, bringing the total number of children living in multidimensional poverty to over 1.2 billion
Sept	17	India reports 97,894 new cases in a single day, the highest of any country since the pandemic began
Sept	17	Confirmed global cases top 30 million
Sept	18	Israel begins a second general lockdown amidst a surge in cases in that country
Sept	18	London announces that they are cancelling their New Year's Eve firework display
Sept	20	The Emmy Award ceremony takes place virtually
Sept	22	Confirmed COVID-19-related deaths in the USA top 200,000 (an average of more than 850 deaths per day since the first death was reported on February 6)
Sept	23	WHO director-general Tedros Adhanom Ghebreyesus states, "Just as COVID-19 has spread around the world, so too have rumors, untruths, and disinformation. And they can be just as dangerous."
Sept	23	The Metropolitan Opera cancels their 2020–21 season due to concerns about the pandemic
Sept	23	An announcement is made that New York City's Times Square annual New Year's Eve ball drop – one of the largest NYE celebrations in the world – will be virtual this year
Sept	25	Confirmed cases in the USA top 7 million
Sept	26	A new report reveals that fewer than 20% of Brits self-isolated after showing key COVID-19 symptoms
Sept	28	Confirmed cases in India top 6 million – it took six months for that country to reach 1 million cases but only two more months to reach 6 million cases
Sept	28	It is announced that the G20 Summit will be held virtually in November
Sept	28	New York State extends residential eviction protections through the end of the year
Sept	28	Confirmed COVID-19-related deaths top 1 million globally
Sept	30	India's vice president, M. Venkaiah Naidu, tests positive for COVID-19
Sept	30	A new report suggests that as many as 60 million people in India might have already contracted the virus
Oct	1	A new survey shows that more than 61% of households in the USA with children under 18 are dealing with increased financial hardship due to the pandemic, with 44% of households reporting spending all or most of their savings during the pandemic
Oct	1	A new study suggests that more than 500,000 additional girls are at risk of child marriage due to the pandemic

Month	Date	Event
Oct	1	Gavi, the Vaccine Alliance approves $150 million to help 92 low- and middle-income countries obtain and deliver a future vaccine
Oct	1	A report suggests that Trump was likely the largest driver of misinformation related to the COVID-19 pandemic
Oct	1	Global clothing retailer H&M announces that they will be closing 250 stores as a result of the pandemic
Oct	2	Donald and Melania Trump both announce having tested positive for the COVID-19 virus – a large number of people who work closely with Trump soon follow with confirmations of having tested positive
Oct	3	Confirmed COVID-19-related deaths in India top 100,000
Oct	3	Poland reports 2,367 new confirmed cases – the highest reported daily increase since the pandemic began
Oct	4	Pope Francis says that capitalism has failed during the pandemic
Oct	5	Confirmed global cases top 35 million – more than half of those cases are in the USA, India, and Brazil
Oct	6	A new report from the WHO suggests that as many as one in ten people on the planet might have already had the virus
Oct	7	The *New England Journal of Medicine* publishes an editorial condemning the Trump administration's response to the pandemic
Oct	7	Canada's weekly average of new COVID-19 cases reaches its highest levels since the pandemic began
Oct	7	More than 1,000 new cases are linked to a single garment factory in Sri Lanka
Oct	8	Confirmed cases in Brazil top 5 million with nearly 150,000 deaths
Oct	8	The World Bank releases a report indicating that as many as 115 million more people could be pushed into extreme poverty by the end of 2020, and as many as 150 million during 2021, as a result of the pandemic
Oct	8	The UK reports 17,540 new confirmed cases – the highest reported daily increase since the pandemic began
Oct	9	China officially joins the COVAX vaccine initiative
Oct	9	Broadway announces that all shows will be suspended through at least May 2021
Oct	9	The United Nations World Food Programme wins the 2020 Nobel Peace Prize in part because of their efforts to combat food scarcity during the pandemic
Oct	9	The WHO reports 350,766 new confirmed COVID-19 cases in a single day – the highest daily confirmed increase by that organization since the pandemic began
Oct	9	Canada reports 2,558 new confirmed daily cases – the highest reported daily increase since the pandemic began
Oct	10	France reports 26,896 new confirmed daily cases – the highest reported daily increase since the pandemic began
Oct	11	Confirmed cases in India top 7 million. The country maintains one of the lowest death rates in the world.
Oct	11	Confirmed death toll in Brazil tops 150,000
Oct	12	Confirmed cases in Latin America and the Caribbean top 10 million – with almost 370,000 confirmed deaths related to the virus
Oct	12	WHO director-general Ghebreyesus speaks out against a "herd immunity" approach as the primary way to control the virus citing, "letting COVID-19 circulate unchecked therefore means allowing unnecessary infections, suffering, and death"

(*Continued*)

(Continued)

Month	Date	Event
Oct	12	Chinese authorities in the town of Qingdao plan to perform 9 million tests on the population over the course of five days after a dozen new cases were reported in the city
Oct	12	Four members of the Swiss Guard, the elite guard that protect Pope Francis, have tested positive for the virus
Oct	12	Confirmed cases in Iran top 500,000 with just over 28,800 confirmed deaths related to the virus
Oct	12	Drug maker Johnson & Johnson pause their advanced clinical trial of a vaccine because of an "unexplained illness" in one of the volunteers
Oct	13	South Korea mandates the use of face masks at all crowded facilities
Oct	13	Fans are able to attend a Major League Baseball game in person for the first time since March
Oct	13	Russia reports 13,868 new confirmed cases – the highest reported daily increase since the pandemic began
Oct	13	Soccer star Cristiano Ronaldo tests positive for the virus
Oct	13	The New York Philharmonic cancels their entire season for the first time in history
Oct	14	A woman in the Netherlands dies after having caught the virus twice, the first reported reinfectiond death
Oct	14	Portuguese Prime Minister, Anotonio Costa, declares a "state of calamity" in that country because of the pandemic
Oct	16	Confirmed cases in the USA top 8 million, another 1 million cases were added in just the last three weeks
Oct	18	Slovakia's Prime Minister, Igor Matovic, announces plans to test every person in that country
Oct	18	Switzerland announces a nationwide mask mandate
Oct	19	Confirmed global cases top 40 million, with more than 1.1 million confirmed deaths as a result of the virus
Oct	19	China announces that their economy expanded by 4.9% from the July-to-September period as compared to one year ago
Oct	19	Portugal surpasses 100,000 confirmed cases though their death toll remains low at just 2,198
Oct	19	Confirmed cases in Argentina top 1 million
Oct	21	Confirmed cases in Spain top 1 million
Oct	21	The UK reports a highset single-day increase so far with 26,688 new confirmed cases; Italy also reports a new daily high with 16,079 cases
Oct	22	Confirmed cases in France top 1 million
Oct	22	The FDA approves Remdesivir as a treatment for hospitalized COVID-19 patients despite that a WHO study found that the drug does not help patients to survive or even recover faster
Oct	22	Macy's announces that Santa Claus will not visit their stores this year, breaking a 159 year old holiday tradition
Oct	23	Uruguay announces that they will close their borders over the summer season to help prevent the spread of the virus
Oct	23	Polish president Andrzej Duda tests positive for the virus
Oct	24	Confirmed cases in Colombia top 1 million
Oct	24	Feeding America, the largest hunger relief organization in the USA, announces that up to 54 million people in that country could soon face food insecurity, 17 million more than before the pandemic
Oct	25	Spain imposes a national nighttime curfew to help curb the spread of the virus
Oct	26	It is suggested that as many as 1 in 5 members of Russia's lower house of parliament have had or currently have COVID-19

Month	Date	Event
Oct	26	A new report suggests that 40-45% of people infected with the virus remain asymptomatic but may account for more than 50% of transmissions
Oct	27	Confirmed daily new cases globally top 500,000 for the first time since the pandemic began
Oct	27	Russia and Portugal both impose a nationwide mask mandate
Oct	27	The Czech Republic reports a record 15,663 new daily cases - it is currently the country with the highest reported cases per million in all of Europe
Oct	28	Confirmed cases in India top 8 million
Oct	28	Taiwan goes 200 straight days without recording any locally transmitted cases
Oct	30	Confirmed global cases top 45 million
Oct	30	Confirmed cases in the USA top 9 million, another 1 million cases were added in just the last two weeks
Oct	30	Confirmed cases in Japan top 100,000
Oct	30	Confirmed cases in Europe top 10 million, with more than 1.5 million cases reported in the last week alone
Oct	31	Confirmed cases in the UK top 1 million alongside an announcement of a new nationwide lockdown
Nov	1	Australia records zero new daily COVID-19 cases for the first time in 5 months
Nov	3	Hall of Fame quarterback John Elway tests positive for the virus
Nov	4	Denmark announces that they will cull all of the 17 million mink in the country in order to avoid the spread of a mutated form of the virus
Nov	4	Severeal European countries report new daily high case counts including Poland (27,143), Germany (19,900), and the Czech Republic (15,728)
Nov	4	The USA confirms 107,771 new daily cases, the first time any country has topped the 100,000 mark
Nov	5	Germany reports a record 21,506 new daily cases
Nov	6	France reports a record 60,486 new daily cases bringing the total to over 1.8 million; Russia also reports a record 20,582 new daily cases also bringing the total to nearly 1.8 million
Nov	6	White House Chief of Staff, Mark Meadows, tests positive for the virus
Nov	7	Joe Biden becomes the 46th president-elect in the USA and announces plans for a new coronavirus task force
Nov	7	Bosnian Prime Minister, Zoran Tegeitija, tests positive for the virus
Nov	7	Britain's Queen Elizabeth is seen in a face mask for the first time during a public ceremony
Nov	7	The USA confirms 126,742 new daily cases, the highest single day increase for any country since the pandemic began
Nov	8	As surges spike all over the world, there are now more than 50 million confirmed cases and more than 1.25 million confirmed deaths as a result of the virus
nd	nd	a successful vaccine is made available to the general public

NOTES ON THE CONTRIBUTORS

Toni Attard is the Founder and Director of Culture Venture, an arts advisory and management firm. He was the first Director of Strategy at Arts Council Malta and served as an advisor to the Ministry of Finance to co-author the Creative Economy Strategy and is one of the authors of Malta's national Cultural Policy. Toni is a regular speaker at international conferences and a visiting lecturer in arts management at the University of Malta. He is a founding member of Opening Doors, an NGO for the artistic development of adults with learning disabilities. Toni chaired the International Programming Advisory Committee for the 8th World Summit for Arts and Culture in Malaysia.

Donna J. Barbie earned a PhD from Emory University and is an associate dean of the College of Arts and Sciences and professor of humanities and communication at Embry-Riddle Aeronautical University in Daytona Beach, Florida. Publications in cultural studies include the monograph *The Making of Sacagawea: A Euro-American Legend*; a chapter concerning Tiger Woods in *Horsehide, Pigskin, Oval Tracks, and Apple Pie*; and two edited anthologies about sports, *The Tiger Woods Phenomenon* and *Athletes Breaking Bad*. She is an avid golfer and has attended golf tournaments around the globe.

Lee Millar Bidwell, Professor of Sociology, has been teaching at Longwood University since 1990. She received a BA in sociology and political science from Maryville College in 1984, and a master's degree (1986) and PhD (1991) from the University of Tennessee, Knoxville. She is the co-author of the textbook *Sociology of the Family: Investigating Family Issues*. Lee is a certified family life educator and specializes in teaching family classes. She is currently involved in a collaborative project designed to enhance parental engagement with children, and is conducting research on the value of project-based learning for undergraduate student learning.

Dinur Blum is a lecturer in the Department of Sociology at California State University, Los Angeles. He received his PhD from the University of California, Riverside. He researches the social causes of mass shootings in the United States (with Christian G. Jaworski) and is publishing a forthcoming book (working title: *School, Sports, or Sleep: Student-Athletes and the College Dilemma*) exploring obstacles student-athletes face to help them in school. Dinur co-hosts the *Learning Made Easier* podcast with Dr. Adam G. Sanford, offering effective learning and teaching techniques. He has been interviewed by various news outlets as an expert on mass shootings.

Pamela P. Chiang received her MSW and PhD from the University of Illinois at Urbana-Champaign. She is currently an associate professor of social work in the Department of Sociology, Anthropology, Criminology, and Social Work at Eastern Connecticut State University. She is passionate about empowering immigrants and their families in their access to services and equity in the United States, particularly those of Asian descent. Her research interests are centered on immigrants' mental health service use, immigrant families in the child welfare system, evidence-based pedagogies of macro practice, and culturally sensitive pedagogies in social work education.

Deborah J. Cohan, Associate Professor of Sociology at the University of South Carolina Beaufort, is the author of *Welcome to Wherever We Are: A Memoir of Family, Caregiving, and Redemption*. A public sociologist, she writes for *Psychology Today*, is a frequent contributor to *Inside Higher Ed*, and is regularly featured in national media including: CNN, MSN, *Teen Vogue*, *USA Today*, *US News & World Report*, *The New York Times*, *The Washington Post*, *The Chicago Tribune*, and *The Atlanta Journal-Constitution*. Deborah is trained in mindfulness and healing work and facilitates Deep River workshops.

Kristen Desjarlais-deKlerk is a public sociologist who teaches sociology full time at Medicine Hat College in Medicine Hat, Alberta. Her academic work has centered on health, stress, and social support with a focus on homelessness and housing. Before completing her doctoral work, she worked at a homeless shelter, and she maintains connections to homeless service agencies.

Jodie Dewey is a professor of sociology and director of the Criminal Justice Program at Concordia University Chicago. Her research interests mainly focus on how gender shapes institutional knowledge and practices used in the field of medicine, psychiatry, and the criminal justice system and how such processes regulate the daily lives of those most marginalized in society. Specifically, Jodie has studied and published on reintegration of the formerly incarcerated, medical and psychiatric decision-making of trans-identified patients seeking gender transition, and more recently, masculinity and the training of police recruits. This latter work informs her development of a certification in policing that connects academic theory with social justice principles and practices to students interested in working within the criminal justice system.

Scott T. Grether was born and raised in Asheville, North Carolina. He earned a PhD in sociology from North Carolina State University in 2018. His primary research interests are in exploring how gender, racial, and class inequalities are reproduced in varying social contexts. He explored this thread of research in recently co-authored projects examining how frames of colorblind racism are produced in film reviews and how HR professionals utilize social media and "googling" to screen job candidates. He's currently working on projects examining the relationship between social support and interracial divorce and how men experience and explain their involvement in housework and child care.

Nazneen Kane is Associate Professor of Sociology at Randolph-Macon College. She received her PhD in sociology and a graduate certificate in women's studies from the University of Maryland. Her research uses qualitative methods to examine intersections of race, class, and gender within US families. Currently, Nazneen is working on a research project that examines state-level maternal mortality review committees and the ways in which their policies and recommendations drive and/ or address practices of obstetric racism. Her recent scholarship can be read in *Contexts*, *Children & Society* and *Sociological Focus*.

John C. Lamothe earned a PhD from the University of Central Florida and is an associate professor of humanities and communication at Embry-Riddle Aeronautical University in Daytona Beach, Florida. He has written and spoken widely about a variety of issues related to athletics, including a chapter in *The Tiger Woods Phenomenon*. He is the co-editor of the anthology *Athletes Breaking Bad* and wrote two chapters for that work. His dissertation, being developed for publication, addresses how culture rhetorically constructs arguments about performance-enhancing technologies in sports.

Steven Master earned an MS from Northwestern University's Medill School of Journalism and is an associate professor of communication and humanities at Embry-Riddle Aeronautical University in Daytona Beach, Florida. Prior to his teaching career, he worked for 20 years as a sports writer for the *Daytona Beach News-Journal*, where he still contributes as a correspondent. His 2006 story commemorating the 40th anniversary of Jackie Robinson breaking baseball's color barrier earned a national award from the Associated Press Sports Writers. Steven also was previously a columnist for *NASCAR Illustrated* and published a chapter in both *The Tiger Woods Phenomenon* and *Athletes Breaking Bad*.

James K. Meeker is an assistant professor of sociology at University of Maryland Eastern Shore. Previously, James was a visiting assistant professor at Miami University, Oxford, Ohio. James graduated from Kent State University with a PhD in sociology in 2019, having been awarded the 2019 Lewis-Benson Outstanding Graduate Teaching Award, the 2018 Outstanding Doctoral Student Award, and the 2017 James E. Fleming Memorial Award in Theory. Currently, James's research investigates the relationship between inequality and cultural production, having most recently published an article examining the role of resistance and misrecognition in hip-hop music in *Critical Sociology*.

Heather L. Mello is a writing instructor at Nazarbayev University, Kazakhstan. She began her career as a military linguist and later earned a master's in sociology from Georgia Southern University and a PhD in linguistics from the University of Georgia. She has taught language and social science courses in academic and community settings in the USA and abroad and worked as a public health researcher and statistician for state and federal agencies. Heather served twice as a US Department of State English Language Fellow in Volga-region Russia. Her research interests include the sociology of language, heritage languages, and language variation.

Melissa A. Milkie is Professor and Graduate Chair of Sociology at the University of Toronto. An author of *Changing Rhythms of American Family Life*, her research centers on links among gender, work-family strains and well-being. With a unique focus on gendered culture, she identifies forces linked to mothering and fathering across time and region. Current projects include analyzing (1) paradoxes within families' time use; (2) trends, ethnic variations, and cross-cultural patterns of parents' paid and unpaid labor, and leisure time; (3) multi-level buffers of work-life conflicts, and (4) parental strains among Syrian refugee mothers. Her research has been supported by SSHRC-Canada and the US-NIH.

Monita H. Mungo, PhD, is an assistant professor in the Department of Sociology and Anthropology and the Associate Director of the First in the Family Center at the University of Toledo. Her research seeks to unearth and disperse the myriad of ways society marginalizes, oppresses, distorts, ignores, silences, destroys, appropriates, and commodifies the voices of people of color generally, and Black folks specifically. Her research interests focus on the inequities of access and success in higher education as well as teaching and learning policies and practices, racial inequality, critical race theory, and roots of social conflict.

JoEllen Pederson, Associate Professor of Sociology, has been teaching at Longwood University since 2013. She received a BA in sociology from Berea College in 2007, and a master's degree (2010) and PhD (2013) from Florida State University. Her research interests include cross-national welfare state comparisons, health care, and aging. In addition to research, JoEllen works with interdisciplinary groups of faculty and students to improve project-based learning with a service-learning focus resulting in multiple publications. She is presently engaged in a multi-year collaborative project focusing on improving parental involvement, as well as research on the health benefits of volunteering.

Marilyn Plumlee earned a PhD in linguistics from the University of Hawai'i. She has taught language and linguistics courses at both undergraduate and graduate levels at universities in the USA, South Korea, and Egypt. She is currently a faculty member of the Writing and Communication Studies program at Nazarbayev University in Kazakhstan. Marilyn served terms as the national president of the professional association of English language teachers in both Korea and Egypt. She has had leadership roles in internationalization projects in both academic institutions and private sector international educational exchange organizations. Her current research interests are in multilingualism, language sociology, and intercultural communication.

Lynnette Porter is a professor in the Humanities and Communication Department at Embry-Riddle Aeronautical University in Daytona Beach, Florida. She has authored or edited more than 20 books. Although she frequently analyzes themes within television series, her most recent publications document more personal concerns. Her memoir, *A Year in the Life of a "Dead" Woman: Living With Terminal Cancer*, describes, in part, her experiences and concerns with US health care. For a forthcoming book, she interviewed beekeepers in the US and Canada to better learn about protecting pollinators; her interviews returned her to her professional roots as a technical communicator.

J. Michael Ryan is an assistant professor of sociology at Nazarbayev University (Kazakhstan). He has previously held academic positions in Portugal, Egypt, Ecuador, and the United States of America. Before returning to academia, Michael worked as a research methodologist at the National Center for Health Statistics in Washington, DC. He is the editor of *Trans Lives in a Globalizing World: Rights, Identities, And Politics* (Routledge, 2020) and *Core Concepts in Sociology* (Wiley, 2019), and co-editor of multiple volumes including *Gender in the Middle East and North Africa: Contemporary Issues and Challenges* (with Helen Rizzo, 2020), *The Wiley-Blackwell Encyclopedia of Social Theory* (with Bryan Turner et al., 2018), and *The Concise Encyclopedia of Sociology* (with George Ritzer, 2011).

Daniel M. Ryu, PsyD, is currently completing a postdoctoral fellowship in the Palo Alto VA Health Care System. Daniel has a strong background in leadership and service in professional and institutional committees oriented toward LGBTQ+ well-being and access to care, including currently serving as a diversity committee member at the Palo Alto VA and previously in the LGBTQ+ Healthcare Equity Committee at the Cambridge Health Alliance/Harvard Medical School, and they co-chaired the Gender and Sexual Diversity Special Interest Group of the Association for Contextual Behavioral Science. Daniel's experience and clinical work is broadly inclusive and diversity focused, and they have experience conducting psychotherapy in both English and Spanish.

Adam G. Sanford, PhD (UC Riverside 2012), is a long-term lecturer in the Department of Sociology at California State University Dominguez Hills. His research focuses on legitimacy assignment, decision-making, viral ideas, and pedagogical methods. Past research centered on socioeconomic status and life expectancy (with Dr. David Swanson), student-athletes' assignments of legitimacy to coach and family demands (with Dr. Dinur Blum), and effective teaching methods. Adam's research interests include the sociology of education, criminology and deviance, pedagogy, social theory, and cognitive studies. He co-hosts the *Learning Made Easier* podcast with Dr. Dinur Blum and has been interviewed by the *Chronicle of Higher Education*.

Matthew D. Skinta, PhD, ABPP, is a board-certified clinical health psychologist and an assistant professor at Roosevelt University. His background is in integrated medical settings, HIV/AIDS-related work, and supervision and training. Matthew has specific clinical expertise working with sexual orientation and gender identity, HIV/AIDS, chronic pain, and chronic depression. His research interests are primarily focused on the interpersonal costs of minority stress upon sexual and gender minority (SGM) individuals. Past research has focused on the efficacy of clinical approaches that might promote vulnerability, acceptance, and self-compassion in ways that nurture social connections and promote health.

Stacy L. Smith, PhD (Kansas State University 2017), is a fixed-term assistant professor in the Department of Sociology at Michigan State University. Her research focuses on meaning making, identity creation, and social cohesion in marginalized groups. Her research on Deadheads (fans of the Grateful Dead) produced seven mechanisms responsible for social cohesion in that subculture. Currently, she seeks to use qualitative methods to understand the complex interaction between sublimated and realized identity among cosplayers. Her research interests include group behavior (subcultures and social movements), sociology of culture, social psychology, emotion, and pedagogy. Her work has also been featured in *Teaching Sociology*.

Angela H. Sun, MA, completed her BA in psychology at UC Berkeley and her MA in Chinese history at the Regional Studies – East Asia program at Harvard University before moving to and working in China for nine years. Her experiences as a first-generation immigrant to the USA and then as an American expatriate living in China have led her to be interested in identity issues and life transition. She is currently pursuing her doctorate in clinical psychology at Roosevelt University and plans to work with diverse and underserved communities in interdisciplinary healthcare settings in the US and abroad.

Magdalena Szaflarski, PhD, is an associate professor of sociology and scientist in medicine and public health at the University of Alabama at Birmingham. Her research interests include immigrant health, religion and HIV, and disparities in epilepsy care. Her most recent study examines health professionals' attitudes toward medical cannabis. Magdalena's research has been funded by the NIH, state agencies, and private organizations. She teaches graduate seminars in medical sociology, contemporary theory, sociology of mental health, global health, and healthcare delivery systems, as well as undergraduate courses in the sociology of mental health, globalization, and social change.

Valerie Visanich, PhD, is a senior lecturer at the Department of Sociology at the University of Malta. Her latest published work is her monograph entitled *Education, Individualization and Neoliberalism: Youth in Southern Europe* (Bloomsbury). She is a co-editor (with Victoria Alexander and Christopher Mathieu) of the forthcoming book series *The Sociology and Management of the Arts* (Routledge). She is one of the authors of Malta's national cultural policy and had occupied the position of chairperson within the European Sociological Association, Research Network Sociology of Art (RN02) between 2017 and 2019. Valerie is the co-founder and current board member of the Malta Sociological Association.

1

COVID-19

Social consequences and cultural adaptations

J. Michael Ryan

The SARS-CoV-2 virus, commonly referred to as COVID-19, is perhaps the greatest threat to life, and lifestyles, the world has known in more than a century. The first case of a "pneumonia with an unknown cause" was reported to the World Health Organization (WHO) by the Chinese authorities on December 31, 2019. The WHO declared COVID-19 a global pandemic some three months later on March 11, 2020 (though they had already labeled it a "public health emergency of international concern" as early as January 30). There are now few, if any, people on the planet that have not in some way been impacted either directly by the virus itself or by the series of lockdowns and preventative measures that have been put in place to control it. It is, with little argument, the pandemic that will mark a generation.

As of mid-October 2020, there were some 40 million confirmed cases of COVID-19 worldwide and more than 1 million confirmed deaths related to the virus. And while more than half of those cases are in just three countries – the USA, Brazil, and India – there is arguably no country on the planet that has not felt the major impacts of the pandemic. This has been the most widely responded to (emphasis on "responded to") global pandemic in generations.

From the time the first case was officially reported to the WHO, it took just over three months for there to be 100,000 confirmed cases of COVID-19 around the world (which happened on March 7); just 12 days to double that number (March 19); and just three more days to reach 300,000 (March 22). Less than two weeks later, confirmed cases topped 1 million (April 2) and less than two weeks after that they topped 2 million (April 15). Just over a month later cases had already reached 5 million (May 21), doubling to 10 million just 38 days later (on June 28), and doubling again to 20 million just 44 days after that (August 10). It took more time for the number of cases to climb from one to 100,000 than it did for them to climb from 10 million to 20 million. From another perspective, while it took more than 180 days to reach 10 million confirmed cases, it took just 44 more days to reach 20 million. The spread of the virus on a global level has undoubtedly been exponential rather than arithmetic.

No doubt by the time this volume appears in print, the numbers will be greater still. It is also important to note the key word of "confirmed," as it is certain that there have been far more cases, and far more deaths, directly related to COVID-19 than official numbers have captured. This is in part due to the ongoing global shortage of COVID-19 testing, the reluctance and/or inability of many counties to properly report accurate numbers (we have, in fact, seen the numbers of many countries increase as testing and reporting improved), and the nearly universal recommendation in light of shortages of testing, hospital accommodations, and other socio-medical deficiencies that those with mild symptoms stay home (thereby not allowing for inclusion in official tallies).

Perhaps more insightful of our status as a global human community than the reported numbers of cases and deaths has been the extreme variation in ways that different communities have responded to the crisis. In addition to being a global medical pandemic, COVID-19 has done much to reveal the ways in which we as human beings sharing a single planet view ourselves in terms of nation-states, races, ages, institutions, political ideologies, social classes, and, indeed, members of a shared humanity. While the pandemic has brought humanity together in some noteworthy ways, it has also laid bare many of the systemic inequalities that lay at the foundation of our global society.

The impact of the virus has spread well beyond the realm of the medical, also heavily affecting social, cultural, economic, political, and quotidian ways of living for nearly every human being on the planet. It has impacted not just the way we live today, but also the ways we will be able to live tomorrow. As a sociologist, I had initially placed calls for contributions to a volume on the sociology of COVID-19. Given the outpouring of interest from researchers across a broad range of fields, I later realized how short-sighted this call was to the humanitarian interests at hand and redirected the focus of the volume to a broader interest in all aspects of the causes and consequences of the virus, and, even more so, to the impact of responses to it. The great number of high-caliber proposals also prompted me to push for the creation of two separate, though highly interrelated, volumes in order to be able to help bring more of this high quality work to print.

This volume, *COVID-19: Social Consequences and Cultural Adaptations*, addresses issues related to institutional adaptations, communal consequences, cultural adaptations, and unveiling social inequalities. The chapters in this volume address such critical issues as the future of institutions of higher learning, local responses to a global pandemic, culture changes related to the call to utilize personal protective equipment, and the impact of the virus on racial, gender, and sexual minority populations.

The companion volume, *COVID-19: Global Pandemic, Societal Responses, Ideological Solutions*, addresses issues related to ethics and ideologies, exacerbating inequalities, and social responses to crisis. The chapters contained within that volume address such critical issues as poverty work amidst the pandemic, environmental impacts, changes in the understanding and application of key social scientific theoretical perspectives, and how the novelty of the virus has increasingly become accepted as commonplace.

Together, these two volumes represent a timely and critical advance in knowledge related to what many believe to be the greatest threat to global ways of being in more than a century. They represent the collaboration of some of the leading social scientists from across the globe, including sociologists, anthropologists, psychologists, political scientists, historians, economists, scholars of race and ethnicity, sex and gender, class and inequality, and the work of leading social activists and scholars committed to social justice. The scholarship in the two volumes represents contributions from nearly a dozen countries across five continents and includes contributions from many well-known, high-profile scholars (e.g., George Ritzer, Bryan Turner, Serena Nanda, and Melissa A. Milkie) as well as top-notch contributions from well-established and up-and-coming researchers from a variety of fields.

It is imperative that academics take their rightful place alongside medical professionals as the world attempts to figure out how to deal with the current global pandemic and how society might move forward in the future. These volumes represent a response to that imperative.

Introduction to chapters

In the second chapter of the volume, Ryan begins by highlighting the important distinction between SARS-CoV-2 as a virus and COVID-19 as a pandemic. He further highlights potential reasons why this particular virus and the associated pandemic are receiving such unprecedented attention. Ryan goes on to discuss the tenuous reasons why this pandemic might contain some silver linings, further unpacks a small portion of the reasons why this pandemic is inarguably a bad thing, and explores some of the as-yet unknowns related to the pandemic as it exists today. Ryan concludes with some thoughts as to potential future impacts and possible directions as to where we, as a global community, can go from here.

In the third chapter, "Rethinking What We Value: Pandemic Teaching and the Art of Letting Go," sociologist Deborah J. Cohan draws on themes gleaned from her memoir that was published less than a month before the pandemic put a chokehold on our lives. Reflecting on the central lessons from the memoir, she creatively uses these to make sense of the pitfalls, priorities, and possibilities of pedagogical shifts in pandemic teaching. As educators around the world seek to find not only new ways of doing their work, but new ways of finding meaning in doing so, Cohan's insights serve as a practical, moral, and therapeutic guide to teaching in the era of pandemic.

The sudden transition to online instruction mid-semester at traditional, residential colleges and universities due to the COVID-19 pandemic created unprecedented challenges for students and faculty. In Chapter 4, "Disruption and Difficulty: Student and Faculty Perceptions of the Transition to Online Instruction in the COVID-19 Pandemic," Lee Millar Bidwell and her co-authors draw on two sets of surveys distributed to faculty and students to analyze faculty and student perceptions and experiences of the abrupt move to online instruction. Their findings indicate that students and faculty agreed that the move to online instruction was necessary and that online learning is less effective than face-to-face instruction; however, they also indicate that faculty misjudged the degree to which students were concerned about balancing work, school, and family obligations and changes to course material. The authors conclude by recommending better emergency planning by and communication from university administrators as necessary to facilitate a more seamless response to unforeseen events.

Building on the aforementioned themes, Adam G. Sanford and his co-authors in Chapter 5, "Seeking Stability in Unstable Times: COVID-19 and the Bureaucratic Mindset," argue that as a bureaucracy, higher education is ill-suited to make rapid changes such as those demanded by COVID-19. They draw on the works of Weber, Lenski, Durkheim, Garfinkel, and Sanford to explain *bureaucraticity*, or the bureaucratic culture and mindset; how its norms of assembly, rules, rule-makers, rule-enforcers, and standards were disrupted by the onset of the international pandemic; and how some types of bureaucratic norms and actors worsened, rather than improved, institutional response to the pandemic. They conclude by suggesting avenues for further research into remedies for bureaucracies when confronted with unavoidable and sudden change, noting that novel problems demand nuanced solutions and that this creates a conflict for bureaucracies, where simple, rapid solutions are the default.

Policing has become a global health crisis. In Chapter 6, "The Solution Is the Problem: What a Pandemic Can Reveal About Policing," Jodie Dewey argues that though global pandemics and police-involved deaths appear to be separate problems, they become interconnected when the government transforms a health crisis into a criminal justice problem. Dewey further argues that the COVID-19 pandemic has revealed enduring health disparities among communities already experiencing the negative effects of aggressive police tactics and shows how protests against police violence and police responses to those protests both help further spread the virus.

During the COVID-19 pandemic, healthcare providers have made stay-at-home orders to help minimize the spread of the virus. This has been a particularly problematic public health intervention for those experiencing homelessness as well as those who provide services to the homeless. In Chapter 7, "Housing as Health Care: Mitigations of Homelessness During a Pandemic," Kristen Desjarlais-deKlerk examines the ways in which three different Canadian cities have responded to the needs of their unique homeless populations and the types of interventions they have enacted. In doing so, she highlights the importance of housing, demonstrates differences in responses, displays the types of risks identified, and cites the ways in which providers have advocated for clients experiencing homelessness.

In Chapter 8, "COVID-19 and Reproductive Injustice: The Implications of Birthing Restrictions During a Global Pandemic," Nazneen Kane draws on a reproductive justice framework to explore obstetric policy in the United States in the wake of COVID-19. Kane examines three core areas of the birth experience that are impacted by the pandemic – birth setting, birth support, and birth services – and explores the ways in which COVID-19 obstetric policies and practices heighten reproductive injustices and how these injustices map onto women's lives in differential ways. Kane's chapter further articulates the importance of considering the ways in which COVID-19 obstetric policies may result in higher rates of maternal mortality for birthing individuals of color.

In Chapter 9, "When Sports Stood Still: COVID-19 and the Lost Season," Donna J. Barbie and her co-authors argue that although sports cannot distract or unite us through a particular tragedy, their suspension does present an opportunity to examine their importance in our culture. They argue that such an opportunity offers a chance to observe how deeply, if at all, we feel the loss, how we manage to cope and work around it, what we are finding to fill the void, and how this unprecedented event might change sports or how we view them and their place in our lives.

In response to COVID-19, nations have implemented a variety of quarantine measures restricting the movement of their population in order to combat the plague. These restrictions to contain COVID-19 are, by and large, universally supported by the global scientific community and healthcare experts. However, in the United States, a series of movements have emerged to protest these quarantine restrictions. In Chapter 10, "The Political Nightmare of the Plague: The Ironic Resistance of Anti-Quarantine Protesters," James K. Meeker argues that these anti-quarantine movements are largely motivated by (a) anti-rational and (b) anti-governmental frames standing in contrast to the governmentality of the modern, rational state. Meeker further argues that the growth of these postmodern frames, as evidenced by quarantine protesters, suggests a political climate that is increasingly hostile to rational, scientific, and medical expertise. Rather than a surprise, therefore, it is consequently anticipated that public healthcare policies, such as implementing quarantines, shall be increasingly met with resistance and noncompliance.

Chapter 11, "Toxic Wild West Syndrome: Individual Rights vs. Community Needs" by Dinur Blum and colleagues, introduces the concept of Toxic Wild West Syndrome – the combination of performative rugged hyper-individualism, a weaponized display of strength, and nationalism framed as patriotism in the United States. The authors argue that citizen responses to COVID-19 have fallen into two general categories: prosocial/flexible and hyper-individualist/inflexible, and that while most people are prosocial: self-isolated, working "essential jobs," or sheltering in place, a highly visible and audible minority falls into the hyper-individualist category: assembling in public to protest public health directives, which disrupt their cherished norms. Although the prosocial response is a larger group, the hyper-individualist response is louder and more visible. The authors call for extensive research into methods of penetrating and mitigating this inflexibility in order to maximize the safety of the population during this and future crises.

Since the 1918 flu pandemic, wearing masks during illness has been uncommon in many parts of the world. With the spread of the COVID-19 virus, however, this practice has been changing. From discouragement to adoption and promotion, the rise of mask-wearing behaviors is an unusually rapid cultural practice change. In Chapter 12, "Innovation Diffusion, Social Capital, and Mask Mobilization: Culture Change During the COVID-19 Pandemic," Heather L. Mello applies a "diffusion of innovations" and "social capital" approach to recent mask mobilization and draws on content and corpus analysis methods to examine the role played by formal and informal social relationships in the adoption and diffusion of mask wearing as a pandemic preventive behavior. Mello argues that widespread mask making, organizing, and distribution, and their cascading communication through social networks, played a positive role in this change and further argues that contradictory messaging by social media networks and change agents played a negative role and contributed to anti-mask attitudes and practices.

The COVID-19 pandemic powerfully altered parents' time schedules and time pressures as their lives shifted in unique and unprecedented ways. In Chapter 13, "Changing Times: New Sources of Parenting Stress and the Shifting Meanings of Time With and for Children," Melissa A. Milkie shows how three central forms of parents' time during the pandemic – time parents spent *with* children, *for* children, and *toward safeguarding* children's futures – was upended. Milkie illustrates how the pandemic transformed these aspects of time, increasing parents' demands. Notably, the increased demands and pressures related to parental time varied by social class and gender. Looking toward the future, Milkie argues that there may be countervailing effects that lessen the blow of pandemic time stressors, as new meanings surrounding the value of spending time with and for children may develop among families and societies.

When home confinement protocols dramatically reduced face-to-face interaction opportunities as the SARS-CoV-2 virus spread around the globe in the spring of 2020, a group of young adult Deaf friends in Kazakhstan created an online WhatsApp group called "Antistress" where they began sharing information and providing mutual support. In Chapter 14, "Sites of Silence: Deaf Online Communication in the Time of Corona," Marilyn Plumlee draws on discourse analysis, augmented by the principles of the ethnography of communication, to analyze the communication within this group. Plumlee finds strong evidence of Deaf in-group solidarity and mutual psychological support as they dealt with pandemic-related uncertainties such as infection rates, lockdown measures, and government subsistence payments, in addition to the stress of extended confinement.

There is a limited understanding of how people in different sociocultural contexts have fared during the COVID-19 pandemic and how they have viewed their societies' responses. In Chapter 15, "People's Experiences and Attitudes During the COVID-19 Pandemic in the United States and Poland," Magdalena Szaflarski compares the perceived threat, governmental response, impacts, and experiences related to COVID-19 in the United States and Poland. Szaflarski finds that COVID-19 perceived threat and impacts (e.g., logistical, psychological) are generally lower in Poland than in the United States, but that views on government responses (e.g., lockdowns) were largely similar. She further finds that conservatives and moderates perceived the COVID-19 threat as lower than did liberals, and that women had a greater fear of the virus than men had.

During the current unprecedented times of uncertainty, workers with insecure income, including artists, are amongst those most prone to experience hardship. In Chapter 16, "Performing Precarity in Times of Uncertainty: The Implications of COVID-19 on Artists in Malta," Valerie Visanich and Toni Attard tackle the shared concerns of artists during the pandemic, particularly on the disruption of their everyday life and their experienced financial loss. The authors draw on a survey addressed to artists in Malta to inform various recommendations, specifically to secure the right for equitable income for artists.

Since the mass outbreak of COVID-19 began, racist attacks, harassment, and hate speech towards people of Asian descent have drastically increased in many parts of the world. In Chapter 17, "Anti-Asian Racism, Responses, and the Impact on Asian Americans' Lives: A Social-Ecological Perspective," Pamela P. Chiang draws on a wide survey sample of adults of Asian descent living in the United States to better understand anti-Asian racism and discrimination experienced by Asians and Asian Americans, their responses to it, and the impact that it has had on their lives during the pandemic. Chiang's chapter also examines approaches that governments and nongovernmental organizations have taken with regard to the rise of anti-Asian racism amid the pandemic.

The COVID-19 pandemic has upended many aspects of daily life across the globe, though orders to shelter in place and fears about the spread of the virus have had a disparate impact on many minority communities. In Chapter 18, "The Impact of COVID-19 on the Lives of Sexual and Gender Minority People," Matthew D. Skinta and colleagues argue that sexual and gender minority peoples have served as a lightning rod for political and religious scapegoating during this era, and increased discriminatory acts against their communities have occurred globally. The authors explore some of the forms of bias that have been amplified by the COVID-19 pandemic, in both the type of actions ostensibly intended to prevent the spread of the virus and the more common phenomena of preexisting sites of discrimination becoming amplified within the context of a pandemic.

The spread of the SARS-CoV-2 virus has bewildered scientists and medical experts as well as the politicians and public officials whom they advise. Because the virus behaves in ways that are novel, its current, short-term, and long-term health effects are only beginning to be discovered. This is also true of the social impact of the virus. In Chapter 19, "Violence, Virus, and Vitriol: The Tale of COVID-19," Monita H. Mungo argues that measures taken, and measures *not* taken, to restrict the spread of the virus have disparate effects on lower socioeconomic groups. Not only is the current pandemic highlighting stark social inequalities, it is also illuminating numerous problems in social infrastructure. Mungo argues that the spread of the virus and the United States' governmental response provides an ongoing case illustrating the concept of structural violence and its grave consequences.

During parts of 2020, many US states issued stay-at-home or quarantine orders for everyone not performing "essential services," as defined by the state. High-risk seniors, as defined by the Centers for Disease Control, were highly recommended to stay indoors and have no contact with anyone other than those with whom they live. In Chapter 20, "High Risk or Low Worth? A Few Practical and Philosophical COVID-19 Issues Surrounding the Isolation of High-Risk Senior Women," Lynnette Porter provides a highly thoughtful analysis about social isolation and loneliness. She further explores questions about the worth and value of high-risk senior women to society and offers valuable insights into life for these women during the pandemic.

Some concluding remarks

The concept of "syndemic" has become increasingly popular during the COVID-19 era. The idea of a syndemic analysis implies examining not only the health consequences of disease interactions but also how they interact with the social, cultural, economic, political, and environmental factors that promote, and worsen, disease. As the chapters in this volume demonstrate, perhaps more than a "pandemic," COVID-19 is better thought of as a "syndemic." The tenuous differentiation between health and society has perhaps never been so fraught.

Environmentalists and epidemiologists – two professions finding increasing contact points recently – agree that this is unlikely to be the last great global pandemic. In fact, as human beings increasingly encroach on our natural habitat, thereby increasing our exposure to "hidden" diseases, such pandemics are largely predicted to become increasingly likely. More than a snapshot in time, the current pandemic speaks to what is likely to become the beginning of a new era in global human–virus relations.

As is evident in the introduction to the chapters, this volume (along with its companion) brings together a remarkable diversity and quality of impassioned scholarship. The contributors included in these pages have contributed novel analysis, insights, and theoretical perspectives that have much to offer not just to an understanding of the ongoing world of COVID-19, but also to helping us (re-)build, and better shape, the world beyond.

2

THE SARS-COV-2 VIRUS AND THE COVID-19 PANDEMIC

J. Michael Ryan

It is important from the outset to distinguish between a virus and a social response to a pandemic. Someone dying due to infection from SARS-CoV-2 is the result of a virus. Someone dying due to starvation or disruption of a global medical supply chain, or as a result of their own hand because of exacerbated mental health issues related to confinement, is the result of a response to the COVID-19 pandemic. I will further discuss these differences later, but it is important to note from the outset the importance of distinguishing a virus from a social response to a pandemic in order to better understand how to combat both.

We also need to consider connectedness. In a territorial sense, the current pandemic has highlighted both the magnitude and the diversity/variety of transglobal connections. Environmentalists and anti-nuclear activists have been making this claim for decades, but the current pandemic, and its rapid global spread, has made that claim all the more difficult to ignore. It has also highlighted the interconnectedness between various social systems, on local, regional, national, and global levels. For example, the virus is a medical issue, but one that has had profound impacts on the connected areas of education, housing, employment, discrimination, food security, and religion, to name but just a few.

This chapter will begin by highlighting the important distinction between SARS-CoV-2 as a virus and COVID-19 as a pandemic. It will also highlight potential reasons why this particular virus and the associated pandemic are receiving unprecedented attention. I will then discuss the tenuous reasons why this pandemic might contain some silver linings, further unpack a small portion of the reasons why this pandemic is inarguably a bad thing, and explore some of the as-yet unknowns related to the pandemic as it exists today. The chapter will conclude with some thoughts as to potential future impacts and possible directions as to where we, as a global community, can go from here.

The SARS-CoV-2 virus and the COVID-19 pandemic

It is important to distinguish between the SARS-CoV-2 virus, the virus responsible for causing the disease more commonly labeled as COVID-19, and broader references to the COVID-19 pandemic. A virus is an entity (whether it is alive is still highly debated – see Astorino and Nicola 2021) that infects living organisms. It requires a host to survive and reproduce. The term "pandemic," on the other hand, refers to the outbreak, occurrence, and spread of a particular disease. In that sense, it has a much more prominent social connotation. There is a clear overlap, but there are also important distinctions. Medical doctors, for example, are primarily responding to the SARS-CoV-2 virus, while politicians, economists, and social scientists are primarily responding to the COVID-19 pandemic.

One way of better understanding the relationship between medical and social factors is to understand the difference between contagion issues and systemic issues. Contagion refers to how likely something is to spread, how easily it spreads, and how quickly it spreads. We can think of the SARS-Cov-2 virus as something that is contagious. A systemic issue refers to something that is an underlying factor in how societies operate, is widespread, and is part of a broader system. We can think of issues of inequality and discrimination as systemic. However, one thing that the COVID-19 pandemic has made clear is that these are not separate issues. In fact, we have clear evidence that systemic issues have directly informed many aspects of contagion – for example, how closely together people live, the type of employment one is/was engaged in, access to information and medical care (whose own unique relationship to each other has also become increasingly clear in recent months), and one's racial and ethnic heritage have all become predictors of one's likelihood of contracting, and spreading, the virus. While medical doctors have historically focused primarily on issues of contagion, social scientists have historically focused primarily on more systemic issues. The COVID-19 pandemic has highlighted the value of both areas of focus, as well as the need for a conversation between the two.

The direct deaths from the SARS-CoV-2 virus have already surpassed those of the number of people killed in a number of major recent wars and conflicts (I will refrain from listing specifics, as those sorts of death tolls are often highly controversial). The loss of so much life is not a thing that can, or should, be taken lightly. That said, the death toll from COVID-19 still pales in comparison to that of a number of other causes. For example, while the virus has already led to the death of more than 1 million people as of mid-October 2020, that is still far below the number of people who died of other diseases in 2019, including diarrheal diseases (roughly 1.4 million), tuberculosis (TB) (roughly 1.5 million), diabetes (roughly 1.6 million), and respiratory cancers (roughly 1.7 million). These are but a few of the arguably highly treatable conditions that not only cause the deaths of millions every year but, more to the argument at hand, millions more than COVID-19. Perhaps most egregiously, global hunger and starvation, issues sure to be exacerbated by current pandemic responses, kill an estimated more than 25,000 people every day. In other words, more people die in a single month due to lack of food than died in the first eight months of the COVID-19 pandemic.

So why has COVID-19 caught the attention of the global community, and the lives of nearly everyone living in it, to such a greater degree than other leading killers whose death tolls are substantially higher? One reason certainly has to do with novelty. The virus is new – in fact, it is sometimes referred to as the "novel" coronavirus – and what is new tends to get more attention. Few would argue that if the virus should persist for many years to come (and many think that it will in some capacity), it would continue to receive the kind of unprecedented global attention that it has. Another factor is that it is dramatic. As the cases of 9/11, Hurricane Katrina, and the sinking of the Titanic highlight, sometimes it is not the death toll but the far-reaching social impact that matters most.

Some might also point to the fact that unlike many of the leading global killers, SARS-CoV-2 is also infecting the relative global elite – the types of people who worry about international jet travel, have no worry of starvation, and have access to medical care to mitigate the other (largely preventable) global infectious killers. For example, when I travel to places with a risk of malarial infection, I simply visit my travel clinic, get the appropriate preventative medicines, and jet off. It is not ironic that the same drug used to treat malaria was suddenly mass-produced to potentially treat COVID-19 (something now discouraged by all leading global medical authorities, even if still defended by the likes of United States president Donald Trump and Brazilian president Jair Bolsonaro). Why was this medicine not produced in 2019 when the year before there were more than 228 million cases of malaria and more than 400,000 deaths as a result of it? Why are millions of doses of this same medication now sitting in storage (for example, Brazil has more than 2 million doses, shipped to them by the USA, sitting in storage [Walsh et al. 2020]), yet hundreds of thousands will still die of malaria this year because they cannot get access to it? Is it because those who die of malaria are overwhelmingly poor and Brown? Is it something else? These are important questions to ask, and their answers could almost certainly lend credence to the arguments of many as to why COVID is getting more attention.

Another potential argument is that COVID-19 is serving as a perfect distraction while many of the world's ultra-rich are getting ultra-richer (for example, Jeff Bezos, Elon Musk, and Mark Zuckerberg – three white men all living in the USA – increased their combined wealth by nearly $200 billion during the first 9 months of the pandemic while the world's billionaires saw their wealth increase by more than 25% during the same time), many of the world's political elite are deflecting from controversies and passing personal agendas (for example, Viktor Orbán in Hungary and Narendra Modi in India), and many of the right-wing groups propping up many of the powers-that-be are seeing a resurgence in their rolls. The ensuing disruption (of the pandemic) to nearly all aspects of our lives has also given politicians newfound reasons to blame each other – nationalists touting anti-immigrant and regionalist arguments, a "reason they were right," and employers a rationale for thinning their work forces. COVID-19 has certainly been a "distraction," and one from which many have clearly benefitted.

The aforementioned potential arguments aside, there are also very real, medically confirmed, scientifically valid reasons COVID-19 should be receiving such potentially disproportionate attention. For one, it is far more easily transmitted than are most infectious diseases, including the seasonal flu to which it is most often (erroneously) compared. It also has an unusually long incubation period and, more egregiously, can be spread by asymptomatic carriers. In fact, it is highly likely that the greatest spreaders of the virus are those who do not even realize that they are infected. COVID-19 has also a range of nasty side effects, many of which we are just beginning to understand, none of which we know the long-term effects of. It also has a higher fatality rate than the seasonal flu, so while far more people are infected with the flu each year (roughly 800 million), a much lower percentage of those infected will die because of it. Perhaps most pointedly, one reason COVID-19 is getting such attention is exactly that we know so very little about it. It is indeed "novel," and the fear of the unknown is often the most powerful fear of all.

To connect the social arguments with the medical ones, one reason COVID-19 has been, and should be, receiving this kind of attention – and the fundamental rationale behind these volumes – is that its impacts extend far beyond the realm of the medical and the scientific (Ryan 2021b). The *SARS-CoV-2 virus* has led to the death of more than one million people and infected tens of millions more, but the *COVID-19 pandemic* has arguably done far worse comparative damage. The latter has also led to radical impacts on the economy, disruptions of global supply chains, including those of basic medical and essential supplies, the lockdown of billions, government expenditures in the multiple trillions, and attention diverted from addressing other social ills. In other words, while the virus is a negative force unto itself, the pandemic has become an amplifier of already existing social ills to a far greater degree than other viruses or pandemics have been in living human memory. With all due respect for the existing death toll, it is the latter that may be of the greatest social significance, especially for the future of a shared, increasingly interconnected humanity.

The good(?), the bad, and the unknowns of the COVID-19 pandemic

The good

It might seem odd to speak of the good coming out of such a widespread and deadly pandemic and yet there have been some positive effects. Most notably, the environment has been a clear (perhaps only?) winner since the pandemic began (see counter-arguments to this later). A worldwide reduction in travel by pollution-emitting forms has led to a dramatic decrease in air pollution levels in most parts of the world. In China, for example, the world's most air polluted country, there was at least a 25% reduction in carbon emissions and at least a 50% reduction in nitrogen oxides emissions. One scientist predicted that just two months of such reductions led to a reduction of more than 77,000 premature deaths from air pollution in China alone (Burke 2020). Those numbers are undoubtedly much higher by the time of writing and when calculated on a global level. A Carbon Brief analysis further suggests, "the coronavirus crisis could trigger the largest ever annual fall in CO_2 emissions in 2020, more than during any previous economic crisis or period of war" (Evans 2020). On a purely aesthetic, yet telling, level, Mount Everest became visible from Kathmandu, Nepal, for the first time in living memory due to a drop in air pollution.

The other "good" aspects of the pandemic are much more personally based, biased, and questionable when taken from the perspective of the social good. For example, while millions lost their jobs, investors in a number of companies (e.g., Facebook, Amazon, Nintendo, Zoom) and industries (e.g., pharmaceuticals) saw their investments soar. Those supporting anti-immigration and anti-asylum policies have no doubt been pleased. And staunch supporters of particular political leaders have no doubt been happy to see them be able to enforce their policies at will without democratic checks and balances.

The bad

As Ryan (2021c, this volume) notes, the negative impacts of the virus have been more far-reaching than simply infection and death toll counts. As the COVID-19 pandemic continues to ravage the world, its people, and its economies, a number of long-standing inequalities are becoming even more pronounced (Nanda 2021). For a brief time, stock markets fell, and then they soared. Unemployment just soared. Billionaires lost spare change, and then made fortunes. Essential workers just lost life and livelihood. The global elite flew off to private islands or sheltered in place in summer homes. The global poor just crowded into hovels, if they even had a hovel to crowd into. The current pandemic is indeed impacting different populations unequally, with the greatest tolls being felt among the already underprivileged.

The number of indirect deaths from the pandemic is not one that has yet been calculated but will no doubt far outstrip the number of direct deaths as tolls are taken into account from multiple factors including increased starvation, lack of access to medication due to disruptions in supply chains, suicides, victims of domestic violence, future deaths from viral complications, and victims of related hate crimes, among others. Further, as individuals who lost income had to spend money intended for medications on items like food, overall inequality levels have widened/are widening, which is a well-known predictor of premature deaths, and as pharmaceutical industries have halted research and production on treatments of other diseases, deaths from those causes will also rise.

The death toll from these interruptions in research, treatment, and attention to other leading global killers as a result of the COVID-19 pandemic is expected to far exceed those of direct deaths from the SARS-CoV-2 virus. For example, a report by the Stop TB Partnership (2020), published in May 2020, estimated that cases of TB in 2020–2025 could increase by more than 600,000 for every month of lockdown and more than 400,000 for every month of restoration. This translates to excess deaths from TB during the same period of more than 125,000 for every month of lockdown and more than 80,000 for every month of restoration. The numbers are staggering. A projection from the WHO and UNAIDS (2020) has further projected that a six-month disruption of treatment of HIV/AIDS could result in an excess number of deaths from complications of that virus of between 471,000 and 673,000 in sub-Saharan Africa alone. They further projected that such a disruption could result in a more than a 100% increase in mother-to-child infections in Uganda alone. Moreover, a report from The Global Fund (2020) has estimated that if healthcare systems collapse or treatment and prevention services are interrupted, the death toll from HIV, TB, and malaria could double over the next year.

Governments around the world have spent many trillions of dollars on research and response related to the COVID-19 pandemic. The USA alone has spent more than $2 trillion, most notably under the CARES Act. The European Union has also invested nearly $1 trillion. All of this has been allotted within roughly six months of the outbreak of the pandemic. These numbers are worth comparing to the investment in other global diseases as a means of understanding the increased attention being paid to COVID-19 vis-à-vis other global killers. For example, between 2000 and 2015, only just over $560 billion was spent on HIV/AIDS research combined, a number that has been declining since 2013 (IHME 2018). HIV/AIDS has already killed more than 33 million people. Global spending on malaria totaled just over $4 billion in 2016, roughly 2/3 of the target set by the WHO (IHME 2019). Malaria kills between 1 and 3 million people each year. Global research on TB did not even reach $1 billion in 2017, though it would only take $2 billion a year to eliminate the disease by 2030 according to research (Makoni 2018). TB kills roughly 1.5 million people every year.

Another potentially under-recognized negative impact could be on the environment. Despite the positive environmental impacts outlined earlier, a number of other negative impacts have also come into play. For example, there are growing concerns about increased water pollution, especially as millions of single-use masks are being discarded, too often simply as litter. Laurent Lombard, director of the French NGO Operation Mer Propre, has warned, "soon we'll run the risk of having more masks than jellyfish in the Mediterranean" (quoted in Kassam 2020). Other environmental hazards are also increasing, particularly as corporations and governments have begun using the virus as a reason to flout environmental law and concerns. For example, deforestation of the Brazilian Amazon increased by more than 50% in the first three months of 2020 compared to just one year before (Simon and El Hammar Castano 2020). A study published in Nature Climate Change (Le Quere et al. 2020) further noted that any positive environmental changes gained under the current pandemic "are likely to be temporary as they do not reflect structural changes in the economic, transport or energy systems" (652).

Educational loss is another side effect of the pandemic. During April 2020, UNESCO reports indicated that more than 90% of the world's students were under lockdown, impacting nearly 1.6 billion learners (UNESCO 2020). Some countries have also already taken longer-term measures that will impact education – for example, Kenya has already declared the school year lost in that country (France-Presse 2020) and Mexico's educational system will be conducted through a home learning program broadcast on television through at least January 2021 (Esposito 2020). In fact, most countries are now considering either nationwide or localized moves to online education, a move that will further exacerbate educational inequalities between students on different sides of the digital divide. The closing of schools means much more than just a loss of education, however, and UNICEF and the World Food Programme (2020) have estimated that up to 370 million children will miss out on meals provided to them to at school.

The role of educators themselves has also been thrown into peril. A number of educational institutions have shuttered entire departments or have simply folded up entirely, others are experiencing severe financial distress, and others are surviving but doing so, in part, by slashing educator salaries while increasing educator workloads. It is also uncertain how the broad moves to online education will impact the future of educators and brick-and-mortar educational institutions, though few predict it will be in a good way.

The aforementioned examples are but just a sampling of the secondary negative impacts of the pandemic; there are, no doubt, many more. For example, there has been a notable increase in the unequalizing principles of neoliberalism, a rise in nationalism, and a resurgence of neoconservative ideologies (Ryan 2021a) and an increase in discrimination, especially hate crimes, targeted at individuals of Asian descent (Chiang 2021, this volume); several countries have taken advantage of the distraction to pass a number of anti-LGBT laws (Skinta, Sun, and Ryu 2021, this volume); companies have gone bankrupt, individuals have lost lives and livelihoods, and future debt burdens have increased across the board; millions more are likely to be pushed into homelessness; and a near-endless list of other factors. The bottom line is an understanding that while SARS-CoV-2 is ravaging the world, so are the impacts of the COVID-19 pandemic.

The unknowns

To speak of the unknowns of the pandemic is almost simply to speak of the pandemic itself. We don't know exact infection or death toll counts. We don't know the full extent of the long-term, or even really the short-term, damages wrought by the virus itself. We are still figuring out the best treatment and prevention methods. In short, we still don't even know what we still don't even know.

One of the more looming unknowns at the moment is when a vaccine might be developed. As of mid-August 2020, there were more than 200 vaccines currently under some stage of clinical testing in countries around the world (including China, the United States, the UK, and Russia). Whether these trials will be successful is yet to be known. Further, there is already a debate emerging as to who will have access to the first batches of the vaccine (Chaturvedi 2020). Will it go to the world's most vulnerable? To citizens of the nation that first develops it? Or, as many predict, to those with the money and social connections to gain access to it? It seems unlikely that a child in the Brazilian Amazon or the poor neighborhoods of the US rural south will have a vaccine before Jeff Bezos, Donald Trump, or most professional athletes will.

Perhaps the unknown that is causing the greatest level of heightened stress among so many is the unknown of tomorrow. What will life be like in 2021? Or 2022? Or 2025? Will we ever go back to having close contact conversations with friends and family where we can actually see their mouths moving? Will international holidays again become possible for the few of us in the global elite with the means to afford them? Will entire populations be culled due to starvation, increased disease, and economic ruin? Will there be more, and potentially more serious, global pandemics in the future, especially as we continue to diminish our natural environment and slash our social welfare systems? These are important questions, and while no one can provide the important answers needed at this time, we can at least begin to consider what we have already learned in an effort to shape what we might know tomorrow.

Determining a global future

The SARS-CoV-2 virus and the COVID-19 pandemic are both calling for increased attention to a number of issues (including issues that are not yet receiving any attention). Alongside medical understandings, there are also calls to better understand the impacts on global, regional, state, and local communities; environmental impacts; social impacts; economic impacts; impacts on state-level and global-level inequality; and a variety of other medical and nonmedical factors. Even abstract academic theoretical understandings are receiving the call for revision under current conditions (see Duzgun 2021; Ritzer 2021; Schaffer 2021).

Mark Lowcock, UN Under-Secretary-General for Humanitarian Affairs and Emergency Relief Coordinator, has called on the world's wealthiest countries to provide $90 billion in relief to aid the world's poorest countries. He claims that amount will help to protect 700 million of the world's most vulnerable people (cited in Mai 2020). A lack of action to protect and assist the most vulnerable among us could lead to up to 12,000 *additional* people dying per day of hunger due to the COVID-19 pandemic (Oxfam 2020), a number that far outstrips the daily death tolls related to the actual SARS-CoV-2 virus. It could also push at least another 100 million into extreme poverty (Mahler et al. 2020). All of this to say nothing of those pushed to greater levels of undue stress and suffering related to housing, education, health care, food security, and a host of other personal troubles and public issues.

Where the world goes now in terms of response to both the SARS-CoV-2 virus and the associated COVID-19 pandemic is still anybody's guess. Ramifications of existing inequalities and discrimination are being increasingly brought to attention, as well as exacerbated, by the current situation. That said, the alarm of such ramifications has also started to sound increasingly louder. Will enough people hear it? Will they hear it in time? Will the virus, or the associated pandemic, be what brings humanity together? Or what tears us further apart? Predictions cannot be made, but hopes can certainly be fostered. It is now up to us, as a global collective (whether we want to be or not), to decide where humanity goes from here.

References

Astorino, Joseph A., and Anthony V. Nicola. 2021. "Making the Invisible Visible: Viral Cloud Moments in the SARS-CoV-2 Pandemic." In *COVID-19: Global Pandemic, Societal Responses, Ideological Solutions*, edited by J. Michael Ryan, 184–96. London: Routledge.

Burke, Marshall. 2020. "COVID-19 Reduces Economic Activity, Which Reduces Pollution, Which Saves Lives." Accessed March 8, 2020. www.g-feed.com/2020/03/covid-19-reduces-economic-activity.html.

Chaturvedi, Amit. 2020. "Who Should be the First in Line for COVID-19 Vaccine? Experts Debate." *Hindustani Times*, August 3. www.hindustantimes.com/world-news/who-will-be-the-first-in-line-for-covid-19-vaccine-experts-debate/story-6FGrW9t6LdjnuRCBIw3KAL.html.

Chiang, Pamela P. 2021. "Anti-Asian Racism, Responses, and the Impact on Asian-Americans' Lives: A Social-Ecological Perspective." In *COVID-19: Social Consequences and Cultural Adaptations*, edited by J. Michael Ryan, 215–29. London: Routledge.

Duzgun, Eren. 2021. "Ecology, Democracy, and COVID-19: Rereading and Radicalizing Karl Polanyi." In *COVID-19: Global Pandemic, Societal Responses, Ideological Solutions*, edited by J. Michael Ryan, 54–67. London: Routledge.

Esposito, Anthony. 2020. "Mexican TV Networks to Provide Home Learning for Students as Schools Stay Shut." *Reuters*. Accessed August 3, 2020. www.reuters.com/article/us-mexico-education/mexican-tv-networks-to-provide-home-learning-for-students-as-schools-stay-shut-idUSKBN24Z1LZ.

Evans, Simon. 2020. "Analysis: Coronavirus Set Cause Largest Ever Annual Fall in CO2 Emissions." *CarbonBrief Analysis*. Accessed April 9, 2020. www.carbonbrief.org/analysis-coronavirus-set-to-cause-largest-ever-annual-fall-in-co2-emissions.

France-Presse, Agence. 2020. "Kenya Declares School Year 'Lost', Classes Back in 2021." *Hindustani Times*. Accessed July 7.2020. www.hindustantimes.com/world-news/kenya-declares-school-year-lost-classes-back-in-2021/story-zpxZsoACtqn4hGtLsPAirJ.html.

The Global Fund. 2020. "Mitigating the Impact of COVID-19 on Countries Affected by HIV, Tuberculosis, and Malaria." www.theglobalfund.org/media/9819/covid19_mitigatingimpact_report_en.pdf?u=637321467815130000.

IHME. 2018. "First Long-Term Study Finds Half Trillion Dollars Spent on HIV/AIDS." Accessed April 17, 2018. www.healthdata.org/news-release/first-long-term-study-finds-half-trillion-dollars-spent-hivaids.

IHME. 2019. "Global Malaria Spending $2 Billion Short of WHO Target, Stifling Progress Toward Eliminating Disease." Accessed April 24, 2019. www.healthdata.org/news-release/global-malaria-spending-2-billion-short-who-target-stifling-progress-toward-eliminating.

Kassam, Ashifa. 2020. "More Masks Than Jellyfish: Coronavirus Waste Ends Up in Ocean." *The Guardian.* Accessed June 8, 2020. www.theguardian.com/environment/2020/jun/08/more-masks-than-jellyfish-coronavirus-waste-ends-up-in-ocean.

Le Quéré, Corinne, Robert B. Jackson, Matthew W. Jones, Adam J. P. Smith, Sam Abernethy, Robbie M. Andrew, Anthony J. De-Gol, David R. Willis, Yuli Shan, Josep G. Canadell, Pierre Friedlingstein, Felix Creutzig, and Glen P. Peters. 2020. "Temporary Reduction in Global CO2 Emissions During the COVID-19 Forced Confinement." *Nature Climate Change* (10): 647–53.

Mahler, Daniel Gerszon, Christoph Lakner, R. Andres Castaneda Aguilar, and Haoyu Wu. 2020. "Updated Estimates of the Impact of COVID-19 on Global Poverty." *World Bank Blog,* June 8. https://blogs.worldbank.org/opendata/updated-estimates-impact-covid-19-global-poverty.

Mai, H. J. 2020. "U.N. Warns Number of People Starving to Death Could Double Amid Pandemic." Accessed May 5, 2020. www.npr.org/sections/coronavirus-live-updates/2020/05/05/850470436/u-n-warns-number-of-people-starving-to-death-could-double-amid-pandemic.

Makoni, Munyaradzi. 2018. "Global Funding for Tuberculosis Research Hits All-Time High." *Nature.* Accessed December 12, 2018. www.nature.com/articles/d41586-018-07708-z.

Nanda, Serena. 2021. "Inequalities and COVID-19." In *COVID-19: Global Pandemic, Societal Responses, Ideological Solutions*, edited by J. Michael Ryan, 109–23. London: Routledge.

Oxfam. 2020. "World on the Brink of a 'Hunger Pandemic': Coronavirus Threatens to Push Millions into Starvation." www.oxfam.org/en/world-brink-hunger-pandemic-coronavirus-threatens-push-millions-starvation.

Ritzer, George. 2021. "McDonaldization in the Age of COVID-19." In *COVID-19: Global Pandemic, Societal Responses, Ideological Solutions*, edited by J. Michael Ryan, 23–8. London: Routledge.

Ryan, J. Michael. 2021a. "The Blessings of COVID-19 for Neoliberalism, Nationalism, and Neoconservative Ideologies." In *COVID-19: Global Pandemic, Societal Responses, Ideological Solutions*, edited by J. Michael Ryan, 80–93. London: Routledge.

———. 2021b. "COVID-19: Global Pandemic, Societal Responses, Ideological Solutions." In *COVID-19: Global Pandemic, Societal Responses, Ideological Solutions*, edited by J. Michael Ryan, 1–8. London: Routledge.

———. 2021c. "COVID-19: Social Consequences and Cultural Adaptations." In *COVID-19: Social Consequences and Cultural Adaptations*, edited by J. Michael Ryan, 1–8. London: Routledge.

Schaffer, Scott. 2021. "Necroethics in the Time of COVID-19 and Black Lives Matter." In *COVID-19: Global Pandemic, Societal Responses, Ideological Solutions*, edited by J. Michael Ryan, 43–53. London: Routledge.

Simon, Evan, and Aicha El Hammar Castano. 2020. "Deforestation of Amazon Rainforest Accelerates amid COVID-19 Pandemic." *ABC News.* Accessed May 6, 2020. https://abcnews.go.com/International/deforestation-amazon-rainforest-accelerates-amid-covid-19-pandemic/story?id=70526188.

Skinta, Matthew D., Angela H. Sun, and Daniel M. Ryu. 2021. "The Impact of COVID-19 on the Lives of Sexual and Gender Minority People." In *COVID-19: Social Consequences and Cultural Adaptations*, edited by J. Michael Ryan, 230–44. London: Routledge.

Stop TB Partnership. 2020. "The Potential Impact of the COVID-19 Response on Tuberculosis in High-Burden Countries: A Modelling Analysis." Accessed May 1, 2020. www.stoptb.org/assets/documents/news/Modeling%20Report_1%20May%202020_FINAL.pdf.

UNESCO. 2020. "Education: From Disruption to Recovery." https://en.unesco.org/covid19/educationresponse.

UNICEF and World Food Programme. 2020. "Futures of 370 Million Children in Jeopardy as School Closures Deprive Them of School Meals." Accessed April 28, 2020. www.unicef.org/press-releases/futures-370-million-children-jeopardy-school-closures-deprive-them-school-meals.

Walsh, Nick Patton, Jo Shelley, Marcia Reverdosa, and Eduardo Duwe. 2020. "The US Sent Brazil Millions of Hydroxychloroquine Doses. Months Later They're Still in Storage." *CNN News*. Accessed August 4, 2020. https://edition.cnn.com/2020/08/04/americas/brazil-us-hydroxychloroquine-doses-intl/index.html.

WHO and UNAIDS. 2020. "The Cost of Inaction: COVID-19-Related Service Disruptions Could Cause Hundreds of Thousands of Extra Deaths from HIV." Accessed May 11, 2020. www.who.int/news-room/detail/11-05-2020-the-cost-of-inaction-covid-19-related-service-disruptions-could-cause-hundreds-of-thousands-of-extra-deaths-from-hiv.

PART I

Institutional responses

3

RETHINKING WHAT WE VALUE

Pandemic teaching and the art of letting go

Deborah J. Cohan

I clearly remember my first day of my Introductory Sociology class on January 13, 2020. I always devote some time during the first session to give students some background on who I am and how I got to be standing in front of them, and I am sure to leave time for questions with which I can start to provide answers that weave in sociological observations and ideas. That day, in front of almost 70 students, I moved a chair in front of a long seminar table, perched myself on the table with my feet on the seat of the chair, and proceeded to hunker down and talk story with them. I have long relied on this setup when I want to be more intimate with my students. This was a group of virtually all first-year students, and the crux of my message was to urge them to think about college as the transformative space it can be if they are open to it, to listen to the still small voice inside themselves, to follow the thread that binds their passions and dreams, and to never, ever give up. Motivated by the practice of yoga that I have been engaged in for some time, I asked my students to pause for a moment and to set an intention, not just for our class but also for the college experience and their futures, over and above earning the degree. My question was to start to get them to think about why we're here and what we want to really do with our time here. I hinted at the fact that the *here* to which I was referring was about much more than class, more than the college experience then, and actually much more about the *here* of this life. I always try to impart versions of that message when I teach, but that particular day I had another reason for wanting to encourage them to consider all of this.

I needed to help them understand why I had already planned to be away a number of days during the term though I am usually never absent, and while there is much I love about teaching, this semester my head and heart would also be somewhere else, and for good reason. I shared with them that for the better part of my life I dreamed of writing a book and that this thing I had been working to make happen for years was finally set to be published on Valentine's Day, and that immediately after that I would be hitting the road to embark on a multi-city book tour. Many students clapped. And I breathed a sigh of relief. It felt liberating to not be so needed. We have all grown accustomed to ideals about availability and access, and I simply could not promise them the same thing I had in years past. What I was less aware of at that moment and am acutely aware of now is how true that would become, how all our promises and plans would look different, and how something good might even come from that, too.

When I had planned my syllabi early the month before, I was worried about having absences from classes and how to minimize the disruption of that for my students. Little did I know how truly upended our semester would become and how all my best-laid plans and contingency plans, of which I always have plenty, would also be out the window. I also had no idea how prophetic the title of my new book would be, *Welcome to Wherever We Are* (Cohan 2020), or how it would come to feel like a slogan for our times. When I wrote this sociological and feminist memoir, I had no idea the current world moment in which it would be launched and that the essential messages of the book might later inform how I would begin to reshape my pedagogy and rethink my life.

My book is about caregiving for my father, a man who was at once adoring and abusive. Central thematic issues anchor the various stories I share in the book, and as I see it now those issues are at the heart of things to consider when thinking about pedagogical shifts in higher education. These include (1) meditating on what we hold onto and what we let go of; (2) how almost nothing is all good or all bad and the narrative of our lives is always blended; (3) how we navigate a labyrinth of unpredictability and ambivalence, resist fragmentation, and make ourselves whole; (4) how we think about a sense of home and place and how we ground ourselves to feel creative and purposeful; and (5) breaking silences and puncturing secrets to reveal deeper truths and to nurture a sense of voice. The very themes that permeate the intimate stories in my memoir now reverberate and guide my thinking about pandemic teaching and learning. My hope is that this chapter provides readers, and those who are educators, with something liberating as we envision what is sacred about teaching in the most tender and vulnerable of moments.

Meditating on what we hold onto and what we let go of

College is a chance for pause and thoughtful reflection, yet that is so often not how it feels, even under normal circumstances. This is the time to do this, more than ever. The more this pedagogy ride keeps spinning, right alongside the relentless, panic-inducing blizzard of information and misinformation about the state of the world, the dizzier and more exhausted I feel. It's simply not the time to fixate on and fetishize methods or to add more content or more to the to-do lists. And things are bound to flop when methods drive and dictate content. A crisis should not prompt us to add more; it should encourage us to distill things to an essence and to model for students how and what to prioritize. Keep busy, they say. Get still and centered, I believe.

In Parker Palmer's landmark book, *The Courage to Teach*, he writes, "The connections made by good teachers are held not in their methods but in their hearts – meaning heart in its ancient sense, the place where intellect and emotion and spirit and will converge in the human self" (Palmer 1998, 11). Doing this requires great compassion for students, for oneself as a teacher, and for the entire learning process. Right now, our hearts and bodies are trembling, and we need compassion for our students and ourselves more than ever.

In the flurry of posts and emails, it's as if the big, important questions have gone missing. So many faculty members are wholly preoccupied with the basics of how to set up an online class with Zoom features, how to narrate PowerPoint slides, what to wear to teach online in a synchronous format, how to condense information into a new format, what videos to choose, how to record lectures with other people at home for students with their own set of responsibilities, how to prevent students from cheating on online exams – the list is truly endless. And, students are emailing about advising and extra credit. It's understandable. When people are nervous, they fixate on the little they can control. This reminds me of when parents of college-bound students go into a buying frenzy before school starts. In all the frantic rushing around and back and forth trips to purchase and return at Bed, Bath & Beyond, Target, and Walmart, some crucial conversations about big life issues seem to go missing. The focus of the administrations is overwhelmingly on social engineering and orchestrating every move of every person, yet what have we learned to date from this pandemic? That we cannot control everything.

The question becomes, for what are we holding space and why? For example, I'm comfortable with abandoning a lot of course content now. So what if instead, students wait and learn some of the concepts in future classes with me? They need not master them in an emergency. As older adults, most of us are scared and uneasy. Making myself busy with technology and loads of assignments to grade and discussion boards to monitor, with far too many students, is not going to accomplish anything for anyone. Instead, my focus will be on easing my fears and those of my students and doing anything that assists our mental and physical health. This is a good lesson in boundary making, a lesson I was slow to learn with in-person teaching but that makes sense now given both the inherent limitations of the online environment and the pandemic.

I want this moment to be an opportunity for my students to pause and think about how they might be better and healthier selves, citizens, and leaders in the face of uncertainty, crisis, fear, and change. I want them to think about how and where they can be of the most service and how they can channel their energy to effect change. I will urge them to think about what they want to hold onto and what they could let go of, and I want them to think about how they want to be remembered. I want to encourage them to dream about how they can chart a course for and about hope, even and especially when it feels like there is none.

Aren't these the eternal questions of the human condition and lessons we want to impart on and off campus? It just might be that this current emergency prompts us to re-evaluate our real purpose in teaching.

Nothing is all good or all bad

I have long been critical of online teaching and learning for a variety of reasons.

Yet, in this current pandemic situation, I accept that online education is good enough. And good enough is actually okay. It is the safest, best option we have. I am willing to forgo all that I cherish most about in-person teaching so that I, and my students and colleagues, will be around long enough to do it again when it's possible. I will do the most good with what I have from where I sit now.

According to sociologist George Ritzer (2012), McDonaldization happens when the principles of the fast-food industry – efficiency, quantification, control, predictability, convenience, and speed – dominate more and more sectors of our lives. If you ever wondered what the McDonaldization of education looks like, here we are. Appealing to issues like ease, convenience, and money, universities have long drawn upon tenets of McDonaldization to market online programs. One university offering online programming says on its website:

> Your well-deserved salary increase is attainable. The ability to better support your family is no longer out of reach . . . you can access your coursework from home or the office . . . or you can pick it up and take it with you to your son's soccer game, your hair appointment or the nearest Starbucks!

And corporations work to bolster this; multiple times a day, I am bombarded with emails from companies across the country trying to capitalize on the recent shift to online teaching and learning because of COVID-19. They are looking to sell their goods and services to educators at a needy and vulnerable moment.

It is profoundly revealing to see that, for years, many of the same higher education institutions that have been pushing the hardest for more students to go online to save or make money now want to insist on face-to-face education in the midst of a health and humanitarian crisis of epic proportions. In and of itself, this rich irony should cause us to question motives. It is nothing short of institutional gaslighting.

During a pandemic, faculty are being expected to rush it all out, fast and hot, and many feel pressured to supersize their content, all in the name of convenience and choice for students to have it their way, especially in the newly touted HyFlex model. I want to step back and ask, is this what we want to make and consume? Is this what will nourish and sustain us? Will this be good for our individual and collective bodies, minds, and hearts?

Education need not be easy and convenient. Even pre-pandemic, education was being sold as something to be as convenient as possible, which in turn has dramatically reduced the credibility of higher education. But perhaps in prioritizing convenience above all, the thing that is most lost is the classroom as a last sacred space for where we can have and enjoy the promise and possibility of certain deep and risky conversations.

How we navigate a labyrinth of unpredictability, resist fragmentation, and make ourselves whole

What are we modeling for students when we engage in a frenzy about teaching methods and tools amid a global crisis that will have epic impacts on health care, economics, politics, and human rights? Instead, what might we *want* to model? What do we really think our students need and want right now? What do we as educators most need and want right now?

For me, my goal while teaching during a pandemic is this simple and this complex: to try my best to be kind to myself as I move in and out of fear. In fact, I even sent that as a message to all of my students via our online learning platform with an announcement that I would continue to provide more information as I learned more, that I planned to streamline and simplify as much as possible, and that I hoped we would share inspiration to help sustain each other during such a challenging time. By doing that, I was trying to convey to students the importance of early and direct communication, our shared humanity, my own sense of vulnerability, and the need for self-care.

Often, at the end of a semester or even years later, when students share with me what they really got out of my class, I hear time and time again how it transcended content and was about how I showed up for and with them in moments of great fear, grief, loss, sadness, and seismic shifts in their lives. It's about how I took them to their farthest edge, stood there with them bearing witness and paying attention, and didn't let them fall off. No amount of Zoom, Google, Moodle, or Blackboard will ever make *that* happen. Students often come to us wanting a degree. Yet when all is said and done, they suggest that they actually yearned for something else: a new lease on life, an alternative approach to how to craft a life worth living. And they look to us as their professors for how to do that. I can't imagine burying myself in all the technical minutiae and especially now.

Worldwide health is too precarious, the world feels too uncertain, and all that dis/ease feels frighteningly loud and overwhelming. I need and want what I instinctively believe my students need and want: reassuring leadership, humor, quiet and rest, joy and beauty, a departure from the mania, and a release to be still.

Motivated by an ethic and pedagogy of care, my message to students will continue to be one where I will tell them: You will learn something here, it may not be exactly what you would have learned had you taken my class in years past, it will be something else entirely, born of this moment in which we find ourselves. I'll have learning objectives and outcomes on the syllabus because it's required, but for the most part, we will deviate from these. I cannot possibly determine these. I never could but I definitely cannot now. This will be a class shaped more by present moment awareness than one I have ever taught before. Guided by current context, temporality, mortality, spontaneity, I, as a lifelong learner, will inhabit this liminal and sacred space with you.

How we think about home and place and ground ourselves to feel creative and purposeful

A global pandemic can leave people feeling frighteningly isolated. Furthermore, in the United States, social unrest around systemic racism is another location of profound disconnection. Oppression itself is deeply dislocating and works by cutting people off from what they most care about and need. These deeply complicated and intersecting issues are further magnified by the fact that online education, as a method, has the tendency to feel more alienating for most educators and students alike.

One thing we can do to give online pandemic teaching a sense of rootedness and place is to really leverage our own discipline to teach about the pandemic. For example, in my own discipline of sociology, we might consider the sociology of the coronavirus, how private troubles are indeed public issues of the social structure, how existing social inequalities deepen the health crisis, and how the health crisis will create deeper social inequality. Or, we might look at topics like domestic violence and how lockdowns and isolation further complicate the experience of entrapment for victims of abuse. Or, we might explore issues of intimacy and dating, or marriage and divorce, to see how these phenomena are shaped and constrained by a pandemic. Students of art, English, theater, dance, and music might consider the creative work that has emerged in response to the rockiest periods in our history. Students in communications would benefit from exploring how to sensitively report on emerging issues from the pandemic like political polarization. Business and hospitality students might consider the role of pandemic crises on the tourism industry and the lingering effects on community building. Surely, every discipline could make some connections here. And at a time when the liberal arts have been dismantled or nearly gutted at many institutions, those of us in the liberal arts have to think about how to collectively and creatively organize to showcase our pivotal role at this time.

Now is also the time for faculty to engage in coalition building on and off campus and within their own states as well as their professional associations on the state, regional, national, and international level. By doing this, faculty can mobilize and strategize and also bring forth creative ideas for the good of the whole. With crisis comes opportunity and change, and faculty can pave the way toward thinking about new ways of constructing knowledge and structuring campus life. It is a time when people may be more open to hearing unusual ideas. For example, I taught a brand-new course online for the university that I had never taught before, titled the Sociology of Food, during a three-week Maymester class; it compelled me to think much more seriously about the merits of a block plan where students take, and faculty teach, only one or two classes during a very condensed period of time. Given that life in a pandemic is stressful and distracting, faculty might have a greater chance of showing students the joy of learning when conditions are cultivated so there is more focused depth and immersion. We inhabit bureaucracies that we made, and we can demonstrate the creativity and ethical conviction to make necessary humane changes in them.

Breaking silences to reveal deeper truths and to nurture a sense of voice

It is important to consider both the emotional life of the classroom (in person or virtual) and our own emotional landscapes as educators in order to foster a more embodied and empathetic learning space. Given that students often disclose to professors about the traumas of racism, violence, and poverty, and since these issues are as explosive as ever at the time of this writing, it makes sense to consider trauma-informed perspectives for teaching.

While not all faculty members have been adequately trained to think about, teach about, and respond to trauma, colleges and universities would always be better off, pandemic or not, to demonstrate a better handle on trauma and should provide ways for faculty and staff to receive better training on this. For example, given the high rate of sexual assault on campus and the extent to which students come forth about issues related to all forms of sexual and dating violence, a comprehensive and coordinated trauma-centered response on campus would always prove helpful. Now, amidst a pandemic, people are experiencing so much loss as well as anxiety and fear around illness and death, grave concerns about their ability to make a living, and the impact on their own mental health, and a trauma-informed perspective in the classroom adds necessary nuance, depth, and meaning. It also functions in a way to help break silences and nurture a sense of voice. As educators, we need to give ourselves permission to create some spaciousness for our students and for ourselves and to hold space for the complexity of emotion so we don't burn out.

The most effective, meaningful, and memorable teaching and learning is about removing the metaphorical masks, rolling up our sleeves and getting our hands dirty, getting up close and personal, being embodied and coming to a place where we don't fear the stranger in our midst. What makes teaching the most magical is the act of tender, curious, and open surrender –by both the teacher and the student. The art of letting go is a worthy pursuit at any time and certainly amidst a pandemic. It's from the chaos, the mess, and the community we cultivate that order, answers, and hope show up.

References

Cohan, Deborah J. 2020. *Welcome to Wherever We Are: A Memoir of Family, Caregiving, and Redemption.* New Brunswick, NJ: Rutgers University Press.

Palmer, Parker. 1998. *The Courage to Teach: Exploring the Inner Landscape of a Teacher's Life.* San Francisco, CA: Jossey-Bass.

Ritzer, George. 2012. *The McDonaldization of Society.* 20th anniversary edition. Thousand Oaks, CA: Sage.

4

DISRUPTION AND DIFFICULTY

Student and faculty perceptions of the transition to online instruction in the COVID-19 pandemic

Lee Millar Bidwell, Scott T. Grether, and JoEllen Pederson

As a result of the increasing spread of COVID-19 in March 2020, college administrators at residential campuses in the United States made decisions that significantly affected students and faculty. In most cases, including the one discussed in this chapter, university presidents and administrators developed strategies for rapidly closing campus and implementing remote teaching based upon changing guidelines from federal and state health agencies and gubernatorial mandates. Understandably, these decisions were made swiftly due to an evolving health crisis. However, faculty and students typically did not have formal input in these decisions, nor is there evidence that officials at most universities relied upon preexisting continuity of operations plans to guide the process.

Faculty and students were suddenly thrust into a new teaching and learning environment that was unplanned and involuntary. Unlike traditional online courses, the type of instruction delivered during the response to the COVID-19 campus closures is best described as "emergency remote teaching" (ERT), which is "a temporary shift of instructional delivery to an alternate delivery mode due to crisis circumstances" (Hodges et al. 2020, under "Emergency Remote Teaching"). The goal of ERT is not to replicate existing educational delivery methods but "to provide temporary access to instruction and instructional supports in a manner that is quick to set up and is reliably available during an emergency or crisis" (under "Emergency Remote Teaching"). The shift to ERT as a result of the pandemic required faculty to decide how to meet students' educational needs while quickly moving to an online teaching format. For students, the implementation of ERT entailed simultaneously moving out of campus housing, adjusting to a variety of online instructional technologies and changes to course syllabi, and managing the effects of an evolving worldwide health crisis to their personal life (e.g., health, high-risk family member, finances, job security).

During times of ERT, it is important to consider how each individual's status within a college or university shapes how they experience the crisis. Generally, colleges and universities are often described as a homogenous entity, an environment with a set of "common, mutually perceived set of conditions that influence the members of the academic community" (Hartnett and Centra 1974, 161). Faculty, students, and administrators (and other stakeholders such as staff), however, experience the institution differently because of the varying levels of power, status, and roles associated with their positions. To better understand what happens on college campuses and universities in times of ERT, the experience of the educational environment should be examined "as seen through the eyes of the student (or faculty member . . .)" (161). The research reported in this chapter examines how the status of faculty and students within a university's organizational structure shaped their perceptions and experiences in the wake of the administration's decision to implement ERT in response to COVID-19.

Background

Colleges and universities are organizations comprised of individuals who have different status positions and roles. Sociologists use the concepts of status and roles to understand how social interaction operates within a society. Status is often defined as the social position a person holds, while roles are behaviors expected from people with a particular status (Macionis 2017). For example, Falchikov (1986) applied these concepts to university classrooms by arguing that students hold less power than faculty because faculty design course syllabi, assign work, and evaluate student performance. Traditionally, those with the status of faculty have the role of the authority figure inside the classroom, giving them the power to decide how to structure interactions and outcomes for their courses (Hirschy and Wilson 2002).

Despite their elevated status within the classroom, faculty members do not hold the highest status within a university. Research from organizational sociology indicates that middle-status actors, like faculty within the context of a university, cannot make decisions without considering their high- and low-status counterparts. High-status actors, such as administrators at a university, have legitimacy assured through their achieved status and have more power to make decisions (Sanford, Blum, and Smith 2021, this volume). The benefits of being high-status within an organization include a sense of security, increased confidence, greater means to control impressions, more visibility, higher compensation, and increased access to resources (Sauder, Lynn, and Podolny 2012). Low-status actors, students in this example, have little to lose by violating norms. Whereas both high- and low-status actors at the university experience some benefits based on their status, "Middle-status actors [faculty] must conform to expectations in order to avoid risking their standing" (Sauder, Lynn, and Podolny 2012, 271).

In times of crisis, people use the roles associated with their status to prioritize actions. "When under time constraints, layering on top of, or copying from, existing or past institutional arrangements is considered as an effective strategy to come up with solutions" (Saurugger 2016, 74). In the case of COVID-19 in the university setting, faculty controlled their course material and how it was transitioned online within the parameters of institutional policies and resources while trying to estimate student expectations. Students, however, did not have the same power to control their experience.

Data and methods

Data were collected at a traditional residential regional state university in spring 2020 through four separate surveys administered at two times. On March 13, the university president announced classes would be offered online for a two-week period while COVID-19 information developed; nine days later the administration declared that classes would remain online for the remainder of the semester. The first set of surveys, one sent to students and another to faculty, was distributed on March 20 (the day after they were notified that in-person classes would not resume), to capture their perceptions and experiences in the initial transition to online instruction. Five weeks later (the last Friday of classes, April 25), a second set of surveys, one to students and one to faculty, was sent to measure respondents' perceptions and experiences at the end of the semester with the administrative decision to close the campus in response to the pandemic. In summary, middle- and low-status actors were surveyed at two different time points. Staff, middle-status actors, and administration, high-status actors, were not surveyed because of time and resource limitations.

Using open- and closed-ended questions, the online surveys of students asked about a variety of issues, including what they found most and least difficult about ERT, whether they agreed with the administration's decision to close campus, the type of online instruction they preferred, how online instruction would affect their learning, and their overall concerns about the pandemic. Online surveys of faculty asked open- and closed-ended questions about their perceptions of ERT, changes they made to their courses and why, how online instruction would affect student learning, and their perceptions of what they believed students would find most and least difficult with the sudden change to ERT.

The student surveys were sent to all faculty teaching classes in sociology, anthropology, criminal justice studies, mathematics, computer science, mathematics education, and music. Faculty teaching these classes were asked to email the survey to their current students (undergraduate only). Departments were chosen using a convenience sample that resulted in students from a variety of disciplines being surveyed. The two student surveys yielded 310 and 87 responses, respectively. We were unable to measure how many students actually received either survey. Differences in the response rate between Time 1 and

Time 2 for the student surveys may be due to fewer faculty sending the survey to students during the last week of class, fewer students checking email regularly at the end of the semester, or students having less time to complete the survey due to new schedules influenced by academic- or pandemic-related issues. A list of 130 faculty was generated by the researchers using convenience sampling. These faculty were sent an email asking for their opinions five weeks apart, yielding 60 responses (46.1%) in Time 1 and 54 responses (41.5%) in Time 2.

Close-ended survey questions were analyzed using descriptive statistics. Faculty and student responses were compared at the Time 1 and Time 2 surveys. The demographic composition of the sample is shown in Table 4.1. Open-ended responses were analyzed utilizing an open-coded approach (Charmaz 2006; Esterberg 2002), whereby codes were created to capture the statements or themes reflected in respondents' writing. After all responses were analyzed, the authors met to discuss which codes appeared frequently in student and faculty responses, which codes overlapped, and which were unique to students and faculty. Of students who

TABLE 4.1 Descriptive Statistics of Sample (Time 1 and Time 2)

	Faculty		Students	
	Time 1	Time 2	Time 1	Time 2
Gender				
Female	55.9%	47.1%	76.9%	83.9%
Male	30.5%	33.3%	21.8%	14.9%
Prefer not to answer/Other	13.6%	19.6%	1.2%	1.1%
Race				
White/Caucasian	78.0%	76.5%	84.1%	79.3%
Black/African American	1.7%	2.0%	12.0%	13.8%
Latino/Latina	1.7%	0.0%	3.6%	3.4%
Asian/Asian American	0.0%	0.0%	1.3%	2.3%
Prefer not to answer/Other	18.6%	21.6%	2.9%	4.6%
Teaching Status (Faculty only)				
Tenured	76.7%	66.7%		
Tenure Track	20.0%	25.5%		
Non-Tenure Track	3.3%	7.8%		
Online Teaching				
No experience	28.3%	35.8%		
1–5 classes previously	36.7%	26.4%		
More than 5 classes	35.0%	37.8%		
Class Status (Students only)				
First-year			23.9%	26.4%
Sophomore			25.6%	23.0%
Junior			33.3%	34.5%
Senior			17.2%	16.1%
N	60	54	310	87

Note: Respondents were asked to "check all that apply" for race, resulting in a total percent > 100.0%.

completed each survey, 84.5% of students answered at least one open-ended question in Time 1, and 73.5% answered an open-ended question in Time 2. Of faculty who completed the survey, 95% in Time 1 and 96% in Time 2 answered at least one open-ended question.

Findings

The data suggest that students and faculty shared three major concerns about the shift to ERT – balancing work, school, and family obligations; changes to course material; and learning less during ERT. Although students and faculty agreed that moving classes online was "necessary" and "unavoidable" and described the shift to ERT using similar words, such as "difficult," "overwhelmed," "stressed," "unhappy," and "worried," the source of their concerns differed depending upon the respondents' responsibilities and degree of authority within the institution. The perceptions and experiences of students and faculty to ERT were shaped by and reflect their status and roles in the university. Students, who are low-status actors, had no control over the decisions made regarding campus policies or changes to course material. Within a very short period of time, students had to move out of campus housing – most of them returning to their homes – where many assumed more family and job responsibilities. At the same time, their courses were being redesigned in various ways by multiple professors. Faculty members, as middle-status actors, on the other hand, were suddenly responsible for changing their mode of instruction without compromising the integrity of their courses, while trying to be sensitive to students' needs.

Balancing work, school, and family obligations

Quantitative and qualitative data indicate that students were extremely concerned about balancing work, school, and family obligations.[1] Although faculty acknowledged these student responsibilities, they underestimated the degree to which students were concerned about adequately meeting these demands.

Figure 4.1 shows what students were most concerned about moving to ERT and what faculty believed were students' greatest concerns. Students were most concerned about balancing work, school, and family obligations in both Time 1 (39.3%) and Time 2 (52.8%). Only a quarter of faculty respondents at Time 1 thought students would be most concerned about balancing work, school, and family obligations, whereas at Time 2 most faculty (57.4%) estimated this would be student's biggest concern moving to ERT. Overall, students were consistent with what they chose as their highest level of concern between Time 1 and Time 2. Faculty, however, were not good at identifying what students were most concerned about. Between Time 1 and Time 2, the percent of faculty who selected "Balancing work/school/family" noticeably changed, as did several of their other responses as noted in Figure 4.1, but not always in a way that reflected student

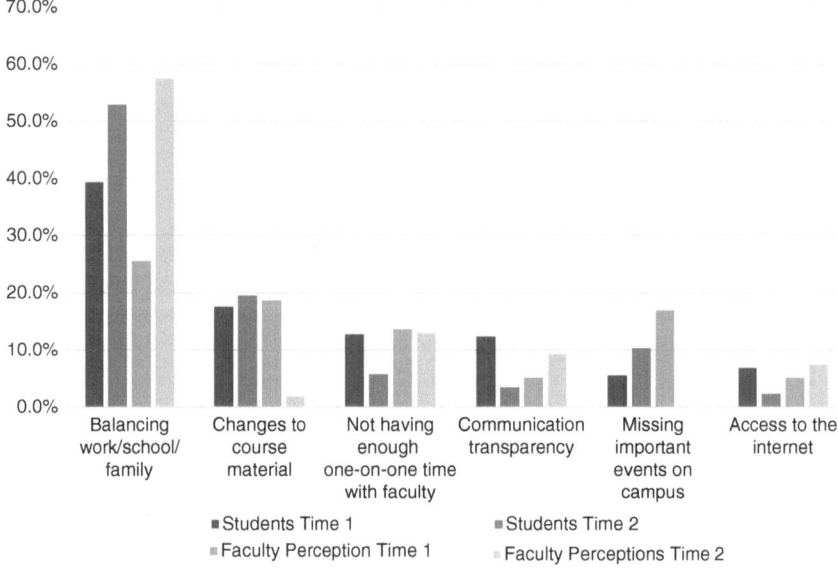

attitudes. The qualitative responses suggest status positions in the university shaped how students and faculty perceived concerns about balancing work, school, and family obligations.

Student experiences

Part of what students experienced during the transition to online learning was having to strike an immediate and intricate balance between completing assigned schoolwork, keeping abreast of frequent announcements and policy changes from the university and faculty, ensuring their loved ones were cared for, and working for pay. Because students occupy a lower-status position within a university setting, they are often the ones who bear the brunt of decision-making from those immediately above them in the university setting (faculty) and those at the top (administration). For example:

> I'm literally super stressed out about this, plus I'm having to work while I am at home to pay my parents [sic] rent. It's just to [sic] much, why can't we just end the semester now and give us the grade we have in the class now.
>
> *(Time 1, Student 025)*

> It is pretty overwhelming and is an unexpected lifestyle and routine change that most students will have to embrace. A lifestyle living at home and away on campus are different in regards to how we get our studies done. Living at home and balancing academics with family and employment affairs is excessive.
>
> *(Time 1, Student 236)*

Moving classes online created additional burdens for students that faculty members and administration, perhaps, did not fully appreciate. As these examples demonstrate, living *at home*, attending online classes *at home*, and completing homework *at home* coalesced to create feelings of stress and exasperation. Additionally, as the aforementioned responses illustrate, some students also had to work during this time period, which, in some cases, was essential for the financial stability of their families. Although the number of students in the sample who were employed is not known, having financial obligations was a substantial source of anxiety and stress for some students.

Indeed, finding a balance between school, work, and home was still a concern for students in the Time 2 survey. Students continued to express that the experience of ERT was challenging partly because they had other responsibilities that were just as important to them as their schoolwork, as indicated by the following:

> I missed a lot of lectures because I needed to find a job to make sure I could pay off my student loans and my rent for my housing.
>
> *(Time 2, Student 066)*

> Most teachers did communicate very well and were flexible but also added way more work once we switched to online which made it incredibly difficult to manage when it wasn't expected. Being at home w[ith] other people who don't understand and having a job, the amount of brand new work assigned made things very difficult.
>
> *(Time 2, Student 085)*

Many students experienced not only an increase to their coursework (Student 085), but also increased uncertainty with how the pandemic would affect their financial well-being (Student 066) and home life (Student 085).

Faculty experiences

Although faculty did not fully perceive the magnitude of students' concerns about balancing work, school, and family, they were sensitive to these issues. Faculty reported making choices about whether to deliver course material synchronously, asynchronously, or in combination to accommodate students' family and work obligations, as evidenced in these statements:

> I believe students have to balance their situations at home (younger siblings they may be taking care of, jobs, etc.) that is not amenable to synchronous learning right now.
>
> *(Time 1, Faculty 026)*

> Several of my students have stated that they have family obligations (such as looking after younger siblings and/or grandparents). I like to give them the time they need to manage their time to their needs. They may not be able to meet with me at 10am as they would on campus (due to internet or family)

so I give them an assignment and a due date and trust them to get it done as their other classes/family/internet allow.

(Time 1, Faculty 051)

Although students did not recognize it, faculty made choices about how to best deliver ERT based on their perceptions of students' needs. Perhaps faculty were not aware of the magnitude of stress students were experiencing suddenly balancing multiple responsibilities and adjusting to significant changes in living and learning circumstances, but they did reshape their courses with students' needs in mind.

Concerns over changes to course material

Students consistently reported that changes to course material caused by COVID-19 was one of their greatest concerns. At Time 1, 17.5% of students reported this was their top concern and 19.5% of students listed course changes as their top concern in Time 2. When classes initially shifted to online format, faculty recognized changes in course material were likely one of students' primary concerns, with 18.6% of faculty selecting this as students' top concern in Time 1. However, only 1.9% of faculty felt that changes to course material would be students' top concern in the Time 2 survey. This noticeable disconnect between students' concern and faculty members' perception of students' concern over changes to course material can be explained several ways. First, the Time 2 survey was distributed on the last Friday of the semester; faculty may have believed that concerns about changes to course material would not be paramount since the class was almost over and students likely had adapted to syllabi revisions. Second, as is evidenced by qualitative responses, faculty perceived that changes they made to courses accommodated students' circumstances and were based on careful assessment of pedagogical priorities and, therefore, should no longer be a significant concern for students.

Student experiences

At Time 1, many students expressed concerns about how their instructors were adjusting the workload for their classes. It seems that many emotions students expressed in their open-ended responses (e.g., stressed, nervous, confused, drained, miserable, overwhelmed) were linked to how their instructors were designing their ERT. For instance:

It's been an emotional roller coaster. I feel like my professors have not given me and other students time to mentally process what's going on. I feel like it was for the best given the situation, but some of my professors could have handled this better. They were more worried about shoving content down our throats versus checking in with us to see if we were okay.

(Time 1, Student 290)

Many students, like Student 290, expressed frustration with a perceived increase to the amount of work being assigned in the shift to ERT.

Even as the semester progressed, students remained steadfast in critiquing the adjustments that instructors made to their courses. Open-ended responses from the Time 2 survey continued to demonstrate that students experienced ERT as being fraught with negative emotions stemming from the heavy workload in their classes. For instance:

> I most likely would've been okay managing one or two classes online, but it was overwhelming. We were in the middle of the semester and a lot of professors are assigning extra activities, sending too many emails at once, and for me it made the process harder.
>
> *(Time 2, Student 011)*

Student 011 captures the sentiment of other students in feeling "overwhelmed" as "extra activities" were assigned in "the middle of the semester" and instructors were "sending too many emails at once." Student 026 believed that the move to ERT led "Professors [to] assign a lot more papers and 'busy work' that they wouldn't normally assign" (Time 2). Reflecting at the end of the semester, Student 014 sums up the experience this way: "It was stressful especially when considering everything else that is happening in the world right now. Ultimately it has worked out but it was tricky managing class loads and work for five different classes."

When considered collectively, the quotes in this section demonstrated that while students accepted the move to ERT, they perceived that more coursework was added during ERT. The academic workload was an ongoing source of frustration and anxiety for students, especially because they were simultaneously managing other affairs at the university – tuition refunds, moving out of on-campus housing, registering for future classes, securing course materials for remote learning, navigating academic policy changes, and determining whether they wanted to return for the fall term – while at home. In this sense, concerns about changes to course material were intricately linked to student concerns about how to balance school, work, and family during an ongoing pandemic.

Faculty experiences

Like students, faculty had no choice in moving to ERT. The emotions created by the sudden transition – feeling "overwhelmed," "frustrated," and "stressed" – described by faculty echoed students' sentiments. Faculty respondent 014 in Time 1 said, "I am just short of all out panic, all day, every day." However, unlike students whose feelings were in response to decisions made by others, faculty emotions were related to their status position as middle-status actors within the university setting. One role of occupying a faculty status was the difficult responsibility of redesigning a formerly in-person class to an online format in just days. As Faculty 019 explained, the shift to emergency remote teaching was "Obviously [a] tough transition in a matter of days and in the middle of the semester with no intention of doing so at the beginning of the semester" (Time 1).

When asked in the first survey to describe the online course delivery methods they were using and why, faculty indicated that the adaptations they made to their classes were designed to maintain the integrity and continuity of the course. Faculty emphasized the importance of fulfilling course objectives and preserving content with as little disruption for students as possible, as these statements suggest:

> This semester I am using synchronous delivery via Zoom because this is the easiest and most seemless [sic] transition in my opinion. We were already doing this, so I felt it best to continue along these lines. This also results in the least disruption to the course schedule. Had we started online, then I would have chosen asynchronous.
>
> *(Faculty 019)*

> [I'm using] synchronous for the upper-level seminar (because it lets us continue very fruitful classtime discussions and even hold onto a slight sense of normalcy).
>
> *(Faculty 035)*

Faculty described tailoring the modifications to course material for the online format based on a myriad of pedagogical considerations, including the discipline, the size of the class, whether the course was for majors or non-majors, entry level or upper level, undergraduate or graduate, and lecture based or experiential based. The following statement illustrates the nuanced factors faculty considered when modifying their courses for ERT:

> I'm using asynchronous and synchronous for my upper division class because I don't want to expect students to be available for every single class with their other obligations and lack of access to internet. But I do think a few synchronous classes are necessary for a more in-depth discussion of the readings. For my lower division [core] classes, I've only used the Discussion Board for posting and they turn in previous assigned assignments.
>
> *(Faculty 060)*

Faculty teaching classes with laboratory, clinicals, simulations, private lessons, performances, or studio time described the difficulty of translating those course components into a virtual experience. Faculty teaching in disciplines that rely more on lecture and discussion often expressed empathy for their colleagues in disciplines that were harder to move online.

I was jealous of my colleagues who had taught similar courses online already, since they already had massive infrastructure in place, and I had to build mine, but at least I was not teaching labs, rehearsals, or anything that cannot be simulated almost 100% through text alone.

(Faculty 001)

Given their status as instructors, the priority of faculty was to deliver the highest quality course to students under the circumstances. Faculty were resourceful in quickly moving classes online and preserving the bulk of course content using a host of technologies including Canvas, FaceTime, Google Slides, Panopto, online polling, publisher-provided products, Skype, Slack, Camtasia, WebEx, and Zoom. Depending on the course, faculty delivered the content either synchronously, asynchronously, or a combination of the two. Decisions about changes to course material were designed to maintain the integrity of the course. However, the fact that faculty were using a variety of course technologies and course delivery methods had the unintended effect of increasing students' perceived workload.

Learning less during emergency remote teaching

One area where student and faculty perceptions were most aligned was in belief that learning was compromised by the sudden shift to online instruction. Students and faculty were asked what they expected students to learn during ERT compared to the same portion of the semester if courses had not been moved online. Faculty and students agreed that students learned less during ERT compared to the intended face-to-face format (See Table 4.2). Specifically, 67.8% of students felt they had learned less in ERT than they would have if classes had continued to be held in person, and the majority (59.3%) of faculty agreed. These results are consistent with other studies that show students (Tichavsky et al. 2015) and faculty (Wingo, Ivankova, and Moss 2017) believe learning in traditional online classes (i.e., not ones created during ERT) is inferior to face-to-face courses.

TABLE 4.2 Perceptions of Learning During the Online Portion of the Semester

	Students	*Faculty*
Learn more	1.1%	0.0%
Learn the same amount	19.5%	11.1%
Learn less	67.9%	59.3%
Unsure	11.5%	29.6%
N	100%	100%

Note: Responses from Time 2, end of semester survey.

Student experiences

Students expressed a range of difficulties at Time 1 associated with online instruction, including changes to the learning environment, a loss of motivation, incompatibility with their learning style, having to "teach myself," and being overwhelmed with the amount of work associated with taking a full course load entirely online. Chief among the perceived difficulties associated with online instruction was that they would learn less than in the classroom. For instance:

> It [ERT] has left me unprepared, decreased my amount of learning, and struggling to keep up with assignments while balancing work and family needs.
>
> *(Time 1, Student 015)*

> I feel my learning will suffer because I am not the kind of person that learns well in online classes. I need the routine and structure of in person classes to have motivation and success.
>
> *(Time 1, Student 013)*

As these quotes illustrate, students perceived they would learn less online due to a combination of factors including time demands, personal learning style, decreased motivation, and lack of classroom structure.

At the end of the semester, students also emphasized in open-ended responses that they were learning less from ERT than from the face-to-face version. For instance: ́

> I honestly think that this was a waste of money. I didn't pay for online classes. I am doing work without even learning any material, honestly. It was possibly the worse [sic] thing that could ever happen.
>
> *(Time 2, Student 058)*

> I understand why it was necessary because health must come first always, but I am barely learning anything and I'm miserable on all fronts. I hate the online format and I hate how sudden it happened.
>
> *(Time 2, Student 070)*

These statements reflect the frustration, regret, and anger many students felt at the end of the semester. While not a prevalent theme in responses, some believed that despite doing the assigned work they were still not learning "any material." Most students realized the pressing health concerns of the coronavirus and accepted the decision of the university to move classes online, but they generally agreed with the sentiments expressed by Student 070 that they were "barely learning anything" and that the experience of ERT made them "miserable on all fronts."

Faculty experiences

Despite the thoughtful ways faculty approached course changes and the many strategies utilized to deliver content, the majority still believed that students learned less in the online environment. In their open-ended comments in both surveys, faculty consistently expressed concern that ERT was not as effective, rich, engaging, or desirable as face-to-face instruction. Faculty remarked that they missed "seeing the students and being able to talk directly to them" (Time 1, Faculty 020) and that because material had to be cut or compressed in the shift to ERT, students literally learned less content. Some respondents worried about the "effect down the road for courses that build on one another, [e]specially in Math, Science, and Languages" (Time 2, Faculty 018).

Given that they chose to work at a residential university that prides itself on teaching excellence in small, in-person classrooms, it is not surprising that many faculty respondents were critical of online instruction in general, as the following statements illustrate:

> [T]here should be no misunderstanding that an online-only education is a sub-par method to create well educated citizen leaders as defined by the campus mission.
>
> *(Time 1, Faculty 040)*

> Online instruction simply isn't as effective or interactive as in-person instruction no matter how good your technology is – especially for technical fields like mine where subtle differences in notation, intonation, and meaning are critical to understanding. Teaching online well requires massive amounts of preparation – none of which we had enough warning to do – and is far more work than teaching in person.
>
> *(Time 2, Faculty 023)*

However, many faculty respondents made a distinction between the instruction being delivered as a result of the pandemic and teaching online courses in general. These faculty, it seems, recognized that they were not offering a true online course, but rather ERT.

> Please remember these are not really online classes or they would have been ready before we started.
>
> *(Time 1, F014)*

> [V]iewing the process as "disaster relief" rather than proper "online teaching" has helped a lot to not worry about the things that aren't quite right because they would need a lot more planning.
>
> *(Time 1, Faculty 032)*

Regardless of their concerns regarding online courses, faculty and students agreed that learning suffered from the remote instruction offered in response to the pandemic.

Conclusion and discussion

This study analyzed how students and faculty at a small, southeastern, public university perceived and experienced ERT during the COVID-19 pandemic. Across four surveys, students and faculty shared three major concerns about the shift to ERT: balancing work, school, and family obligations, changes to course material, and learning less. However, perceptions and experiences of students and faculty to ERT were shaped by and reflect their status and roles in the university. Although this study used a convenience sample and individual responses from Time 1 to Time 2 could not be tracked, three important lessons emerge from the findings.

First, universities should develop or revise policies and procedures in their continuity of operations plan (COOP) based on input from low-, middle-, and high-status actors across the campus using lessons learned during the COVID-19 pandemic experience. Currently, many universities are required to have an annually revised COOP to ensure education continues during disruptions. Inviting middle-status (faculty and staff) and low-status (students) actors into the process of developing or revising crisis response plans would provide a more comprehensive view of how proposed policy changes potentially affect the lives of the people who work and go to school at the institution.

Second, greater guidance for instructional delivery during a crisis must be created by and provided to faculty. The findings of this study indicate that faculty did not receive specific instruction on how best to finish classes during the crisis, increasing their stress and workload and making the process more disruptive and chaotic for students. Despite faculty members' best intentions, collectively, course changes created more perceived barriers for students to excel, additional work they had to manage during a global pandemic, and elicited negative emotions. Given their organizational status, faculty members have a fair amount of discretion to teach classes the way they deem most appropriate, making it difficult to craft policies and procedures that can be applied to all courses. At the very least, however, faculty governance systems can develop basic guidelines and expectations for instructional delivery during times of crisis.

Third, when a crisis necessitates significant changes to course delivery, transparent communication from faculty to students is essential (see Cohan 2021, this volume). Data from this study indicate that students were largely unaware of the reasons why faculty made changes to course material; students simply perceived course changes as more work and highly frustrating and overwhelming. Furthermore, although faculty attempted to accommodate students' needs in restructuring courses, they were not fully aware of what students were experiencing. In future crisis situations, faculty should inquire about immediate and long-term challenges facing their students before modifying their courses. Faculty should then clearly explain to their students how and why they are redesigning assignments, which might help students understand, and perhaps adjust to, course changes.

The COVID-19 pandemic is arguably one of the most disruptive crises of the century. Information gleaned from institutional responses to the disease are invaluable in creating policies and practices that can facilitate more seamless, less disruptive adaptations to future crises.

Note

1 See Smith, Sanford, and Blum (2021) for discussion of how student work obligations during ERT exposed hidden inequities.

References

Charmaz, Kathy. 2006. *Constructing Grounded Theory: A Practical Guide through Qualitative Analysis*. Thousand Oaks, CA: Sage.

Cohan, Deborah J. 2021. "Rethinking What We Value: Pandemic Teaching and the Art of Letting go." In *COVID-19: Social Consequences and Cultural Adaptations*, edited by J. Michael Ryan, 23–30. London: Routledge.

Esterberg, Kristen G. 2002. *Qualitative Methods in Social Research*. Boston, MA: McGraw-Hill.

Falchikov, Nancy. 1986. "Product Comparisons and Process Benefits of Collaborative Peer Group and Self-Assessments." *Assessment and Evaluation in Higher Education* 11 (2): 146–66. https://doi.org/10.1080/0260293860110206.

Hartnett, Rodney T., and John. A. Centra. 1974. "Faculty Views of the Academic Environment: Situational vs. Institutional Perspectives." *Sociology of Education* 47 (1) (Winter): 159–69. https://doi.org/10.2307/2112171.

Hirschy, Amy S., and Maureen E. Wilson. 2002. "The Sociology of the Classroom and its Influences on Student Learning." *Peabody Journal of Education* 77 (3): 85–100.

Hodges, Charles, Stephanie Moore, Barb Lockee, Torrey Trust, and Aaron Bond. 2020. "The Difference Between Emergency Remote Teaching and Online Learning." *Education Review*, March 27. https://er.educause.edu/articles/2020/3/the-difference-between-emergency-remote-teaching-and-online-learning.

Macionis, John J. 2017. *Sociology*. New York: Pearson.

Sanford, Adam G., Dinur Blum, and Stacy L. Smith. 2021. "Seeking Stability in Unstable Times: COVID-19 and the Bureaucratic Mindset." In *COVID-19: Social Consequences and Cultural Adaptations*, edited by J. Michael Ryan, 47–60. Philadelphia: Routledge.

Sauder, Michael, Freda Lynn, and Joel M. Podolny. 2012. "Status: Insights from Organizational Sociology." *Annual Review of Sociology* 38: 267–83. https://doi.org/10.1146/annurev-soc-071811-145503.

Saurugger, Sabine. 2016. "Sociological Approaches to the European Union in Times of Turmoil." *JCMS: Journal of Common Market Studies* 54: 70–86. https://doi.org/10.1111/jcms.12330.

Smith, Stacy L., Adam G. Sanford, and Dinur Blum. 2021. "Spotlighting Hidden Inequities: Post-Secondary Education in a Pandemic." In *COVID-19: Global Pandemic,*

Societal Responses, Ideological Solutions, edited by J. Michael Ryan, 124–38. Philadelphia: Routledge.

Tichavsky, Lisa P., Andrea N. Hung, Adam Driscoll, and Karl Jicha. 2015. "'It's Just Nice Having a Real Teacher': Student Perceptions of Online versus Face-to-Face Instruction." *International Journal for the Scholarship of Teaching and Learning* 9 (2), Article 2. https://doi.org/10.20429/ijsotl.2015.090202.

Wingo, Nancy Pope, Nataliya V. Ivankova, and Jacqueline A. Moss. 2017. "Faculty Perceptions about Teaching Online: Exploring the Literature Using the Technology Acceptance model as an Organizing Framework." *Online Learning* 21 (1): 15–35. https://doi.org/10.24059/olj.v21i1.761.

5

SEEKING STABILITY IN UNSTABLE TIMES

COVID-19 and the bureaucratic mindset

Adam G. Sanford, Dinur Blum, and Stacy L. Smith

Introduction

In the spring of 2020, the academic world was shaken to its foundations by the rapid changes demanded by the appearance of COVID-19. Historically, higher education has changed slowly and incrementally, usually due to external pressure such as new laws or regulations. Higher education's institutions are structured as bureaucracies, and the known inability of bureaucracies to make rapid change (Asatryan, Heinemann, and Pitlik 2016), we argue, is in many cases exacerbated by the culture and mindset bureaucracies create for the actors that work within them – what we here call *bureaucraticity*. We will show that this culture and mindset rest on the idea that bureaucracy creates safety, predictability, and stability and should be protected and preserved. *Bureaucraticity*, or the culture of the bureaucratic mindset, created many additional roadblocks to the quick pivot needed before COVID-19 became a pandemic.

In this chapter, we introduce the concepts of *bureaucraticity, process-oriented* and *outcome-oriented bureaucratic actors*, *decisions through habitus*, *decisions through praxis*, and *stubborn stability*. These concepts, when combined with Weber's theories of bureaucracy, Durkheim's social facts and anomie, Lenski's theories of environmental influences on culture, and Garfinkel's breaching experiments, explain how and why many university systems have been unable to effectively adapt to the rapid changes required by the COVID-19 international pandemic. We start by outlining the ideas of bureaucracy and bureaucraticity, and then discuss what we know about university bureaucracies and their characteristics. After that, we move to a discussion of how bureaucraticity impedes the ability of educational institutions to rapidly adapt to novel situations and sudden change, using the specific example of the COVID-19 pandemic. We conclude by identifying several hurdles that must be overcome if we are to reform academic bureaucracies into flexible systems that can respond, rather than react, to unavoidable and rapid change.

Bureaucracy and bureaucraticity

To understand bureaucraticity, we should start by defining bureaucracy in more detail. For this we turn to Weber's definition: A bureaucracy is an organizational structure with "a clearly established system of super- and subordination in which there is a supervision of the lower offices by the higher ones" (Weber 1978, 957). In other words, there is a chain of command, where people higher up the chain supervise and direct the people who are below them on the chain. Weber identifies several defining characteristics of bureaucracy, as follows:

> The principle of official jurisdictional areas, which are generally ordered by rules . . . this means 1) The regular activities required for the purposes of bureaucratically governed structure are assigned as official duties; 2) The authority to give the commands required for the discharge of these duties is distributed in a stable way and is strictly delimited by rules concerning the coercive means . . . which may be placed at the disposal of officials; 3) Methodical provision is made for the regular and continuous fulfillment of these duties and for the exercise of the corresponding rights; only persons who qualify under general rules are employed.
>
> *(Weber 1978, 956)*

A bureaucracy, therefore, is composed of bureaucratic actors who have the expertise and authority to make decisions in certain defined areas. Under normal conditions, these people hold specific positions associated with specific tasks, rules, and decisions. Bureaucracy's mission is to provide and maintain stability and avoid change unless absolutely necessary. Slow, incremental change over a long period of time is how a bureaucracy functions best. As a result, it often has difficulty dealing with sudden changes demanded or imposed by external conditions, since those changes and conditions may not have defined certifications – that is, there is no bureaucratic position titled "Rapid Change Officer."

Examining these foundational elements of bureaucracy – supervision of lower offices by higher ones, regular activities assigned as official duties, stable distribution and rules concerning authority to command these duties, and the employment of qualified people only – provides an overview of what bureaucracy looks like and how it operates. In the bureaucracies of higher education, administration supervises faculty and staff, while senior faculty supervise junior faculty and senior staff supervise junior staff; regular activities such as teaching, research, and resource management are assigned as official duties; authority is defined by rules and agreements among divisions and departments; and only people with credentials that qualify for these positions achieve and retain employment.

The rules and agreements, expected credentials, and ways in which supervision and power flow up and down the bureaucratic hierarchy are what Durkheim called "social facts" – "ways of acting, thinking and feeling, external to the individual, and endowed with the power of coercion, by reason of which they control him" (Durkheim 1964, 3). Inside a bureaucracy, credentials control what kind of position a person can hold, the authority given by that position, rules that must be followed, who reports to whom, and many other social facts which are taken for granted by the actors inside the bureaucracy. In fact, it can be argued that the social facts create a social environment, which in turn shapes the culture of that social environment. If culture is a "toolkit" (Swidler 1986) and the environment in which a culture develops shapes that culture in ways that a different environment would not (Lenski 2015), then the culture of a bureaucracy – what we are here calling *bureaucraticity* – serves to recreate itself.

We further suggest that bureaucracy's need for a stable, unchanging environment – its *stubborn stability* – is another characteristic that must be taken into account in this analysis. To function well, bureaucraticity depends on stability and predictability, including the stability of the environment in which it operates. It also influences subject actors to make decisions based on the good of the institution rather than the good of individual members. In essence, the social facts of bureaucracy create bureaucraticity, and unless these social facts are somehow breached (broken), they become a taken-for-granted reality and actors generally do not notice their constraints (Garfinkel 1984). More-bureaucratic situations with more-bureaucratic norms and actors will have more difficulty responding to sudden changes in normative standards.

Bureaucratic actors

A bureaucracy contains two kinds of bureaucratic actors, which we here have defined as *outcome-oriented* and *process-oriented*. An academic bureaucracy contains faculty and administrators (as well as students). Outcome-oriented bureaucratic actors (OBAs) are willing to try new methods and processes and tend to prioritize outcomes over process, while process-oriented bureaucratic actors (PBAs) resist new methods, policies, or procedures as inferior to the way things have always been done and tend to focus on process more than outcomes. For example, a PBA faculty member would focus on preserving tried-and-true teaching methods because they are familiar and dependable, while an OBA faculty member would focus on finding teaching methods that produce reliable outcomes in the form of grades, scores, and student feedback. Similarly, a PBA administrator would focus on preserving standards that had been repeatedly used to evaluate faculty progress toward tenure, in the interest of preserving continuity, while an OBA administrator would propose new standards that might better capture what faculty progress looked like in a particular year.

If social conventions (a form of social fact) are broken, their violations can cause mild to intense distress among the social actors who are affected by its breaking.

TABLE 5.1 Types of Bureaucratic Actors

Process-Oriented (PBA)	Outcome-Oriented (OBA)
Resists new methods, polices, or procedures in favor of tried-and-true	Interested in trying new methods, policies, and procedures
Focuses on keeping processes the same	Focuses on creating similar (or better) outcomes
Sees new methods as inferior	Sees new methods as leading to better outcomes
Makes decisions through *habitus*	Makes decisions through *praxis*
Greater distress when faced with sudden change	Moderate stress when faced with sudden change
Watchwords: tradition and longevity	Watchwords: innovation and flexibility

For example, Garfinkel's breaching experiments show these broken social conventions cause people to become bewildered and anxious (Garfinkel 1984, 55), often severely: "[T]he firmer a [person]'s grasp of What Anyone Like Us Necessarily Knows, the more severe should be [their] disturbance when 'natural facts of life' are impugned for [them] as a depiction of [their] real circumstances" (Garfinkel 1984, 54).

The more dependent upon social facts a person is, the more upset and uncomfortable that person will become when the social facts are breached. PBAs, who are more oriented toward processes – "the way things are done" – are more derailed in this situation than are OBAs, who are more oriented toward outcomes and thus more likely to resist situations that would lead to such derailment. Even the breaching of social facts we would consider minor, such as standing facing the back of an elevator instead of the doors, can cause intense distress in a social actor who needs stability and predictability. We can think of process orientation as a security blanket of sorts, and the changing conditions make clinging to the security blanket a defense mechanism, though one not particularly helpful for the institution.

Durkheim's (1964) concept of anomie (the sense of normlessness, or not knowing what the rules are when the rules change suddenly) dovetails with Garfinkel's findings. Anomie describes what happens when a person is confronted with a situation that is unlike any situation they have previously encountered. In this situation, existing norms that usually create stability fail to do so because of the situation's novelty. This failure then creates anomie, requiring social actors to do active cognitive work to manage it, instead of relying on what has always worked in the past. This lack of successful, established norms for the novel situation creates instability and, eventually, social change. Institutions experience anomie as well – the rules that have always worked fail to address the novel situation. This tends to create anomie for all subject actors of that institution – admittedly, some more than others.

Sanford's (2012) work on decision-making – specifically, the decision to treat a situation as legitimate and thus binding on our actions – shows how reactions to anomie differ between PBAs and OBAs. Sanford's findings of *decision-making through habitus* and *decision-making through praxis* map approximately to the ways PBAs and OBAs make decisions and give legitimacy to social situations:

> *Legitimacy through praxis* is that which we treat as legitimate because we have actively, deliberately decided to do so . . . *Legitimacy through habitus* is that which we treat as legitimate because it has always been legitimate. We allow it to bind our actions without conscious deliberation.
>
> *(Sanford 2012, 16–17, emphasis in the original)*

Actors who are able to make decisions using *praxis* – deliberative and purposeful action – are more able to handle novel situations and sudden change than are actors who depend on *habitus* – familiar situations with familiar components – to make decisions. Since bureaucracy depends heavily on rules and credentials defining *what* things get done, *how* they get done, and *who* does them, it creates a perfect *habitus* environment.

Adaptation and change often require deliberation and active decision-making, rather than the habitual decisions bureaucracy is designed to encourage. Given this, PBAs are more likely to have difficulty adjusting to rapid change than are OBAs, and "fixate on the little they can control" (Cohan 2021, this volume). This is not to say OBAs do not also have trouble with novel situations, but they are less likely to experience extreme distress when facing them than are their process-oriented counterparts. OBAs are also embedded in the forms and structures of bureaucracy but are more able to quickly adjust and adapt when faced with novel situations. PBAs, however, cling to their processes and social facts because they do not deal well with novel situations requiring rapid adaptation and change.

Bureaucracy and the academy

Since the early 1990s, many university bureaucracies have been forced to adapt to reductions of state and large donor economic support for university systems, the effects of neoliberalism on the surrounding culture, and the increasing levels of competition between schools for student enrollment. Confronted with these pressures, university bureaucratic structures have reorganized to respond to and manage them. However, these changes have been slow, gradual, and planned, rather than the sudden changes imposed by the pandemic. They have not created new processes to manage rapid change. (Again, there is no "Rapid Change Officer" position!)

Universities have also faced increasing pressures to restructure from a "bureaucratic-collegial" model, where faculty have a lot of input into the various processes and policies of the institution, to a "managerial" model, which is more like a corporate bureaucracy (Bruckmann and Carvalho 2018, 642). In a bureaucratic-collegial model, each part of the university operates more or less independently of administration – an arrangement referred to as "loosely coupled" in organizational theory. In a loosely coupled arrangement, any particular department could close down without harming the overall mission and purpose of the larger institution. The bureaucratic-collegial model was how most colleges and universities were structured prior to the 1990s.

In a managerial model, however, the university is far more "tightly coupled" – that is, each department and division has far more defined lines of managerial control from administration down to faculty and staff. The bureaucratic chain of command is much more in evidence in managerial models than in bureaucratic-collegial ones. Faculty influence on the system has been greatly diminished over the past few decades, as most universities have increasingly moved toward a managerial model (Maasen and Stensaker 2019). Faculty's collegial influence, and therefore their influence in university decision-making more generally, has been significantly reduced.

Perhaps counter-intuitively, the managerial model has a much better chance of rapid adaptation to quickly changing circumstances because the number of decision makers and people with input into the problems has been reduced, streamlining decision-making and response. As such, this model has been somewhat more successful at responding to changing conditions – at least, in terms of "speeding up . . . decision-making processes" (Maasen and Stensaker 2019, 461). However, speeding up decisions does not necessarily mean the decisions create good outcomes for the institutions or their actors – and may actually increase bureaucraticity.

The flexibility offered by the bureaucratic-collegial model serves universities well under *normal* circumstances, because it empowers more faculty. But with the sudden challenges presented by this pandemic, having a clearly defined bureaucratic hierarchy with easily identifiable decision makers allows for more widespread changes to be put into action quickly, although it also imposes a single decision upon all actors, whether those actors find the decision beneficial or not. Faculty who fight for the return of the bureaucratic-collegial model may not see much success, due to the environmental demands imposed on their institutions by the pandemic.

Bureaucracies concentrate power – to make decisions and to make change – at the top. Weber (1978) discusses power as a two-fold concept: having power and exercising it (if those subject to such power agree that its wielders have it). In order to exercise power and make others do as they wish, one must have power. However, merely having power does not guarantee using it, or using it effectively. In higher education situations, bureaucraticity creates power struggles between administration and faculty. These emerge because of the basic nature of bureaucracy: Those who have certifications in certain types of authority have the power to exercise that authority, while those who are not so certified do not. In most universities, faculty are certified as content creators and content communicators, but their certifications are in research and teaching, not administration. Administrators, on the other hand, are certified to manage and make decisions under the conditions normally assumed in a bureaucracy.[1] The problem is the environmental conditions have changed, and, as many people are discovering, the tools that always worked before no longer do, and can even have adverse effects.

On many campuses, especially in the United States, academic bureaucracy has seen a shift in power from PBAs to OBAs, largely due to the neoliberalization of the university (Olssen and Peters 2005, 327, Ryan 2021a) and increasing competition between universities for student enrollment. These situations have pushed the university's bureaucracy in the direction of a much more managerial structure than before. This reorganization has exacerbated the power struggle between PBAs and OBAs within university bureaucracy, with the original process-oriented bureaucrats relying on tradition in trying to keep things the way they always have been, while outcome-oriented bureaucrats push forward with new innovations to make the university more financially stable and competitive.

The power struggle between PBAs and OBAs presents itself through claims (made by PBAs) that the new methods and processes for doing things (proposed by OBAs) are inherently inferior because they do not reproduce the familiar processes that have been used before. By doing so, they assume that tradition and longevity are more important than flexibility, because the tools they use do not lend themselves to flexibility. OBAs argue for similarity of outcomes, but many PBAs insist on similarity of process, as well. This tension between process and results has already been present in institutions of higher education for years, but the institutional response to the pandemic has spotlighted it and exacerbated this tension.

The rule-boundedness of academic bureaucracies is also an impediment to rapid adaptation. Higher education is prone to "bureaucratic legalism," which Kagan (2006) defines as "[a]n administrative decision-making process characterized by a high degree of hierarchical authority and legal formality . . . resemb[ling] the ideal-typical bureaucratic process as analyzed by Max Weber."[2] Legalism creates bureaucratic systems with formalized, regulated, rigorous structures through which there are only one (or possibly two) paths to successful outcomes. For example, in an academic bureaucracy, the successful outcome rests on low attrition and high graduation rates within a normative time frame (typically four years, although a longer time frame is acceptable if the result is graduation), or in the case of two-year institutions, certification, a degree, or successful transfer to a four-year institution. Similarly, the "successful" path for a faculty member is to occupy an increasingly rare tenure line and achieve tenure through a review process conducted by other faculty and the administration. Although higher education relies on non-tenured faculty, these positions typically do not define "success" for faculty. These expectations are built on structures with an inhibiting effect on rapid adaptation and quick responses to outside stressors or changes, because the focus of the bureaucracy "is not about how to respond to rapid changes in societal demands but how to ensure legal certainty" (Lapuente and Suzuki 2020, 456), which, in the Weberian sense, means dependability and repeatability. Innovative and "managerial" bureaucracies have an advantage in adapting quickly to sudden change. The more legalistic and rule-bound the bureaucracy, the less likely it will be able to adapt to rapid social change – because bureaucratic legalism stands in the way of pro-innovation views (Lapuente and Suzuki 2020, 457).

The overall shift toward a more managerial, neoliberal bureaucracy has helped shape a situation where process-oriented bureaucratic actors who oppose these changes feel increasingly unheard, and even betrayed, by the changes happening in spite of their resistance. "[I]n the context of organizations," Sievers (2009, 71) argues, "the introduction of new strategies, policies, and value systems is often experienced as betrayal." Given the ongoing feelings of persistent betrayal they have been experiencing for the last several decades, some process-oriented actors may feel the changes required in a pandemic response are simply a bridge too far and dig in their heels to refuse further change.

The effects of academic bureaucraticity in an international pandemic

According to Ryan, "It is . . . uncertain how the broad moves to online education will impact the future of educators and brick-and-mortar educational institutions" (Ryan 2021b, this volume). Normally, bureaucracy provides its actors with tools that replicate the bureaucracy, *as long as the environment remains stable and the norms remain functional*. Problems arise when the institutional environment changes, the norms no longer function, or both. The response to the pandemic profoundly changed the environment, but many bureaucratic actors continue using the same tools regardless of their effectiveness or potential for harm. For example, the real-time, in-class lecture is a powerful instructional tool – but many instructors discovered, to their chagrin, that holding a real-time lecture over videoconferencing software caused many students to tune out or to struggle far more than they would in an in-person environment. And, of course, some students were unable to connect to the videoconference at all, due to other either demands on their time from families or workplaces, lack of available technology including consistently strong internet access, or both. This not only decreased learning but exacerbated inequity and stress for these students, as discussed by Smith, Sanford, and Blum (2021) in this volume.

Bureaucratic culture lacks any tool to allow it to rapidly change course during abnormal circumstances. Ideally, bureaucratic actors are hired based on specific certifications in specific areas of expertise, regardless of being process or outcome oriented, and they are expected to both wield the authority that goes with those certifications and "stay in their lane." Despite being on the front lines of the situation and knowing the most about the problems they and their students are facing, faculty lack the institutional authority to make decisions and distribute resources directly to help remedy the problems. Instead, they have often been confronted with a bureaucratic process that slows down or even stops getting help where it is needed, when it is needed. This situation creates a power clash between the people who can see the problems and the people who have the authority to solve them.

One of the main ways this struggle showed up, in the first weeks of the move to remote instruction, was administrative requirements (across many institutions) to hold synchronous class meetings over videoconferencing software, despite the inequity issues these meetings created and exposed (Smith, Sanford, and Blum 2021). Although many faculty agreed with this directive, others – especially those who had more experience with online teaching – objected, and were overruled. This attempt to maintain "business as usual" in the face of the pandemic often created more work, stress, and difficulty for students, faculty, staff, and administration.

Many process-oriented faculty – who tend to be more embedded in bureaucraticity – first tried to exert control over the situation by flatly rejecting changes required by the pandemic. We have seen multiple examples of this in higher education discussion groups created in response to the pandemic. First, educators resisted moving online at all. When told they did not have a choice, they then attempted to recreate the in-person environment online, in large part by defending "rigor": increasing students' workload to compensate for the lack of in-class meetings, becoming more rigid about deadlines, insisting on synchronous class meetings through videoconferencing, requiring students to use "lockdown browser" programs to proctor their examinations, extreme concern about academic dishonesty, and a general lack of flexibility. At the same time, these faculty rejected online teaching methods such as recorded lectures, outcome-oriented due dates, and asynchronous approaches to communicating information to students, despite the fact that these methods create better learning outcomes for students in an online or remote environment (Darby 2020). All of these responses to unavoidable change reveal a need to maintain a semblance of normalcy, without taking rapidly changing on-the-ground conditions into account.

In the situation the pandemic has created, bureaucracy's main tools of process, rules, certification, and supervision have failed to produce the desired and expected outcomes. Indeed, the rapid shifting of which qualifications are important and which ones no longer matter – in short, the lack of a certification to manage academic responses to a pandemic – has caused higher education to move into a form of academic triage (Schaeffer 2021), where those "on the ground" are being micromanaged by supervisors who do not have all the information they need to manage the situations effectively. This only worsens the situation, as academic bureaucracy has no effective bureaucratic tools to manage it. This situation has also led to an increase in inequity for students, partly because it has revealed just how much students depend on available computer labs and internet on campus to complete their work (Smith, Sanford, and Blum 2021), and partly because it demands faculty learn and use new pedagogical methods rather than their tried-and-true but now ineffective (and often harmful) teaching tools (Darby 2020).

The bureaucratic nature of higher education is not well suited to adapting to sudden crises. A combination of bureaucratic norms, social facts about education, and a cultural environment reticent to change and designed to prevent change and maintain continuity explain some of the breakdowns caused by the rapid adaptation required by an international pandemic. Bureaucraticity's stubborn stability also impedes institutional adaptation.

Discussion and conclusion

The problems revealed by the COVID-19 pandemic are jarring, and they require quick action and adaptability to cope with them. When COVID-19 first became an international pandemic, and college campuses began the abrupt move from in-person to online instruction, examples of bureaucraticity – and its inability to adapt – started to appear in academic news sources and other literature. These included lists of faculty organization demands of institutions of higher learning (American Association of University Professors 2020) and dire warnings that administrators would "finish what they started" (Berlinerblau 2020). But they also included speculation that modifying bureaucratic operating standards, such as the in-person meeting, might be positive for the university – though losing all bureaucracy would not (Byrnes 2020). Later in the term, universities began considering not just the spring term of 2020, but also how they would manage the new demands of the virus for their summer sessions and the fall term. At this point, articles ranging from cautions against reopening due to serious public health and safety concerns (Sorrel 2020) to descriptions of drastic measures taken by university management to preserve their bureaucratic structures (Furstenberg 2020; Gopalan 2020) and predictions of continued bureaucratic foot-dragging causing university failures and closures (Devinney and Dowling 2020) filled academic news sources, blogs, and magazines. Notably lacking, however, were proposals to make universities more flexible or responsive to rapid change; in fact, the majority of these articles instead proposed reasons to resist it. From these examples, we can see bureaucraticity creates a number of blockades to rapid change.

First, bureaucratic rules, which require getting permissions through a chain of command that may take days, weeks, or even months to produce an answer, cause institutions to be unable to adapt quickly. For example, instructors who wanted to try new methods of teaching during the last half of the spring term of 2020 were often told, as a top-down command, to maintain "normalcy" as much as possible through the use of synchronous videoconferencing, to hold regular classes at the same times they were scheduled before the pandemic closed their campuses. Getting permission to hold asynchronous classes instead could have taken as long as the rest of the term, and in the meantime, instructors had to struggle with Zoom calls, Zoombombings, and other problems that made their jobs much more difficult.

Second, the rule-reliant, hyper-legalistic culture of bureaucracy leads to an over-reliance on process (because process means "following the rules"). Bureaucratic actors assume proper process will lead to correct outcomes, and in a normal situation, this is generally true. The problem appears when the environment changes and the change is not adjusted for. Having to hold synchronous class meetings, when perhaps a third of the students do not have the appropriate tech or internet connection or have other reasons why meeting at 8:30 a.m. from their home is not feasible, shows that bureaucratic process is heavily tied to rules which were developed under specific environmental conditions – such as having a dorm room and access to school computers – which changed the moment students were sent home from campus due to the virus.

Third, stubborn stability – the dependence on an unchanging environment – is so ingrained into the bureaucratic way of doing things that flexibility is seen as weakness. Instead, rigidity, or holding firmly to "how we've always done it," is seen as synonymous with the stability of the entire institution, to the point that trying to insert flexibility into bureaucratic processes, to accommodate the problems of new information and changing environments, is treated as hostile to the institution. This information is then either ignored completely (leading to the other problems already discussed) or fought against – a hopeless process when the new information is a deadly virus. Unfortunately, as the current pandemic has demonstrated, this very rigidity is bureaucraticity's fundamental flaw – "the system becomes so 'rational' that it is, in fact, irrational" (Ritzer 2021).

It is readily apparent that bureaucratic structures in higher education systems are not designed to rapidly respond to threats or changes and have not made much progress in this area, despite outside pressures to develop ways of doing so. "As an organisation [sic]," argues Egero (2006, 43), "a university has a number of particular features that pose structural obstacles to rational responses to a threat." The main issue for universities facing any demand for rapid change is bureaucraticity's stubborn stability. This dependence on an unchanging environment is structural to the system, as much as it is personal for many actors within it, and restructuring the university must be approached with the understanding that such restructuring may negatively affect the many "semi-autonomous entities (departments, institutes, etc.) over whose internal life it has little control" (Egero 2006, 43).

Bureaucraticity motivates actors to push for simple solutions that go "by the book" and follow established procedures and to avoid complex, nuanced ones wherever possible. However, novel problems require nuanced solutions, leading to the construction of new institutional structures and procedures that are less bureaucratic, more flexible, and more dynamic. These changes will improve institutional fitness and adaptability to environmental challenges, both now and in the future. Some of the hurdles that must be overcome, first, include bureaucraticity's resistance to change, even when change is necessary to the survival of the institution; the lack of trust between process-oriented and outcome-oriented bureaucratic actors; and bureaucracy's stubborn stability – its dependence upon the environment remaining stable and unchanging over time.

Byrnes (2020) suggests several ways in which institutions might move toward a reduction in bureaucracy, to enable greater flexibility and responsiveness to the COVID-19 crisis, as well as other situations that may demand rapid change in the future. First, universities must realign themselves with their purpose, or their "why" (Byrnes 2020). Many of the issues caused by bureaucraticity can be traced back to a loss of connection with the ideal purpose of the university, which is to educate students and create both productive members of society and critical-thinking citizens. Universities must look critically at how many of their set processes actually function to serve this goal. Is it central to this goal, for example, to have students be on campus for classes? Does it require synchronous classes, meeting in real time? Is it necessary for students to have in-person meetings with teachers in order to learn?

Second, universities must push to empower every actor – not just administrators but also faculty, students, and staff (Byrnes 2020). This will require PBAs to relax their grip on keeping process the same and become more open to outcome-oriented solutions, while also requiring OBAs to find solutions that honor existing processes, if possible. Identifying issues that get in the way of the university's purpose may be a starting point, as faculty, administrators, staff, and students work to find or innovate processes that can handle these issues.

Finally, bringing respect for all parties to the table will be crucial, in order to establish trust and a sense of working together, rather than against one another (Byrnes 2020). Without real respect for each actor's position and needs, especially as those needs relate to the purpose of the university, we will continue to see stagnation, gridlock, and an inability to move forward without many parties feeling belittled or betrayed.

Academic bureaucracies must, in essence, find ways to make themselves less bureaucratic and more flexible, while still providing stability and dependability to their actors. As Bidwell notes, administrators need "better emergency planning . . . [and] communication . . . to facilitate a more seamless response to unforeseen events" (Bidwell, Grether, and Pederson 2021). Byrnes's solutions should serve as a starting point for researchers, faculty, and administrators who recognize their institutions must develop methods of coping with unavoidable, rapid change – a weakness that has always been present in academic bureaucracies and may doom them, if not resolved.

Notes

1 Administrators who started their careers as faculty may also face issues, as their original certifications were in research and teaching. Many of these administrators may feel they are required to "choose sides" and become fully administrative, up to and including gaining new certifications to qualify them as bureaucratic decision makers and managers.
2 It should be noted that "legalism" here refers to Weber's idea of legalism: high levels of formality and hierarchy, as are often seen in a bureaucracy.

References

American Association of University Professors. 2020. "AAUP Principles and Standards for the COVID-19 Crisis." Accessed June 2, 2020. www.aaup.org/aaup-principles-and-standards-covid-19-crisis.

Asatryan, Zareh, Friedrich Heinemann, and Hans Pitlik. 2016. "Reforming the Public Administration: The Role of Crisis and the Power of Bureaucracy." *European Journal of Political Economy* 48: 128–43.

Berlinerblau, Jacques. 2020. "After Coronavirus, The Deluge." *Chronicle of Higher Education*. Accessed June 17, 2020. www.chronicle.com/article/After-Coronavirus-the-Deluge/248348.

Bidwell, Lee Millar, Scott T. Grether, and JoEllen Pederson. 2021. "Disruption and Difficulty: Students and Faculty Perceptions of the Transition to Online Instruction in the COVID-19 Pandemic." In *COVID-19: Social Consequences and Cultural Adaptations*, edited by J. Michael Ryan, 31–46. London: Routledge.

Bruckmann, Sofia, and Teresa Carvalho. 2018. "Understanding Change in Higher Education: An Archetypal Approach." *Higher Education* 76: 629–47.

Byrnes, Giselle. 2020. "Whither University Bureaucracy Post COVID-19?" Accessed June 2, 2020. www.linkedin.com/pulse/whither-university-bureaucracy-post-covid-19-giselle-byrnes/?articleId=6654848234390986752.

Cohan, Deborah. 2021. "Rethinking What We Value: Pandemic Teaching and the Art of Letting Go." In *COVID-19: Social Consequences and Cultural Adaptations*, edited by J. Michael Ryan, 23–30. London: Routledge.

Darby, Flower. 2020. "Sorry Not Sorry: Online Teaching is Here to Stay." *Chronicle of Higher Education*. Accessed June 2, 2020. www.chronicle.com/article/Sorry-Not-Sorry-Online/248993.

Devinney, Timothy, and Grahame Dowling. 2020. "Is This the Crisis Higher Education Needs to Have?" *Times Higher Education*. Accessed May 14, 2020. www.timeshighereducation.com/features/crisis-higher-education-needs-have.

Durkheim, Emile. 1964. *The Rules of Sociological Method*. Chicago: Free Press of Glencoe.

Egero, Bertil. 2006. "HIV/AIDS on the Campus: Universities and the Threat of an Epidemic." *Eastern Africa Social Science Research Review* 22 (2): 31–50.

Furstenberg, François. 2020. "The University is Failing." *Chronicle of Higher Education*. Accessed June 2, 2020. www.chronicle.com/article/university-leaders-are-failing/248809.

Garfinkel, Harold. 1984. *Studies in Ethnomethodology*. Cambridge: Polity Press.

Gopalan, Mahesh. 2020. "Bureaucracy Forgets It Is Staff and Students that Make a University, Not Exams." *The Wire*. Accessed June 2, 2020. https://thewire.in/education/covid-19-lockdown-university-education-exams.

Kagan, Robert A. 2006. "The Organization of Administrative Justice Systems." Center for the Study of Law and Society Working Papers. Accessed July 4, 2020. https://escholarship.org/uc/item/4k20s5zr.

Lapuente, Victor, and Kohei Suzuki. 2020. "Politicization, Bureaucratic Legalism, and Innovative Attitudes in the Public Sector." *Public Administration Review* 80 (3): 454–67.

Lenski, Gerhard. 2015. *Ecological-Evolutionary Theory: Principles and Applications*. New York: Routledge.

Maasen, Peter, and Bjørn Stensaker. 2019. "From Organised Anarchy to De-Coupled Bureaucracy: The Transformation of University Organization." *Higher Education Quarterly* 73: 456–68.

Olssen, Mark, and Michael A. Peters. 2005. "Neoliberalism, Higher Education and the Knowledge Economy: From the Free Market to Knowledge Capitalism." *Journal of Education Policy* 20 (3): 313–45.

Ritzer, George. 2021. "McDonaldization in the Age of COVID-19." In *COVID-19: Global Pandemic, Societal Responses, Ideological Solutions*, edited by J. Michael Ryan, 23–8. London: Routledge.

Ryan, J. Michael. 2021a. "The Blessings of COVID-19 for Neoliberalism, Nationalism, and Neoconservative Ideologies." In *COVID-19: Global Pandemic, Societal Responses, Ideological Solutions*, edited by J. Michael Ryan, 80–93. London: Routledge.

———. 2021b. "The SARS-CoV-2 Virus and the COVID-19 Pandemic." In *COVID-19: Social Consequences and Cultural Adaptations*, edited by J. Michael Ryan, 9–19. London: Routledge.

Sanford, Adam G. 2012. "Exploring the Decision-Making Process in Relation to Legitimacy Assignment." PhD Dissertation, Sociology, University of California, Riverside.

Schaeffer, Scott. 2021. "Necroethics in the Time of COVID-19 and Black Lives Matter." In *COVID-19: Global Pandemic, Societal Responses, Ideological Solutions*, edited by J. Michael Ryan, 43–53. London: Routledge.

Sievers, Burkard. 2009. "It Is New, and It Has To Be Done! Socio-Analytical Thoughts on Betrayal and Cynicism in Organizational Transformation." *Culture and Organization* 13 (1): 1–27.

Smith, Stacy L., Adam G. Sanford, and Dinur Blum. 2021. "Spotlighting Hidden Inequities: Post-Secondary Education in a Pandemic." In *COVID-19: Global Pandemic, Societal Responses, Ideological Solutions*, edited by J. Michael Ryan, 124–38. London: Routledge.

Sorrel, Michael J. 2020. "Colleges Are Deluding Themselves." *The Atlantic*. Accessed June 2, 2020. www.theatlantic.com/ideas/archive/2020/05/colleges-that-reopen-are-making-a-big-mistake/611485/.

Swidler, Ann. 1986. "Culture in Action: Symbols and Strategies." *American Sociological Review* 52 (2): 273–86.

Weber, Max. 1978. *Economy and Society: An Outline of Interpretive Sociology*. Los Angeles: University of California Press.

6

THE SOLUTION IS THE PROBLEM

What a pandemic can reveal about policing

Jodie Dewey

Policing has become a global health problem. COVID-19 has shed new and brighter light on the health disparities experienced by people of color, and the recent police killing of George Floyd in Minneapolis, Minnesota, showed the disproportionate effect of police brutality on African American bodies. Health and policing converged as people responded to police violence by taking to the street, violating social distancing directives and risking exposure to the virus; these week-long, worldwide protests made it painfully clear that there is not a problem *in* policing as much as there is a problem *of* policing. The pandemic and the killing of George Floyd exposed the government's process of criminalizing people, dehumanizing them, and generalizing them – and one of the most effective ways to do this is by adopting racialized, classed, and gendered constructions that categorize people as (unworthy) victims or perpetrators. Policing risks social health and security when it is used to solve social and health problems.

How we police

The problem of expecting a police agency to enforce health directives, especially during unknown factors presented by a pandemic, is that they will continue to draw upon the narratives and cultural habitus, familiar decision-making based on seeing and constructing situations as equally familiar (Sanford, Blum, and Smith 2021, this volume), that obscure the gendered, classed, and racialized elements of "doing justice." The government, or the state, according to Bourdieu, is "an entity that exists by way of belief . . . a well-founded illusion . . . collectively validated by consensus" (Bourdieu 2014), such as when officers say that they merely "uphold the law" or claim "we don't see race, only crime." The criminal justice system participates in this ethos or habitus that is deeply entwined with other powerful state systems, such as mental health and medical care (Foucault 1977), making policing also a site for "doing health." The structure and mindset of bureaucracies, as well as the people who perform the roles within it, are arranged to maintain stability and reproduce itself and, therefore, are unlikely to respond differently to meet the demands presented by a global pandemic (Sanford, Blum, and Smith 2021, this volume). Overlapping powerful systems ensure criminal justice's longevity, power, and existence (Bourdieu and Wacquant 1992), and through the repetition of messages presented in the field, the processes of "doing police work" that are based on idealized visions of achieving justice conflict with the actual *doing* of justice, which can be reduced to "doing gender," "doing race," and "doing class."

Under a patriarchal system, men enjoy status and material dividends over women, and power is conferred to those who control knowledge and state apparatuses, namely through the use of violence to uphold the law. Narrow, "culturally exalted" (Connell 1987) meanings of masculinity, termed "hegemonic masculinity," are required to sustain a system of patriarchy and can be found in the training of police recruits. Idealized masculine narratives require the subordination of femininity and other forms of masculinity, which is best elucidated in the villain-victim-hero model that is historically powerful and culturally significant in the "new discourse emphasizing a metaphorical and unequal relationship among protective hegemonic masculinity, emphasized femininity, and subordinate masculinity" (Messerschmidt 2016). Therefore, separating people into strong and weak, worthy and unworthy, is required to deliver "justice" (Rios 2009; Gonzalez-Van Cleve 2016). While police ideologies center on policing as a community-engaged institution, their actual practices co-op community interests to police objectives (Gascon and Roussell 2019), and reveal that masculinity and Whiteness are leveraged to achieve power, mostly by demarcating the boundary between the police and the public (Foucault 1977; Dewey, *forthcoming;* Gonzalez-Van Cleve 2016). Construction of an "other," a mythical scapegoat based on perceived inherent inequalities, is required to ensure the ideological, political, and economic success of the state (Ryan 2021, this volume). Immediately following George Floyd's murder, President Donald Trump, in his many disturbing speeches and tweets, aligned masculinity with a show of militarized force against the protesting citizens he pledged to protect, while he dismissed Minneapolis Mayor Jacob Frey's response as weak and indecisive. Such reframing obscures the reality that the "crisis in policing" is really an unexamined "crisis in masculinity" (Connell and Messerschmidt 2005).

How a pandemic makes health problems, criminal justice problems

The World Health Organization (WHO) recorded the first cases of COVID-19 on January 4, 2020 (WHO 2020), and within four weeks, over 7,800 cases were reported in at least 17 countries. As of mid-August, the virus has spread to every continent, with over 23 million cases and 800,000 deaths (CNN Health 2020). While the first reported US case appeared on January 21, by mid-July it had ballooned to over 3.8 million confirmed cases and over 142,000 deaths. It was at this time that while many countries were beginning to flatten the curve of infection, the WHO reported the biggest daily jump in new cases since January, most concentrated in the United States and among the 18–44 age bracket (Mackintosh 2020). Unlike other pandemics, COVID-19 has proven uniquely challenging because a pre-symptomatic person, experiencing no symptoms severe enough to self-quarantine, could potentially infect many people. Contracted through respiratory droplets, the virus easily transfers from person to person during prolonged proximal closeness, essentially making most social interactions, especially those taking place in enclosed spaces, problematic (erinbromage.com).

Beyond the epidemiology of disease of most interest to medical experts, illness also has a social component in which social scientists investigate how virus contagion shapes individuals' lived experiences and their relationship to the people and systems around them (Ryan 2021, this volume). The COVID-19 pandemic highlighted patterns of health disparities that reveal larger structural barriers to quality health experiences and care that already exist (Paradies et al. 2015; Morey 2018; Thomas and Caspter 2019; Kawachi, Daniels, and Robinson 2005; Williams 2003). Where data based on race exists, non-Caucasian ethnic groups are disproportionately more likely to contract and die from COVID-19, such as in Ireland (Gleeson 2020) and the United Kingdom (Bhala et al. 2020). In the United States, African Americans are 2.4 times more likely to contract the virus compared with Caucasians, and while only making up only 13% of the population, African American deaths from the disease account for 25% of COVID-related deaths (APM Research Lab 2020a). In Chicago, for example, African Americans make up 30% of the population but 52% of COVID deaths. Environmental factors most affecting those in lower socioeconomic communities, such as living in congested/multigenerational homes, taking public transportation, and holding essential jobs that do not allow for remote work, exacerbate existing health issues and further increase viral exposure (Bhala et al. 2020). In England and Wales, for example, 34% of those employed in manual work account for 43% of COVID-19 deaths (Daley 2020).

Health disparities are compounded by inequities in police treatment, something made more apparent during a pandemic. In cities where police operate under aggressive tactical policies, continual fear of being stopped, frisked, harassed, and arrested intensifies stress and other health conditions that make one most susceptible to contracting and dying from COVID-19 (Natividad 2020). A global pandemic intensifies problematic experiences with police, which disproportionately impacts communities of color. For example, according to Fryer (2016), Latinos and African Americans are 50% more likely than Caucasians to experience use of force during a police encounter. Although escalated use of force (e.g., displaying/pointing a weapon, handcuffing without being arrested, and using oleoresin capsicum [O.C.] spray) are more rare, African Americans are 21.4% more likely than Caucasians to experience them. While Fryer found that for lethal force, African Americans were 23.8% less likely to be shot at by police, others researchers found that the rate of fatal police shooting disproportionately affects African Americans (Statista 2020) and that African Americans experience police-related injuries five times more frequently than do Caucasians (Feldman et al. 2016).

To limit the spread of COVID-19, many political leaders across the globe initiated stay-at-home orders and social distancing directives, utilizing scientific and medical logic to justify hyper-policing and suspend community-building initiatives and, therefore, transformed a health crisis into a criminal justice problem (NBC Chicago 2020). Policing during COVID-19 has shined a harsh new light on racialized policing practices in many major cities; for example, in the United Kingdom, minorities are 54% more likely to be fined for violating state- and city-mandated pandemic regulations (Mohdin and Dodd 2020). Further, the conflation of race and crime means that citizens who are not Caucasian face increased scrutiny and suspicion when wearing a face mask, forcing them to choose between avoiding contracting a deadly virus and risking the potential physical and psychological damage of being accosted by police who may marginalize their need and right to protection and instead reduce them to stereotypical characterizations of a criminal, gang member, looter, etc. (Natividad 2020).

What can policing reveal about a pandemic?

While a pandemic creates new social conditions in which to evaluate our policing practices, how we police, in turn, impacts our global health. On May 25, 2020, the world saw yet another death of an unarmed African American man caused by the police; using an unapproved tactic in a situation that did not call for such an extreme level of force (the victim, George Floyd, was handcuffed and compliant), now-former police officer Derek Chauvin kneeled on Floyd's neck for 8 minutes and 46 seconds, during which time Floyd fell unconscious and died. While some point to the lack of humanity for the utter indifference of Chauvin and the three other police officers who failed to intervene, it is the police habitus that makes this act so mundane that it must be investigated. Typical use-of-force justifications, such as resisting arrest, fleeing, or weapon possession, were not applicable in Floyd's case.[1] Interestingly, Floyd had contracted COVID-19 weeks earlier, and while his body was successfully fighting off one pandemic, it was forced to succumb to one more insidious (Neuman 2020).

The murder of George Floyd, along with the many other African American lives lost before his, unleashed a groundswell of antiracism solidarity protests in over 350 US cities (Michaels 2020; Mohammad Haddad 2020; Rahim and Picheta 2020). Focused on police brutality, antiracism, and anticolonialism and emerging across the world, from China to Syria, thousands of protesters from various social backgrounds joined together – some after months of pandemic-related self-isolation (Rodriguez-Presa 2020). Often violating state directives meant to contain the virus, many people joined together to protest, including yelling and shouting, which potentially aerosolized and further spread the virus. Mass arrests forced people into close quarters, and officers' use of O.C. spray and tear gas to control protesters forced citizens to remove their masks, cough, and rub their eyes – actions that all help spread the virus. As of mid-June 2020, tear gas has been used in over 100 major US cities and in some places abroad, against its people (APM Research Lab 2020b; Lai, Marsh, and Singhvi 2020). Thus, a militarized criminal justice response to a social crisis intensified a major health problem.

Why police reform will not work

Seeing policing play out during a convergence of a global pandemic and civil unrest due to aggressive police practices sheds light on why discussions about reform may fall short. Due to increasing public dissatisfaction with police practices, various community policing initiatives have been discussed and implemented, originating in the 1970s with the Community Oriented Policing and Problem Solving (COPPS) model. The main goal of this philosophy is to balance power by democratically bringing the police and public together to discuss community-defined problems and solutions (Corsianos 2012), and while many noble ideas have emerged from this concept, these ideas often do little more than weaponize citizens in police expansion rather than alter police practices (Gascon and Roussell 2019). But why is it so challenging for the police and the community they are hired to serve to most effectively work together? Where does this problem in policing originate? And what do our experiences and response to this pandemic, during an intense international cry for improved police relations, reveal about the system of policing more generally? In my own extensive observations of United States police academies, I found that the goals of community policing are unlikely to be reached because recruits are indoctrinated into a "socialized subjectivity" where "rational decisions" (Bourdieu 2014) to follow "the law" are decision-making processes that mask personal and institutional biases and justify force. Further, the perception that they must deal with non-criminal issues results from a history of conflation of policing with state interest in all areas of our lives, especially our health (Foucault 1977). Specifically, this unfolds in police training through three key and interdependent parts: (1) Masculinity shapes police as protectors and heroes, (2) which requires the infantilization and criminalization of the public that (3) is shaped by racialized and classed constructions.

Police as protectors and heroes

Historically, policing has revolved around the image of the (generally male) protector and hero, such as what I witnessed during a police academy graduation where an atheist professor, who was also a rabbi, compared God to the police. He began by saying, "If there is really a god then let him knock me off this stage while I speak. I will give him 15 minutes to do so." The professor continued to speak for five minutes, then he stopped speaking, looked up, and said, "Well, you only have

10 more minutes, so if you exist, then knock me off this stage." The professor continued to speak for another five minutes and nothing happened. Again, the professor said, "Okay, well you only have 5 more minutes, so if you are real, then knock me off this stage." As he began the last five minutes of his presentation, a 6'4", 280-pound, muscular Marine walked up to the professor and punched him so hard that the professor fell off the stage. Bewildered, the professor asked, "Why did you do that?" The Marine responded, "God says he is busy and sent me to take care of it." The audience laughed and applauded.

In addition to protecting the community, police are also perceived to be protecting citizens from each other. During an academy class, an instructor stated, "You are the guardians of our community. You protect my family. You are the warriors, but that word is harsh in our political world right now, but warriors protect the people." Similarly, another academy instructor told the recruits that officers are there to "keep the wolves away from the sheep." When masculinity frames the role and objective of policing, then police feel compelled to interject in the daily affairs of people's lives, which begs the need to decipher who is most in need of police attention and/or protection.

Denigrating and criminalizing the public

Effective policing often relies on the perception that the public is ignorant and/or unintelligent. During an academy course on the law, the instructor stated that if you cannot legally conduct a search, you can seek consent to search, which the officer stated is dependent on the public not being privy to the law because "they are stupid." However, citizen attempts to exercise their rights can often be interpreted as an indication of guilt. For example, during a DUI class, the instructor told recruits, "the only people who are going to refuse to take your (sobriety) test are those who already got arrested for a DUI in the past." Interestingly, in a private conversation earlier that day, that same officer told me that I should always refuse a sobriety test because doing so creates more loopholes that can build a successful defense.

The public is also commonly portrayed as liars and suspects. During a procedures course, one instructor stated, "people lie all the time. Police are often . . .". A recruit chimed in "jaded." "Right," the officer responded. "Police never believe anything they hear because they spend their time being lied to. You will be lied to several times each night. People in your personal life may lie to you." A lecturer who was teaching recruits traffic stop protocols indicated that the officers should be suspicious "when they (citizens) drive past you, and they look surprised to see you or when they intentionally try not to look at you."

As introduced earlier in this chapter, beliefs about race, ethnicity, even religious beliefs, can help influence police suspicion. During a police academy class, when asked for an example of when something is suspicious, a recruit replied, "When a car looks too expensive to be in the area." The instructor nodded in agreement. This exchange demonstrates that, from these police officers' perspective, potential criminality can be dependent on assumptions about class/social status: who should and should not own a particular kind of car and who should and should not inhabit a particular space. During a different class, another academy instructor presented a mock situation of pulling over a man for a suspected DUI; in this example, the officer portrayed both the police officer and the person who had been pulled over. First, the instructor, playing the part of the officer, asked the man how many beers he had consumed. Then, switching to the role of the man who'd been pulled over, the instructor responded, "Oh, sir, I had 28 beers," in broken English and with a Spanish accent. Immediately realizing that using such an accent was problematic, the instructor said to the class, "Now, I know I used that accent, but most of my clients *are* Hispanic." The entire class laughed. In yet another class, an instructor said, "We see a guy in Islamic garb. I don't care if it is politically incorrect (to assume that the person is Islamic) – he's wearing a turban, and he is holding a box that says 'explosives'. Let's keep this simple. Am I wrong here?" The next day, before class, this same instructor approached me and stated that he had to use all "these Abdul and Habib" jokes to get the class to connect to the material.

While most observed instructors were not as blatant when connecting crime to specific ethnicities, race, or religions, such connections were still often implied. During one course, an instructor advised recruits to "get to know the dirt bags. My guys in my town know the dirtbags." He further explained how he handles the "dirtbags" and how an officer can pull them over for failing to reduce their speed while driving through an intersection:

> How many of you actually reduce your speed? No one does but know what is in your toolbox. It is a reason to stop someone. A cheesy reason to stop people, and if they are gang bangers, stop them. If they live here, tell them we are watching them, and if they don't, send them back. I will stop them for a known vehicle code violation and paper them, and if they are criminals, I will tell them to not come back. That is how I clean up a neighborhood. Why can't you do that? What is your job? To deal with crime. You don't do this to everybody, only those that don't support you.

This one example very obviously demonstrates several problems with police conduct that many citizens are regularly subjected to. However, it is also essential to highlight one particularly dangerous concern: In this example, by advising police recruits to tell "criminals" to "not come back" rather than arrest them, what does the word "criminal" really mean here? In this example, is it a legal term for someone who violates an actual law, or is it another word for "undesirable people"?

Another common way that police officers criminalize citizens is by regarding victims as potential perpetrators. During his class, a police academy instructor asked his students,

> Is a call about a heroin overdose a call for help or a crime call? Can be both. If drugs are on the scene, then it is a crime call. If they already used them,

> it is a call for help. But be aware if he gets Narcan they will resist and fight, and so it is a crime call.

The presumptions revealed in this example, particularly with regards to viewing a physiological response to a prescription treatment as a catalyst for a potential criminal act, demonstrate how a call for help can likely result in an arrest – a particularly disturbing policing practice that is commonly observed today. Police are trained to construct people as worthy and unworthy of assistance, framed by racial and classed assumptions that supersede any larger health or safety goals believed to be the objectives of police work during the pandemic.

The possibilities of this moment

The protests stemming from the murder of George Floyd and other police abuses, and officers' response to its citizens to control them, are not new. That these events occurred during a worldwide pandemic, exacerbating the contraction and spread of COVID-19, exposes the length governments would take to knowingly harm their own citizens as, many, simply exercised their constitutional rights. Seeing these similarly extreme responses in cities across the world paraded not just a dilemma in individual police tactics but also a deeper crisis in the process by which states utilize police in non-criminal matters, which must be addressed to produce long-term reform. When a state transforms social and health crises into criminal justice problems, they provide a legal green light for officers to do what they are trained to do: identify and control a threat, forcing cops to construct the public into the criminals they need to justify the very police behavior citizens protest against while exacerbating the very issues they are employed to resolve. Policing under this current pandemic shows us that these are not just social problems in some communities but have become a global health problem that puts all citizens at risk.

As explained in this chapter, the police are often driven by the "obsessive need to solve a paradox" (for example, see the work of Levi-Strauss 1966) between the officer as an enforcer of the state and a public protector and servant (for example, see the work of Vitale 2018). When making an arrest is the main objective of policing, then the public must be constructed as arrestable; it is *whom* the officer initially *chooses* to focus their attention on that reflects the hidden bias. When a threat is successfully constructed, then "protective violence becomes not simply justifiable, but imperative" (Messerschmidt 2016), even when it may violate constitutional rights or intensify a health crisis. Until community leaders and their citizens comprehensively examine and rewrite the narratives that support these abuses, communities will likely only continue to support solutions that become another part of the ultimate social problem.

So, how can these dangerous police narratives that continue to be socially problematic be rewritten? To see true reform, we cannot work within the existing structure. First, we must evaluate the state's overreliance on police systems to handle its non-criminal problems because what the pandemic has shown us is that using the police to address health concerns transforms citizens in need to criminals to be confronted. Further, we must connect the reality that our concern for the public's health that is harmed by police brutality and aggressive uses of force that compel people to take to the streets, even during a global pandemic, literally puts them in the crosshairs of a system that only knows how to treat them as enemy combatants, justifying tactics that spread COVID and, hence, continue to put the health of its citizens at risk. While the call to dismantle the police appears to be an effective way to address this problem, it does not recognize how policing is connected to larger state goals and political systems. The larger community and the organizations and institutions that they make up must also be honest about and confront their existing racial biases regarding their citizens. They must also evaluate how limited meanings around masculinity shape the policies and processes of their organizations in ways that can further harm people as, for example, when the culture, objectives, and training of officers align with narrow meanings around masculinity, officers must construct citizens as either worthy or unworthy of assistance but do not see them as equals whose experiences and expertise are valued. Only when we can engage in this intense critical reflection can the community be seen and respected as true social leaders capable of building a community-led police system. Then, community-shared policing goals need to be redefined, which should drive how officers are hired, trained, and promoted to leadership positions. Deconstructing police systems into the people and processes that each part contributes to is crucial to rebuild a more equitable, functioning system. Further, when we situate how systems, such as policing, can impact other systems, such as health care, it is then that we can critically analyze when one response, such as police response to protests, can further harm its people during a global pandemic. By grasping this full-picture approach, we will more effectively and humanely recognize and respond to issues as they arise and better respond to the shared health, social, and criminal standards envisioned by all.

Note

1 As of June 3, Minneapolis Police Chief Arradondo has fired all four officers, claiming they were "complicit" in the death of George Floyd (www.cnn.com/2020/06/03/us/george-floyd-officers-charges/index.html).

References

APM Research Lab. 2020a. "The Color of Coronavirus: COVID-19 Deaths by Race and Ethnicity in the U.S." *APM Research Lab*, June 10. www.apmresearchlab.org/covid/deaths-by-race Associated Press.
———. 2020b. "Police Fire Tear Gas at Paris Protesters as George Floyd Demonstrations Spread Across Globe." *Associated Press*, June 2.
Bhala, Neeraj, Gwenetta Curry, Adrian, Martineau, Charles Agyemang, and Raj Bhopal. 2020. "Sharpening the Global Focus on Ethnicity and Race in the Time of COVID-19." *The Lancet* 395 (10238) (May 30): 1676. www.thelancet.com/journals/lancet/article/PIIS0140-6736(20)31102-8/fulltext.

Bourdieu, Pierre. 2014. *On the State: Lectures at the Colege de France.* Cambridge: Polity Press.

Bourdieu, Pierre, and Loic Wacquant. 1992. *An Invitation to Reflexive Sociology.* Chicago: Univeristy of Chicago Press.

Connell, R.W. 1987. *Gender & Power: Society, the Person, and Sexual Politics.* Cambridge: Polity Press.

Connell, R.W., and James W. Messerschmidt. 2005. "Hegemonic Masculinity". *Gender & Society* 19 (6): 829–859.

Corsianos, Marilyn. 2012. *The Complexities of Police Corruption: Gender, Identity, and Misconduct.* New York: Rowman and Littlefield.

Daley, Beth. 2020. "Coronavirus Class Divide-the Jobs Most at Risk of Contracting and Dying from COVID-19." *The Conversation,* May 19. https://theconversation.com/coronavirus-class-divide-the-jobs-most-at-risk-of-contracting-and-dying-from-covid-19–138857.

Dewey, Jodie. (forthcoming) "'People Are Stupid': How Academy Training Thwarts Community Policing Objectives." *Justice Quarterly.*

Feldman, Justin, Jarvis Chen, Pamela Waterman, and Nancy Krieger. 2016. "Temporal Trends and Racial/Ethnic Inequalities for Legal Intervention Injuries Treated in Emergency Departments Us Men and Women Age 15–34, 2001–2014." *Journal of Urban Health* 93 (5): 797–807.

Foucault, Michel. 1977. *Discipline and Punish: The Birth of the Prison.* New York: Vintage Books.

Fryer, Roland. 2016. "An Empirical Analysis of Racial Difference in Police Use of Force." https://law.yale.edu/sites/default/files/area/workshop/leo/leo16_fryer.pdf.

Gascon, Luis Daniel, and Aaron Roussell. 2019. *The Limits of Community Policing.* New York: New York University Press.

Gleeson, Colin. 2020. "White Irish in England Half as Likely to Die from Covid-19 Than Minorities." *The Irish Times,* May 7. www.irishtimes.com/news/social-affairs/white-irish-in-england-half-as-likely-to-die-from-covid-19-than-minorities-1.4246823.

Gonzalez Van Cleve, Nicole. 2016. *Crook County: Racism and Injustice in America's Largest Criminal Court.* Stanford: Stanford Law Books.

Haddad, Mohammad. 2020. "Mapping US Cities Where George Floyd Protests Have Erupted." *Aljazeera,* June 2. www.aljazeera.com/indepth/interactive/2020/06/mapping-cities-george-floyd-protests-erupted-200601081654119.html.

Kawachi, Ichiro, Norman Daniels, and Dean Robinson. 2005 "Health Disparities by Race and Class: Why Both Matter." *Health Affairs* 24 (2): 343–52.

Lai, Rebecca, Bill Marsh, and Anjali Singhvi. 2020. "Here are the 100 U.S. Cities Where Protesters Were Tear-Gassed." *New York Times,* June 18.

Levi-Strauss, Claude. 1966. *The Savage Mind.* Chicago: University of Chicago Press.

Mackintosh, Eliza. 2020. "What You Need to Know About Coronavirus on Monday, June 22." *CNN,* June 22. www.cnn.com/2020/06/22/world/coronavirus-newsletter-06-22-20-intl/index.html.

Messerschmidt, James W. 2016. *Masculinities in the Making.* Lanham, MD: Rowman & Littlefield.

Michaels, Samantha. 2020. "Brionna Taylor is One of a Shocking Number of Black People to see Armed Police Barge into Their Homes." *Mother Jones,* May 20. www.motherjones.com/crime-justice/2020/05/breonna-taylor-is-one-of-a-shocking-number-of-black-people-to-see-armed-police-barge-into-their-homes/.

Mohdin, Aamna, and Vikram Dodd. 2020. "UK Protesters Accuse Police of Targeting Black People During Lockdown." *The Guardian,* June 1. www.theguardian.com/world/2020/jun/01/uk-police-accused-of-targeting-black-people-during-lockdown.

Morey, Brittany. 2018. "Mechanisms by Which Anti-Immigrant Stigma Exacerbates Racial Ethnic Health Disparities." *American Journal of Public Health* 108 (4): 460–63.

Natividad, Ivan. 2020. "Among the Reasons COVID-19 is Worse for Black Communities: Police Violence". *Berkeley News*, April 23. https://news.berkeley.edu/2020/04/23/one-reason-covid-19-is-worse-for-black-communities-police-violence/.

NBC Chicago. 2020. "'We Are Not Playing Games:' Lightfoot, CPD, Step Up Enforcement of Stay at Home Orders." *NBC*, May 2. www.nbcchicago.com/news/coronavirus/as-weather-warms-up-officials-warn-residents-to-continue-adhering-to-covid-19-restrictions/2265595/.

Neuman, Scott. 2020. "Medical Examiner's Autopsy Reveals George Floyd HD Positive Test for Coronavirus." *NPR*, June 4. www.npr.org/2020/06/04/869278494/medical-examiners-autopsy-reveals-george-floyd-had-positive-test-for-coronavirus.

Paradies, Yin et al. 2015. "Racism as a Determinant of Health: A Systematic Review and Meta-Analysis." *PLoS ONE* 10 (9): e0138511. https://doi.org/10.1371/journal.pone.0138511.

Pettersson, Henrik, Byron Manley, and Sergio Hernandez. 2020. "Tracking Coronavirus' Global Spread." *CNN Health*, August 22. www.cnn.com/interactive/2020/health/coronavirus-maps-and-cases/.

Rahim, Zamira, and Rob Picheta. 2020. "Thousands Around the World Protest George Floyd's Death in Global Display of Solidarity." *CNN*, June 1. www.cnn.com/2020/06/01/world/george-floyd-global-protests-intl/index.html.

Rios, Victor M. 2009. "The Consequences of the Criminal Justice Pipeline on Black and Latino Masculinity." *The Annuals of the American Academy* 623.

Rodriguez-Presa, Laura. 2020. "'This is a Step Back.' Latino Activists Speak out About Racial Tension with Black Chicagoans on Southwest Side Amid George Floyd Fallout." *Chicago Tribune*, June 3. www.chicagotribune.com/lifestyles/ct-life-chicago-latino-neighborhoods-gangs-floyd-protests-20200603-dsui2w2dabdy7cgxxkbz7a3c3q-story.html.

Ryan, J. Michael. 2021a. "COVID-19: Global Pandemic, Societal Responses, Ideological Solutions." In *COVID-19: Global Pandemic, Societal Responses, Ideological Solutions*, edited by J. Michael Ryan, 1–8. London: Routledge.

———. 2021b. "The SARS-CoV-2 Virus and the COVID-19 Pandemic." In *COVID-19: Global Pandemic, Societal Responses, Ideological Solutions*, edited by J. Michael Ryan, 9–19. London: Routledge.

Sanford, Adam, Dinur Blum, and Stacy Smith. 2021. "Seeking Stability in Unstable Times: COVID-19 and the Bureaucratic Mindset." In *COVID-19: Global Pandemic, Societal Responses, Ideological Solutions*, edited by J. Michael Ryan, 47–60. London: Routledge.

Statista Research Department. 2020. "Number of People Shot to Death by the Police in the United States from 2017 to 2020, by Race." *Statista*, June 5. www.statista.com/statistics/585152/people-shdddot-to-death-by-us-police-by-race/.

Thomas, Stephen, and Erica Casper. 2019. "The Burdens of Race and History on Black People's Health 400 Years After Jamestown." *American Journal of Public Health* 109 (10): 1346–347.

Vitale, Alex. 2018. *The End of Policing*. New York: Verso.

Williams, Gareth. 2003. "The Determinants of Health: Structure, Context and Agency." *Sociology of Health and Illness* 25: 131–54.

World Health Organization. 2020. "WHO Timeline-COVID-19." *World Health Organization*, April 27. www.who.int/news-room/detail/27-04-2020-who-timeline – covid-19.

7

HOUSING AS HEALTH CARE

Mitigations of homelessness during a pandemic

Kristen Desjarlais-deKlerk

The social determinants of health perspective has long argued that social elements impact health and wellness by enhancing or detracting an individual's health and well-being (Link and Phelan 1995). Housing, as a social determinant of health, has garnered particular attention as governments and policy makers across the Western world have advocated for housing first: an approach that houses individuals before resolving other social issues (Tsemberis, Gulcur, and Nakae 2004).

Housing impacts many other social conditions. Individuals who are inadequately housed have limited access to clean water and healthy nutrition and are exposed to various elements, including inclement weather and street violence (Wenzel et al. 2004; Frankish, Hwang, and Quantz 2005). Despite the evidence, housing first programs have found limited support, and homelessness persists in most of Canada (Padgett et al. 2013), with homeless shelters continuing as predominant community responses to homelessness. Selecting shelter as the predominant response has become particularly problematic during the COVID-19 pandemic.

With health advocates advising all citizens to social distance, leaving two meters (six feet) between individuals, shelters and homeless advocates have had to improvise solutions to prevent mass spread amongst homeless populations. These solutions have varied in scope. Some cities have seconded hotel rooms to accommodate homeless individuals – whether symptomatic or not. Others have opened more shelter space in order to accommodate bodies in a highly institutionalized setting. Others still have spray painted lines in parking lots to show homeless individuals where to sleep. Policy makers that have elected to open more shelter space when hotel rooms were available have garnered critique, and they have defended their choices by citing the prevalence of bed bugs, mental health disorders, and potential suicidal ideation brought on by loneliness as reasons for their decision.

In this chapter, I will examine some of these responses and the arguments presented by advocates of these responses. The data cited throughout this piece is all publicly available information via social media (specifically Twitter) and news outlets and has allowed me to examine the ways in which homelessness service providers have responded to the problem and the ways in which advocates perceive these responses. In doing so, I take a critical theoretical perspective and examine the ways in which different types of power are reflected in the narratives. Alongside this, I examine the ways in which housing has become a central component of health care alongside social distancing and social isolation.

Methods

To understand the responses to homelessness during COVID-19, I searched mainstream news sites from Canada and focused on reporting around homelessness between March and May 2020. While this does not represent all publications or responses to homelessness during the COVID-19 pandemic, it does demonstrate many of them and provides an important foundation for discussing and considering what homelessness means during a pandemic, the ways in which advocates, providers, and politicians are talking about individuals experiencing homelessness, and the strategies to circumvent any potential outbreaks amid homeless populations. I have also examined publicly available tweets from known homelessness advocates to demonstrate critiques of responses or their inadequacies. In order to facilitate a focused discussion on these data, I have opted to focus on comparing and contrasting the responses to homelessness in Calgary, Toronto, and Vancouver. While I briefly mention other municipalities, my scholarship and expertise has been in Canadian homelessness, and, consequently, this chapter focuses on Canadian cities. Furthermore, before the pandemic, these three cities have aimed to move away from shelter-based solutions to homelessness and towards housing first models (which I will discuss later). Consequently, all are positioned as being in line with a social determinants of health philosophy towards homelessness. This means that they aim to provide housing to those experiencing homelessness, consequently bolstering their health and well-being. Lastly, all are relatively large Canadian cities in very different provinces. Their responses to homeless individuals amid the pandemic were variable and require deconstruction.

There are some obvious limitations to this data. Reporting, while the best source of this kind of public information, can be one-sided and not reflective of individuals' and organizations' genuine perspectives on an issue. Consequently, organizations' responses and explanations may not be wholly accurate and may not reflect issues in their entirety; however, they do demonstrate important types of governance and the risks inherent to homelessness during a public health crisis.

Furthermore, the sample is not representative. The news search focused on large-scale Canadian media sources rather than smaller news outlets, and while I aimed to find all stories about responses to homelessness across these three Canadian cities, it is entirely possible that I missed some.

Homelessness and shelter living

Before describing the responses to homelessness amid COVID-19, it is necessary to examine homelessness and shelters in Canada. There are two key considerations when thinking about homelessness. First, "the homeless" are not a primordial group with unifying characteristics (Canadian Homelessness Research Network 2017). That is, anyone can experience homelessness; it is not limited to people of any particular race/ethnicity, gender, sexuality, or creed, although those in marginalized statuses are more likely to experience it, and the more marginality an individual experiences, the less likely they are to successfully exit homelessness (Slesnick, Zhang, and Brakenhoff 2017). Second, homelessness is not a static status; most people who experience it drift in and out of homelessness throughout their life course (Canadian Homelessness Research Network 2017). Consequently, homelessness is better considered on a continuum. It includes rough sleepers (those that sleep outside without shelter), shelter users (those that dwell in large-scale homeless shelters), the precariously housed (like couch surfers who live on friends' and relatives' couches), and the provisionally housed (those currently residing in government-provided housing who could be made homeless through change in government). Each of these statuses exists in a state of ongoing marginality and vulnerability. This chapter predominantly examines those residing in shelters as well as rough sleepers and community and governmental responses to these individuals.

Homeless shelters are remarkably variable, yet their similarities are also striking. Shelters typically employ a warehouse design in which individuals sleep on mats (or cots) on an easy-to-wash cement floor. In most facilities, little space exists between users in order to maximize the number of sleeping spaces available. Many shelters provide men's and women's sections in which to sleep, but ultimately garner little privacy between shelter users. Shelters have also been known to use regimented rules that inhibit choice in the environment (Larsen, Poortinga, and Hurdle 2004) and have been called total institutions (DeWard and Moe 2010) because of their often-dictatorial focus on maintaining order. In doing so, many establish rules and routines that limit agency. For example, shelters often have specific hours when shelter users can access beds, food, and sometimes even their own belongings.

That said, shelters exist to protect individuals from the elements and limit the vulnerabilities associated with homelessness. They became particularly important in Canada in the 1960s as a response to homelessness, mostly because inclement weather had rough sleepers freezing outside overnight; the goal of homeless shelters was to limit such exposure. At the time, other responses were considered enabling and consequently had less political will than warehousing people into shared spaces. Recently, however, shelters have been acknowledged as expensive public health risks (Gaetz 2012), especially as shelter living contributes significantly to addictions, violence, and other physical and mental health issues, all of which are treated in ambulatory care situations, and advocates have argued the adoption of a housing first model.

Housing first sees homeless individuals moved into apartments before addressing other personal issues (Tsemberis, Gulcur, and Nakae 2004). Housing first is consistent with Maslow's hierarchy of needs (Greenwood, Stefancic, and Tsemberis 2013) by providing basic needs before addressing higher-level ones, and suggests that shelter barely satisfies survival needs, thereby limiting individuals' abilities to ever move beyond shelter life. It does this by limiting exposure to others and allowing individuals agency, including when, where, and what to eat, when to sleep, and other basic freedoms.

Responses to COVID-19

While many governments were relatively slow to respond to COVID-19, overwhelmingly citizens in most countries were urged to stay home (Flanagan 2020). Messaging focused on language that urged people they were "safe at home" and were helping healthcare workers by staying home and distant from other people. This was true for much of Canada, where outbreaks were met with shelter-in-place orders (Wu et al. 2020). This created vast complications for those without homes to shelter in and begged for new responses to homelessness (Nanda 2021). Political jurisdiction around homelessness continues to be an avenue of debate, but in Canada, responses to homelessness are primarily local and involve partnerships between municipalities and other levels of government (Gaetz 2010). In some cases, federal jurisdiction applies; however, this chapter focuses on both municipal and provincial responses and rhetoric around homelessness amid COVID-19.

During COVID-19, these responses varied from one locale to the next. In most of Canada, shelters were mandated to distance sleeping spaces (to a minimum of two meters) and help residents practice social distancing through markings on floors. These measures were immediately criticized as insufficient by multiple advocates who insisted that those experiencing homelessness needed the ability to isolate from others and drew attention to empty hotel rooms across municipalities as potential spaces for shelter users and rough sleepers. Some municipalities, such as the City of Toronto, seconded hotel rooms to that end (Casey 2020a; Herhalt 2020), while continuing to maintain their shelter spaces; others, such as the City of Calgary, opted to second other buildings such as churches and events centers to spread shelter beds farther apart (Anderson 2020). And while it is not the focus of this chapter, I think it is important to note that other cities in the USA and Canada had troubling responses to the pandemic, and Las Vegas opted to shut down their shelters altogether, opting to paint lines on parking lots mandated for homeless individuals to sleep (Dittrich 2020).

Furthermore, despite online narratives to the contrary (predominantly on social media), unsurprisingly considering COVID-19 is a novel virus, homeless individuals do not seem to have immunity to the virus (Schulte 2020). Research on homelessness, alongside discussions about health systems and marginalization in these systems, suggests that outbreaks amongst homeless populations are likely underreported. Despite this presumed underreporting, the US Centers for Disease Control and Prevention conducted a study amongst shelter populations in four cities and found that 25% of the shelter dwellers tested were COVID-19 positive (Mosites et al. 2020), indicating that homeless populations have no special immunity to COVID-19. Any suggestions otherwise only serve to mask the systemic vulnerabilities that COVID-19 has laid bare (Chiang 2021, this volume; Mungo 2021, this volume; Nanda 2021; Porter 2021, this volume; Schulte 2020; Skinta, Sun, and Ryu 2021, this volume).

The variability in pandemic homelessness responses were met with narratives about shelter users, rough sleepers, and illnesses spread amongst homeless populations that labelled those experiencing homeless as problematic potential carriers. But equally important were the ways in which advocates and providers supported, or did not support, these responses. In the following sections, I discuss the responses exercised by Toronto, Calgary, and Vancouver. What I have cited is by no means exhaustive. I have highlighted the responses I think particularly relevant and pertinent to the pandemic; however, there are many cities across Canada that are not documented here.

Toronto

Overcrowding has been a concern for Toronto's shelter system for years, and on a typical night Toronto shelters house roughly 7,000 people (Casey 2020b). Alongside those living in shelters, approximately another 1,715 (according to Toronto's last homeless count in 2018) rough sleep (homelesshub.ca 2019). While shelter overcrowding is a well-identified problem, amid COVID-19, advocates, service providers, nurses, and physicians in Toronto have argued that hotel rooms should be available to those experiencing homelessness to enable social distancing (Casey 2020b). Shelter conditions already described hardly allow distance between individuals while sleeping and could not be sustained by shelter spaces available at the start of the pandemic. By mid-April 2020, the City of Toronto managed to secure 1,200 hotel rooms for shelter users, leaving approximately 5,800 individuals who lived in shelter still requiring shelter; consequently, shelters remained open but had increased sleeping spaces between shelter dwellers (Casey 2020a; Herhalt 2020).

Alongside making some hotel rooms available, Toronto also opened recovery sites for homeless individuals diagnosed with COVID-19 (Pelley 2020), aptly called "COVID hotels" by both workers and shelter residents. Unsurprisingly, critics have argued that these sites, while important to minimize transmission to healthy shelter users, do not provide enough support, and housing is the only long-term health solution for those experiencing homelessness. Since the first COVID-19 case in Canada on January 27, 2020 (Toronto.com 2020), advocates have moved the argument toward the general benefits of housing and specifically into the epidemiological practice of social distance (also known as physical distancing) whereby space reduces infection.

While homeless advocates did not suggest that the city eliminate all shelter beds, a lawsuit was launched against the City of Toronto on April 25 for not offering enough social distancing in shelters (Herhalt 2020; Knope 2020). Advocates sought all avenues to protect shelter residents, and these efforts resulted in more apartments made available to shelter users and rough sleepers. The lawsuit reached a settlement in mid-May, with the city agreeing to physically distance shelter beds in all shelter spaces, provide space to all clients in the system, offer support services to those living in encampments and the shelter system, and regularly report on its progress (CBCNews.ca 2020d). By mid-May, Toronto shelter administration purported to have moved 2,425 people into housing (CBCNews.ca 2020b) and felt that they had achieved physical distancing. Shelter administration did not draw attention to the lawsuit; however, advocates believe rapid action happened because of the lawsuit launched by community stakeholders.

According to officials, the pandemic also increased the number of homeless encampments around Toronto as shelter users sought distancing measures (Casey 2020b). Many rough sleepers living in encampments have stated that shelters are too crowded and see COVID-19 as a reason to risk inclement weather and potential street violence. These encampments have met predictable conflicts with city officials (who cite safety issues, such as fire safety), and police have forcefully taken many down (Casey 2020b).

Provincially, Ontario has experienced the second highest number of case counts in Canada (Shah 2020). And while Toronto has been lauded by some for its response to its homeless population, Rima Berns-McGowan, the critic on poverty and homelessness for the Ontario Legislative Assembly, has argued that shelter dwellers and workers in Ontario are 35% more likely to contract COVID-19 than the general population is (Berns-McGowan 2020). These arguments have been forwarded by advocates and shelter workers alike and demonstrate the vulnerability still experienced by Toronto's shelter dwellers, despite responses to COVID-19. Housing for shelter dwellers, Berns-McGowan suggests, is the only effective COVID-19 prevention strategy.

Calgary

In response to COVID-19, all of the shelters in Calgary have reduced the number of shelter beds available in each location, with the largest reducing its shelter beds from 675 to 227 (Anderson 2020; Smith 2020). Shelter overflows have opened in events centers and large churches across the city. According to shelter workers, all shelter dwellers who check in are accommodated at shelters or overflows or are housed in government-supported apartments, but as COVID-19 spreads, much like in Toronto, individuals do not want to stay in shelters and are opting to sleep outside instead (Graveland 2020). While rough sleeping limits an individual's exposure to other people and enhances social distancing, it makes it harder to track potential outbreaks amongst homeless populations and exposes individuals to other potential health risks (such as inclement weather and street violence).

Other alternatives have been proposed to the shelter overflows available. For example, the City of Calgary offered to find hotel rooms for shelter users, but according to CBC News at least one homeless shelter rejected the idea, citing bed bugs and potential property damage to areas surrounding hotels as a risk of such measures (Anderson 2020). Other providers and politicians suggested social isolation itself posed a mental health threat and expressed concerns for potential suicides (Anderson 2020).

Alongside issues of social distancing in shelter, many Calgary-based homeless advocates have highlighted the problems with closing public spaces (Smith 2020). While eliminating public washrooms may seem like a necessary public health measure to those who have housing, it becomes a justice issue for those who experience homelessness, and if shelter policies limit access to the shelter and its services during the day, shelter dwellers may experience more marginalization and increased vulnerability (Smith 2020). In one case, highlighted in CBC News, a man rented office space so he would have a space to stay during the day and access to a washroom (Anderson 2020). Office space in Calgary amid a global pandemic and a downturn in oil and gas is relatively cheap, particularly when compared to apartments. Furthermore, provincial social assistance may provide enough funds to cover an office space but not a down payment on an apartment.

While outbreaks in Calgary shelters have been relatively contained, with the largest one only consisting of eight cases, a single local hotel accommodates those that need to self-isolate (Anderson 2020; CBCNews 2020c). While only one hotel has been seconded to this end, the hotel has not yet reached capacity as of mid-August 2020 – 100 rooms – allocating, thus far, appropriate space for individuals to isolate.

Provincially, Alberta's premier has claimed that homeless individuals have immunity to COVID-19 (Braid 2020). He was not alone in this claim, and many USA news sources have fact checked this multiple times (Schulte 2020) and have called this claim false. Low infection rates amongst Alberta's homeless population have been presented as evidence as to why Alberta is no longer in a public health emergency and should, therefore, lift pandemic-related restrictions (Braid 2020). In this case, the homeless have been highlighted as a reason to reopen Alberta's economy.

Vancouver

While Toronto and Calgary have seen increases in rough sleepers, Vancouver's homelessness and housing minister aimed to close all homeless encampments by May 9 (Little 2020). The province planned to move all camp residents into temporary housing, including both apartment- and hotel-style accommodations, to slow the spread of COVID-19. Some former encampment residents, however, claimed they still had nowhere to go following the dissolution of their camps, and so created a tent city in the port of Vancouver parking lot (Miljure 2020; Steacy and Bernard 2020). The tent city being established at the port of Vancouver almost immediately had an injunction filed against it to force campers to move (Proctor 2020). Like Toronto and Calgary, the City of Vancouver seconded multiple hotels to allow their homeless population to self-isolate. While shelters remained open (CBCNews.ca 2020a), they reportedly have been taking no new intakes, thereby increasing the number of rough sleepers in the Vancouver area (Saltman 2020).

Many Vancouver services and service providers have shut down amidst the pandemic, which has seen movement away from the city's core into its outlying areas, resulting in increases in encampments in the greater Vancouver area (Saltman 2020). Mobile outreach workers have reported finding 80% increases in service populations, most of which, they claim, are related to COVID-19 and shelter dwellers' desires to both distance and self-isolate. Increased worries around distancing have seen many residents shy away from enclosed spaces and move to rough sleeping and camping, albeit outside now-enclosed encampments, making them more difficult to find and count. Furthermore, many meal programs for homeless individuals have ceased, meaning that those experiencing homelessness have fewer nutrition options (Saltman 2020).

COVID-19, homelessness, and risk

The Canadian Public Health Association (n.d.) asserts that politics are an important social determinant of health. The responses to homelessness, reactions, and rhetoric described previously demonstrate the importance of politics in the management of a pandemic and its impact on the health and well-being of some of society's most vulnerable and marginalized individuals. Toronto, where homeless service provision appears to predominantly be the work of the municipality itself, had a relatively robust response, and where it failed, advocates sued for better reactions and responses. Calgary and Vancouver, where permanent shelter and service provision are the work of nonprofit organizations, have had more varied responses and have worked to maintain community relations in ways that suggest donors are as important as those being serviced. Furthermore, reporting on responses was far easier to find for Toronto, somewhat more difficult for Calgary, and even more difficult for Vancouver. This may relate to the public nature of Toronto's service provision as well as Calgary's former focus on responses and reductions in homelessness and homeless numbers over the last 12 years (CCTEH 2008).

Conclusion

While globally many labs have devoted resources to developing a vaccine for COVID-19, virology experts have emphasized that plagues and pandemics are likely to continue because of global travel, urbanization, and human encroachment into natural spaces. That is, even once COVID-19 becomes less of a concern, global society remains vulnerable to pandemics and widespread illness. This is particularly concerning to those without homes and those who live in inadequate housing.

Research recognizes that resolving homelessness would make communities less vulnerable to both pandemics and plagues. Homeless people live in public spaces generally open to all members of society. This means that when outbreaks occur amongst homeless populations, they have the potential to impact entire communities. Furthermore, with public health advocates and epidemiologists recommending individuals stay home, the importance of housing has never been so stark.

Efforts to eliminate homelessness have had little traction, even when social, health, and economic evidence has demonstrated the importance of housing, yet COVID-19 has exposed the vulnerabilities in systems that continue to marginalize the already vulnerable (Mungo 2021, this volume; Nanda 2021). Homelessness advocates have become louder, and the Canadian Alliance to End Homelessness has started a campaign called "Recovery for All" to bring attention and focus to homelessness as Canada reopens its economy. The campaign commits to funding public housing and eliminating homelessness as part of the country's economic recovery. It is possible that these efforts will be met with a lack of political will, yet thus far it has found support from housing advocates and some members of the business community (recoveryforall.ca).

The idea of providing housing to those experiencing homelessness is not new. Affordable publicly funded housing has been available in Canada since 1935, and new housing intended to reduce homelessness has been created in recent years, yet new builds are inadequate in meeting demands, especially as older units across Canada have fallen into disarray and require massive renovations to make them tenable (Housing Services Corporation 2013). Affordable, safe, public housing bolsters the health and well-being of communities (Gaetz 2012) and limits the transmission of COVID-19. Housing protects all citizens, but only politics and political will can make that level of inclusion and physical protection a reality. While Link and Phelan (1995) posited poverty as a central social determinant of health, I suspect politics may be equally important. COVID-19 has laid bare the vulnerabilities of shelter systems, and responding to the needs of society's most marginalized is imminently important for all of society's health and well-being.

References

Anderson, Drew. 2020. "Self-Isolation Rooms for Calgary's Homeless Open in Hotel." *CBC-News.ca*. Accessed May 22, 2020. www.cbc.ca/news/canada/calgary/calgary-homeless-hotel-self-isolation-covid-19-1.5526437.

Berns-McGowan. 2020. "Public Twitter Account." https://twitter.com/beyrima/status/12 65974956116135937?s=20.

Braid, Don. 2020. "Braid: Kenney Begins to Normalize COVID-19 as a Risk Mainly to the Elderly, Almost Zero Danger to the Young." *Calgary Herald*. Accessed May 29, 2020. https://calgaryherald.com/opinion/braid-kenney-begins-to-normalize-covid-19-as-a-risk-mainly-to-the-elderly-almost-zero-danger-to-the-young.

Calgary Committee to End Homelessness (CCTEH). 2008. "Calgary's 10 Year Plan to End Homelessness". *Calgary, AB*. Accessed June 20, 2020. http://calgaryhomeless.com/con tent/uploads/10-Year-Plan-Update.pdf.

Canadian Homelessness Research Network. 2017. *Canadian Definition of Homelessness*. Canadian Observatory on Homelessness: Homeless Hub. www.homelesshub.ca/resource/canadian-definition-homelessness.

Canadian Public Health Association. n.d. "What Are the Social Determinants of Health?" Accessed May 29, 2020. www.cpha.ca/what-are-social-determinants-health.

Casey, Liam. 2020a. "Largest Outbreak Reported at Willowdale Welcome Centre, Where 11 Residents and 12 Staff Tested Positive." *CBCNews.Ca*. Accessed May 15, 2020. thwww.cbc.ca/news/canada/toronto/homeless-population-toronto-covid-19-1.5532300.

———. 2020b. "Standoff Between Homeless, City Officials at Downtown Toronto Encampments." *CTV News*. Accessed May 29, 2020. https://toronto.ctvnews.ca/stand off-between-homeless-city-officials-at-downtown-toronto-encampments-1.4941268.

CBCNews.ca. 2020a. "14 People Arrested After Occupying Vancouver Elementary School." *CBC News*. Accessed May 29, 2020. www.cbc.ca/news/canada/british-columbia/home less-activists-occupy-vancouver-school-covid-1.5537589.

———. 2020b. "Advocates Mourn 1st Person to Die of Covid-19 in Toronto's Shelter System." *CBCNews.ca*. Accessed May 22, 2020. www.cbc.ca/news/canada/toronto/first-covid-19-death-shelter-system-toronto-identified-homelessness-1.5567272.

———. 2020c. "COVID-19 Outbreak at Calgary Alpha House Reaches 8 Cases." *CBC-News.ca*. Accessed May 22, 2020. www.cbc.ca/news/canada/calgary/alpha-house-covid-calgary-outbreak-cases-alberta-health-1.5567998.

———. 2020d. "COVID-19 in Toronto: Lawsuit Shelved as City, Advocacy Groups Come to Agreement." *CBC News*. Accessed May 22, 2020. www.cbc.ca/news/canada/toronto/covid-19-in-toronto-may-19-1.5574993.

Chiang, Pamela P. 2021. "Anti-Asian Racism, Responses, and the Impact on Asian Americans' Lives: A Social-Ecological Perspective." In *COVID-19: Social Consequences and Cultural Adaptations*. London: Routledge.

DeWard, Sarah L., and Angela M. Moe. 2010. "'Like a Prison!': Homeless Women's Narratives of Surviving Shelter." *The Journal of Sociology and Social Welfare* 37 (1): 115–35. https://scholarworks.wmich.edu/jssw/vol37/iss1/7.

Dittrich, Valerie. 2020. "Las Vegas Turns Parking Lot into Makeshift Homeless Shelter, Complete with Social Distancing Grid." *National Post*. Accessed March 31, 2020. https://nationalpost.com/news/las-vegas-turns-parking-lot-into-makeshift-homeless-shelter-complete-with-social-distancing-grid.

Flanagan, Ryan. 2020. "Canadians Have Been Told to Stay Home During the Pandemic. Are We Listening?" *CTV News*. www.ctvnews.ca/health/coronavirus/canadians-have-been-told-to-stay-home-during-the-pandemic-are-we-listening-1.4912468.

Frankish, C. James, Stephen W. Hwang, and Darryl Quantz. 2005. "Homelessness and Health in Canada: Research Lessons and Priorities." *Canadian Journal of Public Health* 96 (2): S23–S29.

Gaetz, Stephen. 2010. "The Struggle to End Homelessness in Canada: How We Created the Crisis, and How We Can End It." *The Open Health Services and Policy Journal* 3 (1).

———. 2012. *The Real Cost of Homelessness: Can We Save Money by Doing the Right Thing?* Toronto: Canadian Homelessness Research Network Press.

Graveland, Bill. 2020. "Calgary Homeless Sleep Outdoors Over Fears of Catching COVID-19." *CBCNews.ca*, May 25. Accessed May 29, 2020. www.cbc.ca/news/canada/calgary/homeless-calgarians-calgary-covid-health-1.5583097.

Greenwood, Ronni Michelle, Ana Stefancic, and Sam Tsemberis. 2013. "Pathways Housing First for Homeless Persons with Psychiatric Disabilities: Program Innovation, Research, and Advocacy." *Journal of Social Issues* 69 (4): 645–63.

Herhalt, Chris. 2020. "City of Toronto Sued by Homeless Advocates Arguing Shelter Spacing Violates Charter." *CTV News*. Toronto. Accessed May 15, 2020. https://toronto.ctvnews.ca/city-of-toronto-sued-by-homeless-advocates-arguing-shelter-spacing-violates-charter-1.4911890.

Homelesshub.ca. 2019. "Toronto Homelessness Community Profile." Accessed July 14, 2020. www.homelesshub.ca/community-profile/toronto.

Housing Services Corporation (HSC). 2013. *Canada's Social and Affordable Housing Landscape: A Province-to-Province Overview.* Accessed June 15, 2020. https://www.homelesshub.ca/sites/default/files/attachments/531-Canada-Social-Housing-Landscape_2014.pdf.

Knope, Julia. 2020. "Toronto Groups File Legal Action Against City Over Its Response to COVID-19 Outbreaks in Shelters". *CBCNews.ca*. Accessed April 30, 2020. www.cbc.ca/news/canada/toronto/toront-legal-action-city-covid-19-shelters-homeless-population-1.5545070.

Larsen, Larissa, Ernie Poortinga, and Donna E. Hurdle. 2004. "Sleeping Rough: Exploring the Differences between Shelter-Using and Non-Shelter-Using Homeless Individuals." *Environment and Behaviour* 36 (4): 578–91. DOI: 10.1177/0013916503261385.

Link, Bruce G., and Jo Phelan. 1995. "Social Conditions as Fundamental Causes of Disease." *Journal of Health and Social Behaviour* (Extra Issue): 80–84. DOI: 10.2307/2626958.

Little, Simon. 2020. "'The Park Is Going to Close:' B.C. to Vancouver Homeless Campers Who Refuse COVID-19 Housing." *Globalnews.ca*. Accessed May 30, 2020. https://globalnews.ca/news/6923569/bc-coronavirus-homeless-camps/.

Miljure, Ben. 2020. "Last Camper Moves Out of Oppenheimer Park as Cleanup Begins." *CTV News*. Accessed May 20, 2020. https://bc.ctvnews.ca/last-camper-moves-out-of-oppenheimer-park-as-cleanup-begins-1.4932676.

Mosites, Emily, Erin M. Parker, Kristie E. N. Clarke, Jessie M. Gaeta, Travis P. Baggett, Elizabeth Imbert, Madeline Sankaran, Ashley Scarborough, Karin Huster, Matt Hanson, Elysia Gonzales, Jody Rauch, Libby Page, Temet M. McMichael, Ryan Keating, Grace E. Marx, Tom Andrews, Kristine Schmit, Sapna Bamrah Morris, Nicole F. Dowling, Georgina Peacock, and COVID-19 Homelessness Team. 2020. "Assessment of SARS-CoV-2 Infection Prevalence in Homeless Shelters – Four US Cities, March 27-April 15, 2020." *Centers for Disease Control and Prevention*, May 1. Accessed May 29, 2020. www.cdc.gov/mmwr/volumes/69/wr/mm6917e1.htm#T1_down.

Mungo, Monita H. 2021. "Violence, Virus, and Vitriol: The Tale of COVID-19." In *COVID-19: Social Consequences and Cultural Adaptations*, edited by J. Michael Ryan, 245–55. London: Routledge.

Nanda, Serena. 2021. "Inequalities and COVID-19." In *COVID-19: Global Pandemic, Societal Responses, Ideological Solutions*, edited by J. Michael Ryan, 109–23. London: Routledge.

Padgett, Deborah K., Tran Smith, Bikki, Derejko, Katie-Sue, Henwood, Benjamin F., and Emmy Tiderington. 2013. "A Picture Is Worth . . . Photo Elicitation Interviewing with Formerly Homeless Adults." *Qualitative Health Research* 23 (11): 1435–444. DOI: 10.1177/1049732313507752.

Pelley, Lauren. 2020. "Homeless, Pregnant, COVID-Positive – And Bearing the Brunt of the Pandemic." *CBC.ca*. Accessed May 22, 2020. www.cbc.ca/news/canada/toronto/homeless-pregnant-covid-positive-and-bearing-the-brunt-of-a-pandemic-1.5575982.

Porter, Lynette. 2021. "High Risk or Low Worth? A Few Practical and Philosophical COVID-19 Issues Surrounding the Isolation of High-Risk Senior Women." In *COVID-19: Social Consequences and Cultural Adaptations*, edited by J. Michael Ryan, 256–69. London: Routledge.

Proctor, Jason. 2020. "Port of Vancouver Seeks Injunction to Remove Homeless Camp Near CRAB Park." *CBCNews.ca*. Accessed May 29, 2020. www.cbc.ca/news/canada/british-columbia/port-vancouver-homeless-injunction-1.5575454.

Saltman, Jennifer. 2020. "Mobile Outreach Workers Seeing More Homeless During COVID-19 Pandemic." *Vancouver Sun*. Accessed May 29, 2020. https://vancouversun.com/news/mobile-outreach-workers-seeing-more-homeless-during-covid-19-pandemic.

Schulte, Laura. 2020. "Fact Check: No, Homeless People Are Not Immune from Catching COVID-19." *USA Today*. Accessed May 29, 2020. www.usatoday.com/story/news/factcheck/2020/05/02/fact-check-no-homeless-people-not-immune-covid-19/3070058001/.

Shah, Maryam. 2020. "Canada Now Has More Than 95,000 Coronavirus Cases – More Than 34K Are Active." *GlobalNews.ca*. Accessed June 6, 2020. https://globalnews.ca/news/7035839/canada-coronavirus-cases-june-6/.

Skinta, Matthew, Angela H. Sun, and Daniel M. Ryu. 2021. "The Impact of COVID-19 on the Lives of Sexual and Gender Minority People." In *COVID-19: Social Consequences and Cultural Adaptations*, edited by J. Michael Ryan, 230–44. London: Routledge.

Slesnick, Natasha, Jing Zhang, and Brittany Brakenhoff. 2017. "Personal Control and Service Connection as Paths to Improved Mental Health and Exiting Homelessness Among Severely Marginalized Homeless Youth." *Children and Youth Services Review* 73: 121–27. https://doi.org/10.1016/j.childyouth.2016.11.033.

Smith, Alanna. 2020. "Supports for Homeless Calgarians Slim Amid COVID-19 Pandemic." *Calgary Herald*. Accessed May 29, 2020. https://calgaryherald.com/news/supports-for-homeless-calgarians-slim-amid-covid-19-pandemic.

Steacy, Lisa, and Renee Bernard. 2020. "Tent City Set Up in Port of Vancouver Parking Lot After Oppenheimer Evacuated." *News 1130*. Accessed May 29, 2020. www.citynews1130.com/2020/05/09/tent-city-crab-park-port-of-vancouver/.

Toronto.com. 2002. "Timeline: How the Coronavirus Outbreak Unfolded in Toronto: A Six-Month History of the Covid-19 Lockdown." *Toronto.com*. Accessed July 14, 2020. www.toronto.com/news-story/10023259-timeline-how-the-coronavirus-outbreak-unfolded-in-toronto/.

Tsemberis, Sam, Leyla Gulcur, and Maria Nakae. 2004. "Housing First, Consumer Choice, and Harm Reduction for Homeless Individuals with a Dual Diagnosis." *American Journal of Public Health* 94 (4): 651–56. DOI: 10.2105/ajph.94.4.651.

Wenzel, Suzanne L., Joan S. Tucker, Marc N. Elliott, Katrin Hambarsoomians, Judy Perlman, Kirsten Becker, Crystal Kollross, and Daniel Dolinelli. 2004. "Prevalence and

Co-Occurrence of Violence, Substance Use and Disorder, and HIV Risk Behaviour: A Comparison of Sheltered and Low-Income Housed Women in Los Angeles County." *Preventive Medicine* 39 (3): 617–24. DOI: 10.1016/j.ypmed.2004.02.027.

Wu, Jiachuan, Savannah Smith, Mansee Khurana, Corky Siemaskzo, and Brianna DeJesus-Banos. 2020. "Stay-at-Home Orders Across the Country: What Each State Is Doing – Or Not Doing – Amid Widespread Coronavirus Lockdowns." *NBC News*. Accessed May 24, 2020. www.nbcnews.com/health/health-news/here-are-stay-home-orders-across-country-n1168736.

8

COVID-19 AND REPRODUCTIVE INJUSTICE

The implications of birthing restrictions during a global pandemic

Nazneen Kane

In March 2020, after seven birthing women tested positive for COVID-19 in a single New York hospital, healthcare administrators at two New York hospitals quickly responded by modifying long-standing hospital policies surrounding pre-natal care, labor, and delivery. In two cases, at least 20 healthcare workers were exposed to risk of infection by obstetric patients who presented to the hospital as asymptomatic but developed symptoms during and shortly after delivery (Breslin et al. 2020). With the safety of obstetrical providers and patients in mind, the policy change included prohibiting laboring individuals from being accompanied by a birth support companion, including intimate partners and doulas. To varying degrees, similar policies have spread across healthcare delivery systems throughout the United States.

Yet as restrictions and modifications to reproductive health care spread, so too has resistance to these policies. As over 600,000 New Yorkers petitioned for policy reversal, obstetricians have also demanded access to universal coronavirus testing and personal protective equipment (PPE). Defending their policy stance, obstetricians and hospital administrators argue that coronavirus policies result from lack of PPE and lack of access to universal and rapid COVID-19 testing. They maintain that if parturient women and birth support persons were able to be rapidly tested and if all hospitals had equal access to PPE, these policies would not be necessary (Berghella 2020). In this way, lack of preparation and inaction at the federal level during the early weeks of the COVID-19 pandemic has impacted US women's access to birth justice.

The relationship between the state and reproductive health unfolds differently across the lives and experiences of pregnant and birthing women. Reproductive stratification, a term coined by Colen (1995), refers to the ways in which reproductive health varies by social class, race, public/private insurance, and other dimensions of women's lives. COVID-19 policy modifications exacerbate existent patterns of reproductive stratification (see Nanda 2021 and Ryan 2021 for broader discussions on inequality and COVID-19) because marginalized women, particularly women of color and those who are reliant upon public insurance, are often less able to navigate newly imposed restrictions. This research uses a *reproductive justice paradigm* to examine obstetric policy in the wake of the COVID-19 pandemic and examines its implications for birthing individuals.

Reproductive justice

Reproductive justice (RJ) is an intersectional theoretical and methodological framework that was first mapped out by an alliance of Black women, including the widely influential scholar and activist Loretta Ross, in 1994. Reproductive justice is guided by three core values – the right to have a child, the right not to have a child, and the right to safe and dignified parenting (Ross and Solinger 2017, 65). Birth justice advocates and scholars further extended this model by focusing specifically on the birthing process, arguing that pregnant individuals have the right to safe and dignified birth and elucidating the disproportionate violence experienced by birthing individuals of color (Oparah 2016). Birth justice highlights the ways in which provider racism drives birth trauma and includes a critique of disproportionate cesarean surgeries, irreversible sterilization, and birth trauma amongst women of color (Oparah 2016).

Safe and dignified birthing, a core component of birth justice, necessitates that all women have access to the full spectrum of reproductive services and supports. The RJ framework understands barriers to these services as a violation of human rights. While COVID-19 birthing policies are being implemented to protect healthcare workers and patients, their design undermines safe labor and delivery for birthing women and their neonates by restricting access to vital components of obstetric care. However, the consequences of these restrictions are not the same for all pregnant and birthing individuals.

The reproductive justice framework provides key tools and an analytic lens for exploring the differential impact of COVID-19 reproductive policies on pregnant and birthing women. The RJ framework allows us to consider that pregnant and birthing individuals who have financial and social resources are able to circumvent restrictions by procuring alternative care that is situated outside traditional delivery systems (see Milkie 2021, this volume, for discussion on the relationship between COVID-19, SES, and parental investments in children). It also requires understanding and exploring how COVID-19-related policy decisions build upon and advance historically segmented forms of race and class inequality in obstetric care. As Ross and Solinger argue, "When politicians, judges, and policy makers make decisions that affect our lives, for example, by enacting or upholding laws that restrict access to various kinds of reproductive health care, they are building on the past" (2017, 5). The history of reproductive injustices illustrates that reproductive policies have always been applied and exercised differently across different groups of women. Black, Indigenous, and some groups of Hispanic women have the highest rates of maternal morbidity and mortality in the US (Howell 2018); their maternal health outcomes are already in crisis. It is important to examine the implications of COVID-19 birthing restrictions and the ways in which they heighten that crisis.

Birth setting, birth support, and birth services: the impact and implications of COVID-19 birthing restrictions

Fears of contracting coronavirus while birthing, of being separated from a new-born, of being forced to wear a mask while birthing, and of birthing without a support partner are driving expectant women to modify their birth plans (Thayer and Gildner 2020). Additionally, standard obstetric services are changing in response to COVID-19, often without communication between providers and patients (Thayer and Gildner 2020), leaving women without the quality and level of care that they need for optimal birth during a global pandemic. Through an RJ lens, this section examines the impact and implications of institutional responses to the COVID-19 pandemic on birth setting, birth support, and birthing services.

Birth setting

Due to the coronavirus response, demand for out-of-hospital birthing options such as freestanding birth centers and homebirths with certified midwives is surging. Many pregnant individuals are being turned away as nontraditional birthing centers and midwives are unable to meet the growing demand (de Freytas-Tamura 2020). Further, while some birthing individuals are able to opt out of technomedical birthing altogether, most cannot financially access alternative birthing locations and services such as home birth delivery with a certified midwife.

Poor women and women of color have limited access to out-of-hospital birth alternatives for two related reasons. First, in the 1990s when the natural birth movement garnered greater legitimacy, it increasingly marginalized midwives and birth workers of color. The movement also framed birthing choice and birthing rights such as birth setting and provider options as a commodity for purchase, as opposed to a right that should be accessible to all women (Oparah 2016). While this framing was useful for garnering legislative approval, it sidelined groups of women without financial resources as well as the birthing justice concerns of communities of color. Despite the rich history of midwifery in African American, Indigenous, and Latinx communities (Hays 2016), midwifery in these communities continues to be scarce and under-resourced.

The framing of natural birth in the terms of consumer choice also meant that natural birthing was constructed as a luxury commodity for out-of-pocket purchase and not one that should be covered by healthcare insurance (Oparah 2016). Consequently, poor and low-income women, disproportionately women of color, often do not have the financial resources to cover the expense of obstetric services that sit outside traditional healthcare delivery systems. Public insurance, which covers nearly half of all US births (MACPAC 2020), is particularly limiting, leaving economically oppressed women with the fewest resources for navigating COVID-19 restrictions. In comparison to private insurance holders, Medicaid beneficiaries are limited to a narrow pool of birth settings and providers. While Medicaid coverage is increasingly expanding to cover services rendered at freestanding birth centers, this is not true of all state networks (see Kaiser Family Foundation 2018). Further, because of low reimbursement rates and challenging licensing restrictions, many centers limit Medicaid patients or decline to participate (Courtot et al. 2018). These barriers leave many groups of marginalized women with few birth setting options.

Embodied systemic racial and class discrimination is a second barrier to out-of-hospital birthing. Non-Hispanic Black women, Native Americans, and some groups of Hispanic women have elevated levels of pregnancy-related mortality and morbidity, the common explanation being that these women have elevated rates of chronic illness (Howell 2018). An expanding body of literature demonstrates that these illnesses are embodied manifestations of inequality that are driven by structural racism, including provider racism, experienced by these groups of women (Bridges 2011; Davis 2019).

These embodied manifestations of inequality create the conditions under which disadvantaged women are more likely to have high-risk pregnancies (Holzman et al. 2009), further limiting their care options. Even in hospitals with practicing midwives, women who are categorized as high risk are assigned to obstetricians (Bridges 2011). Midwife teams offer greater flexibility but due to high-demand during the current pandemic are generally only taking low-risk patients with a previous birthing experience. This leaves the most marginalized women to birth in what many pregnant individuals are referring to as "COVID hospitals" (de Freytas-Tamura 2020). Booked birthing centers and the combined fears of obstetric racism and COVID-19 transmission in hospitals is driving many rural Black women to birth unassisted at home (Simpson 2020). Beyond such restrictions to birth setting, perhaps most devastating to birthing individuals are the restrictions limiting continuous birth support persons during labor and delivery.

Birth support

Birthing individuals and their infants have better outcomes when they have access to continuous birth support (Bohren et al. 2017). In US hospitals, continuous care from birth workers is highly exceptional. Consequently, the need for continuous, culturally appropriate support is typically met by a partner or family member and, increasingly, by a doula. Pandemic-related hospital policies place restrictions on, or entirely eliminate, women's access to continuous care. In many cases, women are required to choose between a doula and a partner.

Research demonstrates that support persons, particularly doulas, improve birth outcomes in hospital settings by minimizing unnecessary medical interventions that place women at greater risk of birthing complications (Gruber, Cupito, and Dobson 2013). Doulas also play an especially vital role in shielding women of color from obstetric racism (Oparah et al. 2018). Obstetric racism, defined by Davis (2019) as the racism experienced by women during maternal healthcare processes, comes in many forms, including "critical lapses in diagnosis, being neglectful, dismissive, or disrespectful; causing pain; and engaging in medical abuse through coercion to perform procedures or performing procedures without consent" (Davis 2019, 562). Doulas can provide a vital buffer between birthing women and providers by supporting mothers in self-advocacy (Oparah et al. 2018; Wint et al. 2019). Benefits to doula-assisted births include a decreased risk of cesarean surgeries and birthing complications, a decrease in reported birth trauma, and greater likelihood of initiating breastfeeding (Gruber, Cupito, and Dobson 2013). Doulas also serve as witnesses for women of color, often the only birth workers to report incidences of obstetric abuse during labor and delivery (Morton et al. 2018).

Doulas can also facilitate improved communication between providers and patients, including lifesaving language translation. According to the COVID-19 and Reproductive Effects (CARE) study, 40% of women reported that their care provider had not communicated with them regarding the impact of COVID-19 on their labor and delivery (Thayer and Gildner 2020). This lack of communication is particularly negatively impactful for non-English-speaking pregnant individuals whose relationships with prenatal caregivers are already strained by culturally inappropriate care and lack of communication (Bridges 2011). Non-English-speaking women often rely upon birth supports with skills as translators, preferably who are also trained in birthing support, to make informed decisions about their care.

Black women and Indigenous women, who have the highest rates of maternal mortality in the United States, are especially at risk when vital reproductive supports are denied. They are disproportionately poor and most likely to report adverse experiences with medical providers. In this way, Black mothers are most likely to benefit from birth support persons such as doulas and from the postpartum visits that are often bundled into doula services (Hays 2016). Banning women from doula support during deliveries comes at a particularly inopportune time – when several states have expanded Medicaid to cover doula services and when birth justice activism has led to a rise in demand and support for midwives and doulas of color (Silliman et al. 2016).

Birth services

While pregnancy is not a medical condition, access to quality prenatal care is critical. Quality prenatal care that is culturally appropriate and that involves positive relationships with providers can offer maternal support, reassurance, and practical advice and reduce the risk of maternal and infant mortality (Oparah et al. 2018).

Particularly for those individuals with higher-risk pregnancies, prenatal care can save the lives of mothers and babies. Pre-eclampsia, eclampsia, and gestational diabetes are all potentially life-threatening health conditions that are identified and treated through prenatal care (Oparah et al. 2018). Despite these known benefits, many practitioners are reducing, modifying, and cancelling prenatal services due to risk of disease transmission. In-person maternity tours, birthing and maternal education classes, support groups, and in-person prenatal visits are being cancelled, particularly in COVID-19 hotspots. While COVID-19 presents a need for providers to offer alternative delivery approaches, it is important to think through the implications of such alternatives for different groups of pregnant individuals.

The loss of prenatal services is particularly disadvantageous for pregnant individuals of color, who already face structural barriers to accessing and persisting with prenatal care. Rural women, women of color, Medicaid beneficiaries, and women who do not speak English are particularly prone to disruptions in care because they overwhelmingly experience subpar prenatal care, culturally irrelevant care, and obstetric racism and/or disrespectful care (Bridges 2011; Oparah et al. 2018). Further disruptions to their prenatal care due to COVID-19 puts these groups of women and their fetuses at particular disadvantage, especially for those women in their third trimester.

In addition to reducing prenatal visits, many practices are digitizing prenatal care by using internet technologies. The rise of telemedicine and telephonic appointments for prenatal care minimizes risk of disease transmission but disadvantages pregnant individuals without electronic devices and/or who live in rural areas or otherwise go without access to reliant high-speed internet. In most states, Medicaid does not cover telemedicine services for prenatal care, leaving beneficiaries outside the scope of telehealth services (Weigel, Frederiksen, and Ranji 2020). In conjunction with telemedicine, many practitioners are asking pregnant women to self-monitor their health.

Vital measures such as blood pressure, fetal heartbeat, and maternal glucose levels are increasingly being assessed by pregnant individuals at home. Despite that self-monitoring enables obstetricians to continue profiting and practicing under the pandemic, the cost of devices such as blood pressure cuffs and fetal monitors are most often passed along to pregnant women, as not all private insurance plans cover these devices for pregnancy. Further, only some states report temporary flexibilities that include Medicaid coverage for these devices (Goligoski 2020). With maternal mortality rates as high as they are in the US, the slow response of states to the rapidly changing nature of prenatal care under COVID-19 is alarming.

Many women are also reporting interruptions to postpartum maternal care. Hospital restrictions are the most stringent, with a host of media stories detailing the experiences of COVID-19-positive women having forced inductions and cesareans, birthing by cesarean alone, and/or being separated from their newborn infants (Carmon 2020; Mitchell et al. 2020). This practice of separation persists despite the recommendation of the World Health Organization to keep COVID-19-positive mothers and infants in close contact (WHO 2020) and despite that separation may not prevent infection and disrupts both newborn physiology and immune protection via breastfeeding (Stuebe 2020). Some hospitals are separating mothers and newborns until COVID-19 tests return with negative results, also against WHO recommendations. Ironically, women birthing in public hospitals are often those who need the most support but where policies are likely to be the most oppositional to birth justice and where reproductive resources are most lacking.

Conclusion

By centering the birthing experiences of marginalized women, RJ scholars and birth justice activists have and continue to work to improve birthing conditions for all pregnant and birthing individuals. Pandemic policies that restrict birth support persons and birth services undermine this work and are particularly harmful to publicly insured women, women of color, and economically oppressed groups of women who have the fewest options for quality obstetric care, leaving them at higher risk of birth trauma, disease transmission, obstetric violence, and even death. While states such as New York have responded to these challenges by creating a maternal health task force to identify and create midwife-led birth centers and by rapidly expanding Medicaid to cover a wider range of birth options (New York State 2020), this is the exception. While the delivery of obstetric services should necessarily change amidst a dangerous pandemic, services should not suffer due to lack of resources and federal government undersight.

The United States is already facing a maternal mortality crisis manifested by high rates of maternal mortality and morbidity. Rescinding services and supports for birthing individuals due to lack of PPE and access to virus testing only heightens this crisis. COVID-19 has resulted in an array of economic, emotional, and mental health stressors, all of which can negatively impact pregnancy. A pandemic is not the time to strip birthing rights from women – it is a time to intensify efforts to ensure that reproductive justice is being achieved safely and intentionally.

References

Berghella, Vincenzo. 2020. "NOW! Protection for Obstetrical Providers and Patients." *American Journal of Obstetrics and Gynecology MFM* 2 (2) (May): 100109. https://doi.org/10.1016/j.ajogmf.2020.100109.

Bohren, Meghan, G. Justus Hofmeyr, Carol Sakala, Reiko K. Fukuzawa, and Anna Cuthbert. 2017. *Cochrane Database Systemic Review* 7 (7): CD003766. https://doi.org/10.1002/14651858.CD003766.pub6.

Breslin, Noelle, Caitlin Baptiste, Russell Miller, Karin Fuchs, Dena Goffman, Cynthia Gyamfi-Bannerman, and Mary D'Alton. 2020. "Coronavirus Disease 2019 in Pregnancy: Early Lessons." *American Journal of Obstetrics and Gynecology MFM* 2 (2) (May): 100111. https://doi.org/10.1016/j.ajogmf.2020.100111.

Bridges, Khiara. 2011. *Reproducing Race: An Ethnography of Pregnancy as a Site of Racialization.* Berkeley: University of California Press.

Carmon, Irin. 2020. "'They Separated Me from My Baby': Hospitals are Keeping Newborns from Their Parents Over Coronavirus Fears." *The Cut*, April 7. www.thecut.com/2020/04/coronavirus-newborns-hospitals-parents.html.

Colen, Shellee. 1995. "'Like a Mother to Them': Stratified Reproduction and West Indian Child Care Workers and Employers." In *Conceiving the New World Order: The Global Politics of Reproduction*, edited by Faye D. Ginsberg and Rayna Rapp, 78–102. Berkeley: University of California Press.

Courtot, Bridgette, Caitlin Cross-Barnet, Ian Hill, Sarah Benatar, Jenny Markell, Sarah Thornburgh, and Eva Hruba Allen. 2018. "Midwifery and Birth Center Care Under State Medicaid Programs." Accessed June 26, 2020. https://appam.confex.com/appam/2018/webprogram/Paper27539.html.

Davis, Dana-Ain. 2019. "Obstetric Racism: The Racial Politics of Pregnancy and Birthing." *Medical Anthropology* 38 (7): 560–73. https://doi.org/10.1080/01459740.2018.1549389.

de Freytas-Tamura, Kimiko. 2020. "Pregnant and Scared of 'Covid Hospitals' They're Giving Birth at Home." *New York Times*, April 21. www.nytimes.com/2020/04/21/nyregion/coronavirus-home-births.html.

Goligoski, Emily. 2020. "Prenatal Care May Look Very Different After Coronavirus." *New York Times*, April 28. www.nytimes.com/2020/04/28/parenting/pregnancy/coronavirus-prenatal-care.html.

Gruber, Kenneth, Susan Cupito, and Christina F. Dobson. 2013. "Impact of Doulas on Healthy Birth Outcomes." *Journal of Perinatal Education* 22 (1): 49–58. https://doi.org/10.1891/1058-1243.22.1.49.

Hays, Ruth. 2016. "Birthing Freedom: Black American Midwifery and Liberation Struggles." In *Birthing Justice: Black Women, Pregnancy, and Childbirth*, edited by Julia Chinyere Oparah and Alicia D. Bonaparte, 166–75. New York: Routledge.

Holzman, Claudia, Janet Eyster, Mary Kleyn, Lynne Messer, Jay S. Kaufman, Barbara A. Laraia, Patricia O'Campo, Jessica G. Burke, Jennifer Culhane, and Irma Elo. 2009. "Maternal Weathering and Risk of Preterm Delivery." *American Journal of Public Health* 99 (10): 1864–871. https://doi.org/10.2105/AJPH.2008.15189.

Howell, Elizabeth A. 2018. "Reducing Disparities in Severe Maternal Morbidity and Mortality." *Clinical Obstetrics and Gynecology* 61 (2): 387–99. https://doi.org/10.1097/GRF.0000000000000349.

Kaiser Family Foundation. 2018. "Medicaid Benefits: Freestanding Birth Center Services." Accessed July 2, 2020. www.kff.org/other/state-indicator/medicaid-benefits-freestanding-birth-center-services/.

MACPAC. 2020. "Medicaid's Role in Financing Maternity Care." Accessed June 16, 2020. www.macpac.gov/wp-content/uploads/2020/01/Medicaid%E2%80%99s-Role-in-Financing-Maternity-Care.pdf.

Milkie, Melissa. 2021. "Changing Times: New Sources of Parenting Stress and the Shifting Meanings of Time With and for Children." In *COVID-19: Social Consequences and Cultural Adaptations*, edited by J. Michael Ryan, 152–64. London: Routledge.

Mitchell, Kate, Hagar Palgi Hacker, Tejumola Adegoke, and Katharine Hutchinson. 2020. "Hospitals are Separating Mothers and Newborns During the Coronavirus Pandemic – With Little Evidence it Will Help Slow the Spread of Disease." *Boston Globe*, May 9. www.bostonglobe.com/2020/05/09/opinion/hospitals-are-separating-mothers-newborns-during-coronavirus-pandemic-with-little-evidence-it-will-help-slow-spread-disease/.

Morton, Christine, Megan Henley, Maria Seacrist, and Louise Marie Roth. 2018. "Bearing Witness: United States and Canadian Maternity Support Workers' Observations of Disrespectful Care in Childbirth." *Birth* 45: 263–74. https://doi.org/10.1111/birt.12373.

Nanda, Serena. 2021. "Inequalities and COVID-19." In *COVID-19: Global Pandemic, Societal Responses, Ideological Solutions*, edited by J. Michael Ryan, 109–23. London: Routledge.

New York State. 2020. "Governor Cuomo & COVID-19 Maternity Task Force Chair Melissa DeRosa Announce Increased Access to Midwife-Led Birth Centers Amid COVID-19." June 16. Accessed July 4, 2020. www.governor.ny.gov/news/governor-cuomo-covid-19-maternity-task-force-chair-melissa-derosa-announce-increased-access.

Oparah, Julia Chinyere. 2016. "Beyond Coercion and Malign Neglect: Black Women and the Struggle for Birth Justice." In *Birthing Justice: Black Women, Pregnancy, and Childbirth*, edited by Julia Chinyere Oparah and Alicia D. Bonaparte, 1–23. New York: Routledge.

Oparah, Julia Chinyere, Helen Arega, Dantia Hudson, Linda Jones, and Talita Oseguera. 2018. *Battling Over Birth: Black Women and the Maternal Health Care Crisis*. Amarillo: Praeclarus Press.

Ross, Loretta, and Rickie Solinger. 2017. *Reproductive Justice: An Introduction*. Berkeley: University of California Press.

Ryan, J. Michael. 2021. "The Blessings of COVID-19 for Neoliberalism, Nationalism, and Neoconservative Ideologies." In *COVID-19: Global Pandemic, Societal Responses, Ideological Solutions*, edited by J. Michael Ryan, 80–93. London: Routledge.

Silliman, Jael, Marlene Gerber Fried, Elena R. Gutierrez, and Loretta Ross. 2016. *Undivided Rights: Women of Color Organize for Reproductive Justice*. Chicago: Haymarket Books.

Simpson, April. 2020. "Fearing Coronavirus, Many Rural Black Women Avoid Hospitals to Give Birth at Home." *Stateline*, April 17. www.pewtrusts.org/en/research-and-analysis/blogs/stateline/2020/04/17/fearing-coronavirus-many-rural-black-women-avoid-hospitals-to-give-birth-at-home.

Stuebe, Alison. 2020. "Should Infants Be Separated from Mothers with COVID-19? First, Do No Harm." *Breastfeeding Medicine* 15 (5): 351–52. https://doi.org/10.1089/bfm.2020.29153.ams.

Thayer, Zaneta, and Theresa Gildner. 2020. "COVID-19 and Reproductive Effects (CARE) Study: Research Results." Accessed June 17, 2020. https://sites.dartmouth.edu/care2020/research-results/.

Weigel, Gabriela, Brittni Frederiksen, and Usha Ranji. 2020. "Telemedicine and Pregnancy Care." *Women's Health Policy*, February 26. www.kff.org/womens-health-policy/issue-brief/telemedicine-and-pregnancy-care/.

Wint, Kristina, Thistle I. Elias, Gabriella Mendez, Dara D. Mendez, and Tiffany L. Gary-Webb. 2019. "Experiences of Community Doulas Working with Low-Income, African American Mothers." *Health Equity* 3 (1): 109–16. https://doi.org/10.1089/heq.2018.0045.

World Health Organization. 2020. "Pregnancy, Childbirth, and COVID-19." Accessed June 22, 2020. www.who.int/emergencies/diseases/novel-coronavirus-2019/question-and-answers-hub/q-a-detail/q-a-on-covid-19-pregnancy-and-childbirth.

9

WHEN SPORTS STOOD STILL

COVID-19 and the lost season

Donna J. Barbie, John C. Lamothe, and Steven Master

It was a typically vibrant, electric scene inside Chesapeake Energy Arena on the evening of March 11, 2020. The Oklahoma City Thunder and Utah Jazz, talented young teams in the thick of the NBA's Western Conference playoff race, were seconds away from tip-off. Starters had been introduced. And as players stretched and "Zombie Nation" blared over the speakers, a packed arena began turning its attention to mid-court for a tip-off that never tipped off.

Moments earlier, team medical personnel learned that Jazz center Rudy Gobert had tested positive for COVID-19, setting off a bizarre chain of events for fans inside the arena. It took another 90 minutes for the fans to understand the magnitude of the moment.

At 8:30 p.m. that evening, the National Basketball Association (NBA) made the startling announcement that it was suspending its season indefinitely. A season approaching its crescendo was frozen in time. And so, ultimately, was the sports world as we knew it, a once-unthinkable shock to a country in the early stages of an equally unthinkable pandemic.

For many sports fans, the seriousness of the COVID-19 pandemic did not fully register until this day. The NBA was the first major sports league to announce the indefinite suspension of play, though the signs of a shutdown had arrived even earlier that day. Hours earlier, the NBA's Golden State Warriors announced they were closing home games to fans due to a California ban on gatherings of 1,000 or more. The National Hockey League's (NHL) Columbus Blue Jackets made a similar declaration at the same time. For college sports fans, the news was equally grim. The NCAA announced that March Madness, the NCAA basketball tournament, would be played without fans.

Even that was wishful thinking.

In reality, it was all done. Within 24 hours, the NHL had put its season on hold, Major League Soccer (MLS) had suspended its campaign, and March Madness was canceled . . . not postponed; canceled. And on it went. In short order, fans would learn that, for the foreseeable future, they would be without major sports leagues, high school sports, and everything in between.

No Masters. No Wimbledon. No Kentucky Derby. Even the Olympic Games, scheduled for summer 2020 in Tokyo, were called off.

In the grand scheme of things, of course, the suspension of sports hardly registers as tragic when compared to the lives lost, economic hardships, and social upheaval caused by COVID-19. For much of the world's population, the pandemic has been the most significant global tragedy in their lifetimes.

Yet the absence of sports is notable in that they have historically served an important function during tragedy. They both distract us from our troubles and unify us in our resolve. Monday Night Football returning to New Orleans a year after Hurricane Katrina, President Bush throwing out the first pitch in Yankee Stadium after 9/11, the first Boston Bruins game after the Boston Marathon Bombings: these emotional events were all marked as both catharsis for our pain and as a return to some sense of normalcy. Franklin D. Roosevelt knew this when, following Pearl Harbor, he convinced baseball commissioner Kenesaw Landis to keep the sport going to distract citizens from the war. "But even sports can't get us through this," veteran sports journalist Rick Reilly (2020) wrote in a March 20 *Atlantic* article, noting that he missed sports so much he'd "give my left pinkie toe just to cuddle up with a cold beer and the Valero Texas Open golf tournament."

Although sports cannot distract or unite us through this particular tragedy, their suspension during the summer of 2020 presents an opportunity to examine their importance in our culture. It offers a chance to observe how deeply, if at all, we feel the loss, how we manage to cope and work around it, what we are finding to fill the void, and how this unprecedented event might change sports, or how we view them and their place in our lives.

The significance of play

With all the suffering and chaos brought on by the pandemic, why is the loss of sports worthy of analysis? Dutch historian Johan Huizinga (1955) begins to answer that question in his seminal work, *Homo Ludens*, which translates to *Man, the Player*. As Huizinga argues, play is an essential element of culture, "more than a mere physiological phenomenon or a psychological reflex" (1). He notes that "Play is distinct from 'ordinary' life," enacted in "temporary worlds within the ordinary world" (4). Reinforcing Huizinga's notion, French sociologist Roger Caillois (1961) writes in *Man, Play and Games* that play is "essentially a separate occupation, carefully isolated from the rest of life" (4). Sports fans understand and relish that separation. As Tyler Spence (2010) writes in *Bleacher Report*,

> for us fans, sports is our escape . . . our pain killer. When we are having a bad day or have our mind on stuff . . ., it seems we forget about it after watching our team, or reading up on mock drafts or rumors.

Many sports fans, especially the most fanatical ones, show a "super abundant vital energy" (Huizinga 1955, 1) in this isolated, "consecrated space" (4). They don giant wedges of orange foam "cheese" and scream at the top of their lungs. They paint their faces and chant. Even when removed from the immediacy of the competition by television screens, fans experience exhilaration and despair, sometimes swearing and throwing pizza crusts when disgusted with the official or exasperated by poor play. People who do not count themselves as fans might say all of this is excessive. It is only a game, after all. Fandom, however, is not about logic or reasoning but emotion, and often too much of it. Ardent sports fans eagerly hop on the roller coaster.

A long-time student of sports fandom, psychologist Daniel Wann developed the Sport Spectator Identification Scale (SSIS), an instrument that measures the intensity of a person's involvement with one or more sports. According to Wann et al. (2001), "highly identified" fans establish and maintain significant emotional responses for a variety of reasons, including the need for affiliation, enjoyment of the game's aesthetic, desire for entertainment, and thirst for eustress (30). Often referred to as "positive stress," eustress produces excitement and arousal that the average person may seldom experience in ordinary life.

The SSIS measures, among other aspects of sports identity, the significance that fans place on physiological and psychological stimulation while watching a competition. They found that male participants relish greater suspense because of the resulting higher levels of eustress (Wann et al. 2001, 46). Another study concluded that fans achieve the most gratification when their team wins and they can engage in "BIRGing," or "basking in the reflected glory" of their team or player (Van Leeuwen, Quick, and Daniel 2002, 100). Even before the pandemic, Rachel Anne Williams (2019) noted the significance of escape and emotion when watching sports,

> On its face, the world is a pretty grim place. At the same time the world is falling apart, sports fans everywhere take joy in their teams winning and wallow in their losing, investing a tremendous amount of emotional energy into sports.

Williams had no idea that the "world falling apart" could extend to a sudden sports stoppage in 2020.

Coping with loss

So, what happens to fans when that roller coaster disappears? When asked what impact COVID-19 could have on sports fans, Wann said,

> Fandom assists in our need to belong, our need for uniqueness and our meaning in life. . . . You're taking away an activity that helps people meet

overall general basic psychological needs. . . . It matters to people in deep, profound, and impactful ways.

(Greever 2020)

In 2020, sports fans worldwide, who would normally achieve a sense of belonging by watching and following a particular sport, team, or athlete, are finding they are instead unified in their profound sense of loss.

Katy, a college student-athlete from south Florida, went home for spring break in March and never returned to campus. Her heartbreak of losing her playing season was only deepened by the loss of something so deeply woven into the fabric of her life. "Normally sports is the only thing on in my living room," she said. "In summers, we switch back and forth between different baseball games." She sheepishly admitted that her family tuned to professional wrestling for its "sports time," but anticipated feeling the loss more acutely in April when baseball's opening day passed with empty stadiums nationwide. "I am beside myself that I won't be able to go to a Marlins game any time soon," she said.

Similarly, Gregory, a 50-something financial services professional in Boca Raton, Florida, claimed the breadth of the pause in sports impacted him the most. He said he could have handled the cancellation of one or two sports/events, but having it all disappear deprived him of some of the great joys and traditions in his life. He noted this was the first time in 34 years he did not attend a spring training game, which he described as an "extreme loss . . . an actual void."

Many fans have turned to online sports forums to air their pain among community members who are feeling the same loss. Users on Sportsjournalists.com share a passion for sports media but, more generally, sports. Several concurrent threads on the site laid bare the impact that freezing of sports had on some of the more passionate fans. While many reported not missing sports as much as they thought they would, others shared a deep sense of loss. "I have to say, now more than ever, I wish I could watch a goddamn baseball game today," user Bigpern 23 wrote on April 4. "I understand the sadness," 3_Octave_Fart wrote on April 14. "I miss baseball so much it makes my heart hurt."

Roberta, a college athlete studying in the United States but from Croatia, returned home when her university switched to all online classes after the coronavirus outbreak. Sports were shut down in Europe as well, yet even in the absence of live games, Croatians managed to find joy in revisiting recent triumphs. Roberta reported that Croatian television reran the national men's soccer team's improbable run to the World Cup finals in 2018. "In the place where I live, all the neighbors went out on their balconies and cheered," Roberta reported. Franco, another international student studying in the US, reported a similar experience when he returned to his home country of Argentina. The networks began rebroadcasting the 2014 World Cup where Argentina advanced to the final, and Franco watched the entire run. Although he enjoyed reminiscing in his country's previous accomplishments, he said he longed for other aspects of live sporting events: "I've missed

the post-game talks with my family and friends, as well as the culture that sur-
rounds it, the passion and dedication to the team as if it was your own country."

Although sports would begin to return – shadows of their former selves – by the
middle of the summer, fans scrambled to replace the loss. Activities that six months
earlier would have seemed unthinkable became the nourishment for a ravenous
sports fandom.

Filling the void

Before the COVID-19 pandemic, watching live sports consumed a significant portion of the average sports fan's time. Whether watching a two-hour soccer match
or a four-day golf tournament, or any combination in between, sitting on the
couch with eyes glued to the television required an investment of time not much
less demanding than what a sports fan would spend on sleeping, working, or eating
during the week. When the lights went out in stadiums, tracks, courses, and other
sporting venues around the globe, sports fans were left with a void that needed to
be filled. Veteran sports columnist Thomas Boswell (2020) mused in *The Washington Post*,

> Not much about a pandemic is instructive. But how we use our time in its
> wake, where we invest our passion – even if we just change the tilt of our
> heads a few degrees in the way we see the world – will be an education to us.

Wann said it is very possible that many lowly identified sports fans may move
away from sports during the pandemic, using their newfound time for other things,
and he feels that believing they will all come back when sports resume is a faulty
assumption (Schaerlaeckens 2020). However, most experts agree that moderate
and highly identified fans have little interest in replacing that time with something
other than sports. Andrew Billings, executive director of the Sports Communication program at the University of Alabama, claims that fans see "sports fandom as the epitome of what society is missing [during the pandemic]: a common
shared kinship and interaction" (Schaerlaeckens 2020). Sports fans, therefore, have
attempted primarily to replace the time they typically spend on live sports with
other (albeit, far less satisfying) sports viewing.

Probably the most common replacement, especially in the spring and early
summer, was watching sports events that were being rebroadcast. Marian, a
92-year-old woman who lives in a care center in Bismarck, North Dakota, is an
avid golf fan. In December 2019, she spent nearly two hours recording the names
and locations of the 2019–20 tournaments into her new calendar. Needless to say,
that little exercise went for naught. Starting in March 2020, Marian was entirely
"locked down" in her room, no visitors, and only occasional conversations with
staff members. She has not felt an acute sense of loss of sports, nonetheless, because
she was able to watch tournament replays. As she says, "It's OK because I don't
remember who won."

The same memory lapses cannot be reported of Chris, a sports fanatic who typically watches just about any sport. He knows the names of all the basketball, soccer, and football players and has such a sharp eye that he can make the calls even before the official throws the flag or pulls the card. He was bereft when sports stopped. Like Marian, he resorted to watching years-old competitions, all of the commentaries he could find, and stayed up late into the night to watch the first virtual NFL draft. These strategies helped him cope.

In the absence of sports, Michael watched all five of Duke's NCAA men's championship games as well as the classic Duke–Kentucky 1992 Elite Eight game. "I tried watching some of those ESPN competition shows, like the ultimate dodgeball and the ridiculous cannonball diving or whatever the heck it was called. I was amused for 5–10 minutes, then gave up," he said, adding that watching replays of old games can be enjoyable but no replacement for a "real, live" competition where the outcome is unknown.

Another popular diversion during the months of April and May was the ten-part documentary about Michael Jordan titled *The Last Dance*, which garnered huge ratings and sparked conversations within mainstream media, not just sports outlets. Chris eagerly tuned into every episode, as well as the many commentaries afterward, and Evan, a recent college graduate, reveled in the series, claiming it "satisfied me in a different way than live sports do." Despite the documentary's depth and quality, it is interesting to speculate whether it would have captivated so many if it had been released prior to the pandemic when there were still live sports.

Events beyond the mainstream sports – most of which typically would have been relegated to 3:00 a.m. timeslots – have found their way into primetime programming as sports networks struggle to fill the absence of live sports. ESPN started airing old Classic Tetris Championships, Cherry-Pit Spitting Competitions, and the World Axe-Throwing League (Good 2020). They even showed the 51st National Stone Skipping Competition in a 9:30 a.m. timeslot. Sportsjournalists.com user Bitteryoungmatador2 noted that a three-day challenge of professional pool players was drawing 3,000 viewers a day on Facebook Live. However, he, like others, relied on more traditional ways of filling the void. He wrote he was "having so much fun watching old sports again that I really don't need new ones." Noting that he had watched Game 6 of the 1979 World Series, followed by the final round of the 1997 Masters, he cited the comfort of nostalgia. "We all get to be little kids again," he wrote.

Even many veteran sports journalists fed their desire for sports with previously recorded events they most likely had previously watched live. Boswell admitted that he viewed highlights and games from the 1978 baseball season, as well as PGA events from 2019. But not everyone had a desire to rewatch old events. Joe Gisondi, a 20-year veteran sports reporter and author of *Field Guide to Covering Sports*, said he had absolutely no interest in watching events where he could know the outcome. "I don't go back and watch the classics. Yeah, I don't care," he said. For Gisondi, watching old games would just remind him of what he is not watching: live sports. "If I were watching it, the whole time I would be thinking, 'Why am I not watching the Yankees or Angels or anybody else?'" and Gisondi does not want the reminder.

Some fans even see the sports stoppage as a potential blessing as it might force the sports industry to reimagine itself. For these fans, the perceived purity of sports has eroded over the years, as corporate greed and rapid expansion in the ESPN age has sterilized the industry, to some degree, and priced out the middle class from attending events in person. Due to these factors, Sportsjournalist.com user Alma (2020) wrote, "not having sports for a while is actually kind of refreshing." Another user, Azrael, agreed, sort of, noting, "It was past time for a huge sports culture/sports industrial complex reset . . . And this is almost the only way imaginable we'd ever get it. We've certainly lost sight of what's important in and around sports. Mostly because of money." However, Azrael went on argue that sports will survive this reckoning, as they always have, because of their deep roots in our culture. Poignantly, he wrote, "Sports – not only the games, but the telling of the story of those games – are an important part of our humanity. And have been for thousands of years."

Feeding the need to gamble

Although many turned to watching old, classic games and oddball events during the pause of sports, other sports fans turned their attention to an unlikely venue, the stock market. With sports shut down, avid sports gamblers needed an outlet to replicate the adrenaline rush of having a financial stake in the outcome of a game or, in the case of fantasy sports, performances of individual athletes.

Sports gambling has existed for generations yet has seen massive growth in the US in recent years as states have loosened restrictions and fantasy-sports sites such as Draft Kings and FanDuel have come online. As a testament to the growth of sports betting in general and pay-to-play fantasy sports specifically, Draft Kings went public with its initial public offering in April – oddly enough during the heart of the pandemic – and saw its stock price double in two months. At a 2019 investors' event sponsored by Morgan Stanley, experts predicted the sports betting industry could bring in $8 billion in revenue by 2025 (Associated Press 2019).

Betting on a sporting event, and fantasy sports especially, has proven extremely valuable to the sports leagues in generating interest and viewership. Though fandom literature points to the personal stake loyal fans have for their teams, having a financial stake – "skin in the game" – can be equally powerful. When sports paused, so did the adrenaline rush for sports gamblers and fantasy sports players. And many, it seemed, turned to day trading in the stock market, a controversial and potentially perilous activity that provided the closest thing to that buzz provided by sports betting. A May 22 headline in *Barron's* read, "Day Trading Has Replaced Sports Betting as America's Pastime" (Forsyth 2020). A June 14 *New York Times* article featured a teacher from suburban Philadelphia who withdrew all of his funds from his sportsbook accounts and "turned to one of the last places in town for reliable action –

the stock market" (Phillips 2020). The exchanges had been driven into bear-market territory by the shutdown of the economy and, for many, the drop represented an opportunity to make a quick buck on drastically oversold stocks. In fact, some credited sports gamblers who turned to sports betting using stock-trading platforms like Robinhood as, in part, responsible for the market's comeback. Many day traded with their federal stimulus or unemployment checks. *The Times* quoted one strategist at a brokerage firm as having "zero doubt" the conversion of sports bettors to stocks played a role in the market turnaround (Phillips 2020). Others were doubtful but admitted it could have played a role in making particular stocks move, such as Robinhood favorites Go-Pro, American Airlines and Carnival Cruise Lines (Brokamp, Frankel, and Southwick 2020).

The most high-profile symbol of this shift from sports betting to day trading was David Portnoy (2020), multi-millionaire president of the "raunchy, irreverently juvenile and wildly popular sports and gambling web site, Barstool Sports." With no more sports/sports gambling to cover, he started live streaming his stock trading during the last hour of the trading day, attracting a half-million viewers (Brokamp, Frankel, and Southwick 2020). Portnoy drew the attention of the financial news media for the massive amount of money he was day trading (which amounted to only a small fraction of overall wealth), his influence over his fans (many of whom followed his lead into day trading), and his bluster. He criticized legendary investor Warren Buffett as "washed up" (Langlois 2020) and proclaimed he was "just printing money" (he was not; at one point he was down almost $700,000) and tweeted "stocks only go up" (Portnoy 2020). "I like betting in sports," he told *Business Insider*. "Sports ended, and this was something I could do during the day" (Flanagan 2020).

Games resume . . . without the fans

In late May and early June 2020, roughly two months after sports stood still due to the global pandemic, some events started to trickle back. In the US, it began with the sports that seem the most ideal for making a transition to the new normal: NASCAR racing and PGA golf. Both sports are held outdoors and in situations where the athletes can easily maintain distance from their fellow competitors. Internationally, all eyes turned toward sports leagues not typically in the limelight, such as the South Korean Baseball (KBO) league, and several regional or country-specific soccer leagues, such as the Bundesliga in Germany and the Danish Super-liga in Denmark.

As sports hesitantly started to resume, one thing was glaringly absent – the fans.

In order to prevent the virus's spread, sporting events were held in empty stadiums, tracks, and courses. If COVID-19 has no other long-term impact on sports, it exposed the vital role that fans play in creating the modern sporting event. Those in the sports community and even sports scholars have long acknowledged the effect that fans have on athletic performance. The oft-cited "home field advantage" has been shown in numerous studies to be more than simple superstition, and athletes often praise the fans after a team has a particularly stellar performance. During COVID-19, the athletes recognized and acknowledged the fans' absence. In a sport where the athletes cannot possibly hear the crowds over the roar of their engines, NASCAR driver Kevin Harvick emerged victorious from his car immediately upon winning the first event back after the COVID-19 pause and said, "I didn't think it was going to be that much different, and then we win a race, and it is dead silent out here, so we miss the fans" (Associated Press 2020).

However, COVID-19 brought attention to the impact that fans and crowds have on how we experience sports. Just as games were starting back, Gisondi expressed his concerns that an event without fans would feel inauthentic:

> As much as I'd like to think it's going to be "Wow, this is normal," I think it's going to be a situation where I'm constantly reminded during the game that no one is there. If I'm listening to a baseball game, there's that hum of the crowd that you can hear over the TV. You can hear it on the radio. You can see the people in the stands. Think about all the shots of the stands in a normal game that they just won't have anymore. So it's going to feel a little vacant. I'm still going to embrace it, and I'm sure that I'll watch it, but I wonder how much I'm going to feel like things are abnormal instead of normal when I'm watching it.

Gisondi's concerns appeared justified as sports leagues scrambled to adjust to a sporting environment without fans. The world of professional soccer is an interesting case study in the evolution that occurred in broadcasts during the restart. South Korean soccer was one of the first leagues to start back, and they did so with *nearly* empty stadiums. One club, FC Seoul, attempted to add some more "life" to the stands with the addition of mannequins. Much to their dismay, media outlets revealed that the mannequins were actually sex dolls, and the club was slapped with a record fine (Garger 2020). When Germany's Bundesliga started back in mid-May, it did so with most of the stadium seats covered and broadcasters using a variety of tighter-angle shots to avoid showing the stands as much as possible. The problem, however, was with the audio, not the visuals. Chris was looking forward to "real sports," but when he witnessed the reopening of the Bundesliga that was being broadcast in the US, his enthusiasm waned considerably. He watched for a few minutes, but then said, "You can hear everything, grunts and the coaches yelling." He added, "There is no energy. It is too much like when I used to practice. I hate it." He turned the channel, something he would never have done prior to the pandemic.

As the games went on, Bundesliga began using artificial crowd noise, a mix of sounds recorded from the two teams' previous matches. They even began pumping the sounds into the stadiums. The Danish Superliga experimented with a virtual zone to give fans a stadium-like experience (Lee 2020). They allowed up to 10,000 fans to register for a Zoom meeting, even letting them to choose their "seats" when they signed up and organizing the fans into meeting rooms based on where they were "sitting." However, audio was still problematic as there was a delay between the live actions on the field and when fans were able to react.

When the English Premier League (considered by many to be the world's foremost soccer league) restarted in June 2020, it adopted many of the techniques attempted by other leagues, including the artificial crowd noise. They did not broadcast the sounds into the stadium, but fans could tune into their favorite teams and hear the team-specific chants and songs they would normally hear when watching or attending a live event. The soundtracks were created from audio shared by EA Sports, which has a database of 1,300 tracks they use within the FIFA soccer game series (Hudson 2020). Of course, when the camera would happen to show the empty stadium, the suspension of disbelief could be shattered, but for many fans, hearing a more realistic sporting event was reassuring. According to Bundesliga fan Hunter Fauci, "Anything is better than hearing the echoes around a quiet stadium. Silence would make a lot of fans depressed" (The Daily James 2020). In an opinion article for *USA Today*, author Nate Scott (2020) claimed,

> Yes, it can feel a bit uncanny to hear crowd noise and then look up and see empty seats. But soccer is a game that relies on atmosphere as much as anything. Your eyes are on the field for the most part, so you don't notice the disparity much. With the chants, it *feels* like a soccer game.

However, fans have been somewhat divided over the artificial sounds. Many have expressed their disgust, and networks now are offering ways for fans to tune in without the added noise. The National Football League (NFL) has expressed interest in using artificial crowd noise if fans are not able to attend games when the season begins in the fall, but famed Hall of Fame coach and commentator John Madden has urged against it (Kerr 2020). Instead, Madden believes broadcasters should attempt to capture the sounds from the field – players, coaches, etc. – which is the soundtrack he became accustomed to during his coaching career.

Dr. Glenn Cummins, a professor at Texas Tech University who studied the effects of crowd noise on our perceptions of sporting events, claims that social cues from audio, including artificial crowd noise, make watching the event more enjoyable. "We pay so much attention to camera shots and replays and slow motions, but I think sound and crowd noise is such a big part of how we perceive and respond to the competition," he said while being interviewed on "Hawksbee and Jacobs," a UK sports radio program (ttu_comc 2020). Because COVID-19 has brought the importance of crowd noise more to our attention, Cummins feels that sports broadcasts in the future will allow fans to have more say in what sounds they hear. "We've got to remember that [sports fans] are not just a homogenous unit. . . . I think we're eventually going to enter a day and age where people are going to be able to create their own custom-tailored broadcasts," he said.

The next chapter in sports

As Azrael argues, "Sports are no more or less meaningless than art or music or poetry. In a utilitarian sense, they might be *useless*, but we fill them with meaning and derive meaning from them" (2020). These testimonies show us that sports are indeed significant to many people. They also serve to remind us how far off we are from the halcyon days of sports, from the physiological and psychology highs and lows we feel as sports fans. Only months ago, we could watch one of hundreds of sports channels that broadcast nearly 24/7, all year long. We could debate with our friends, over bottles of beer, whether Michael Jordan is the greatest of all time. Most of all, we could go to arenas and stadiums without worrying about catching a life-threatening disease. Williams envisions a utopian life where "we would be playing games . . . focusing on the simple pleasures of athleticism and fandom." A self-proclaimed sports fanatic, she asserts, "Sports is both an escape from reality and an attempt to create a new reality, a reality of pure joy" (2020).

Will we experience that pure joy again? Must we find eustress in other ways, or might we have to settle for less intense stimulations? During the summer of 2020, no one could say for certain, but we can hope.

References

3_Octave_Fart. 2020. "Comment on Will COVID-19 be the Needle That Finally Bursts the sports Bubble." April 14.

Alma. 2020. "Comment on Will COVID-19 be the Needle That Finally Bursts the Sports Bubble." April 4.

Azrael. 2020. "Comment on Will COVID-19 Be the Needle That Finally Bursts the Sports Bubble." April 4.

Associated Press. 2019. "Sports Betting Market Expected to Reach $8 Billion by 2025." *MarketWatch*, November 4. Accessed June 27, 2020. www.marketwatch.com/story/firms-say-sports-betting-market-to-reach-8-billion-by-2025-2019-11-04.

———. 2020. "Kevin Harvick Wins NASCAR Return with No Fans, Lots of Masks, Other Precautions." *Tampa Bay Times*, May 17. Accessed June 1, 2020. www.tampabay.com/sports/auto-racing/2020/05/17/nascar-returns-with-no-fans-lots-of-masks-other-precautions/.

Bitteryoungmatador2. 2020. "Comments on Will COVID-19 be the Needle That Finally Bursts the Sports Bubble." April 4 and 14.

Bigpern 23. 2020. "Comment on Will COVID-19 be the Needle That Finally Bursts the Sports Bubble." April 4.

Boswell, Thomas. 2020. "Living without Sports Will Teach Us Something About How Much We Really Need Them." *The Washington Post,* March 30. Accessed Month day, 2020. www.washingtonpost.com/sports/2020/03/30/living-without-sports-will-teach-us-something-about-how-much-we-really-need-them/.

Brokamp, Robert, Matthew Frankel, and Alison Southwick. 2020. "The Rise of the Robinhood Trader." Produced by The Motley Fool Podcasts. *Motley Fool Answers,* June 23. Podcast, 36:14. www.fool.com/podcasts/answers/2020-06-23-the-rise-of-the-robinhood-trader.

Caillois, Roger. 1961. *Man, Play and Games*. Translated by Meyer Barash. Urbana: University of Illinois Press.

Chris. Conversations with author. March 28, April 8, June 27.

"Covid and Sports Discussion." *Canvas* Course Discussion Board, COM 268: Sports Communication. https://erau.instructure.com/courses/107760/discussion_topics/1797818.

The Daily James. "Fake Crowd Noise at Sports Events Divides Fans." *The Daily James Online*, June 16. Accessed June 28, 2020. https://thedailyjamesonline.com/fake-crowd-noise-at-sports-events-divides-fans/.

Flanagan, Graham. 2020. "Barstool Sports Founder Switches from Gambling to Day Trading During Coronavirus – And He Says He's Down $647,000." *Business Insider,* April 20. Accessed June 27, 2020. www.businessinsider.com/barstool-sports-founder-dave-portnoy-tries-day-trading-and-loses-2020–4.

Forsyth, Randall W. 2020. "Day Trading has Replaced Sports Betting as America's Pastime. It Can't Support the Stock Market Forever." *Barron's,* May 22. Accessed June 25, 2020. www.barrons.com/articles/day-trading-has-replaced-sports-betting-as-americas-pastime-it-cant-support-the-stock-market-forever-51590174899.

Franco. Email to author. May 27, 2020.

Garger, Kenneth. "South Korean Soccer Team Gests Record Fine for Filling Stadium with Sex Dolls." *New York Post*, May 21. Accessed May 22, 2020. https://nypost.com/2020/05/21/south-korean-soccer-team-fined-for-filling-stadium-with-sex-dolls/.

Gisondi, Joe. Conversation with author. May 14, 2020.

Good, Owen S. "With Sports Shut Down by Coronavirus, ESPN Turns to Tetris and Golden Eye." *Polygon*, March 21. Accessed July 1, 2020. www.polygon.com/tv/2020/3/21/21189256/sports-coronavirus-espn-8-the-ocho.

Greever, Tyler. "Feeling Lost without March Madness? Here's How the Absence of Sports Affects Fans' Psychology." *WHAS11.com.* March 26. Accessed June 28, 2020. www.whas11.com/article/sports/how-the-absence-of-sports-affects-fans-psychology/417-342b663d-0faf-4cdb-8f95–7980216b65b4.

Gregory. Email to author. May 17, 2020.

Hudson, Molly. 2020. "Fake Crowd Noise That Has Divided Fans." *The Times*, June 19. Accessed June 24, 2020. www.thetimes.co.uk/article/fake-crowd-noise-that-has-divided-fans-bh0jfgjbl.

Huizinga, Johan. 1955. *Homo Ludens: A Study of the Play-Element in Culture*. Boston, MA: Beacon Press.

Katy. 2020. "Comment on Covid and Sports Discussion." April 13.

Kerr, Jeff. "John Madden against Networks Adding Artificial Crowd Noise at Games if There Are No Fans." *CBS Sports*, June 1. Accessed July 1, 2020. www.cbssports.com/nfl/news/john-madden-against-networks-adding-artificial-crowd-noise-at-games-if-there-are-no-fans/.

Langlois, Shawn. 2020. "Barstool Sports Founder Believes He's A Better Investor Than Warren Buffett and Has Determined Day Trading Is 'the Easiest Game' There Is." *MarketWatch,* June 13. Accessed June 29, 2020. www.marketwatch.com/story/warren-buffett-is-an-idiot-says-investor-who-claims-daytrading-is-the-easiest-game-ive-ever-played-2020–06–09.

Lee, Alex. "The Premier League's Return Will Be Met with a New Era of Crowd Noise." *Wired*. June 14. Accessed June 16, 2020. www.wired.co.uk/article/football-crowd-noise.

Marian. Conversation with author. March 30, 2020.

Phillips, Matt. 2020. "Trading Sportsbooks for Brokerages, Bored Bettors Wager on Stocks." *The New York Times,* June 14. Accessed June 26, 2020. www.nytimes.com/2020/06/14/business/sports-gamblers-stocks-virus.html.

Portnoy, David (@stoolpresidente). 2020. "Say it with Me . . . Stocks Only Go Up. Only Losers Take Profits." *Twitter*, June 4. https://twitter.com/stoolpresidente/status/126854 2454086750208?lang=en.

Reilly, Rick. 2020. "I Miss Sports So, So, So Much." *The Atlantic,* March 20. Accessed April 27, 2020. www.theatlantic.com/ideas/archive/2020/03/what-are-we-going-do-without-all-sports/608416/.

Roberta. 2020. "Comment on COVID and Sports Discussion." April 14.

Schaerlaeckens, Leander. 2020. "When Sports Return After Coronavirus Pandemic, Fans Will Have Changed – If They Even Come Back at All." *Yahoo Sports,* May 6. Accessed June 15, 2020. https://sports.yahoo.com/when-sports-return-after-coronavirus-pan demic-fans-will-have-changed-if-they-even-come-back-at-all-145618338.html.

Scott, Nate. 2020. "Opinion: German Bundesliga Broadcast Uses Fake Crowd Noise, and It's Actually Great." *USA Today*, May 24. Accessed June 28, 2020. www.usato day.com/story/sports/ftw/2020/05/24/bundesliga-broadcast-uses-fake-crowd-noise-and-its-actually-great/111859288/.

Spence, Tyler. 2010. "Sports Are the Sweet Escape of Life." *Bleacher Report*, February 27, 2010. Accessed April 18, 2020. www.bleacherreport.com/articles/353707-sports-are-the-sweet-escape-of-life.

ttu_comc (Texas Technology University, College of Media Communication). 2020. "Does Fake Crowd Noise Work?" *YouTube Video*, 7:36, June 3. www.youtube.com/watch?v=qNbgFbNFT5E.

Van Leeuwen, Linda, Shayne Quick, and Kerry Daniel. 2002. "The Sport Spectator Satisfaction Model: A Conceptual Framework for Understanding the Satisfaction of Spectators." *Sports Management Review* 5: 99–128.

Wann, Daniel, Merrill Melnick, Gordon Russell, and Dale Pease. 2001. *Sports Fans: The Psychology and Social Impact of Spectators*. New York: Routledge.

"Will COVID-19 be the Needle That Finally Bursts the Sports Bubble." *SportsJournalists.com*. "Sports and News." www.sportsjournalists.com/forum/threads/will-covid-19-be-the-needle-that-finally-bursts-the-sports-bubble.134462/.

Williams, Rachel Anne. 2019. "Sports as an Escape from Reality." *Medium*, July 17. Accessed May 15, 2020. https://medium.com/@transphilosophr/sports-as-an-escape-from-reality-ad21461bfdd.

PART II

Communal consequences and cultural adaptations

10

THE POLITICAL NIGHTMARE OF THE PLAGUE

The ironic resistance of anti-quarantine protesters

James K. Meeker

On January 5, 2020, the World Health Organization (2020a) published a report outlining an outbreak of pneumonia of unknown origin occurring in Wuhan City, China. Within three weeks, cases of this new disease were being reported in Japan, Thailand, the Republic of Korea, and the United States (Wallach and Myers 2020). This new pathogen, genetically related to the 2003 SARS virus, was designated as coronavirus disease, COVID-19 (World Health Organization 2020b). Despite early identification of the pandemic, COVID-19 spread globally due to its high rates of transmission between persons, reaching 90% of all countries within four months of the initial outbreak (Badr et al. 2020).

Due to the imminent threat of COVID-19, the United States launched a Coronavirus Task Force in late January of 2020 (Wallach and Myers 2020). In spite of its urgency, the development of testing kits and other preparations for combatting COVID-19 in the United States was delayed by more than a month due to disorganization and lack of political priority, preventing health officials from containing and localizing outbreaks (Shear et al. 2020). On March 9, 2020, President Trump downplayed the dangers presented by COVID-19, tweeting

> last year 37,000 Americans died from the common Flu. It averages between 27,000 and 70,000 per year. Nothing is shut down, life & the economy go on. At this moment there are 546 confirmed cases of CoronaVirus [sic], with 22 deaths. Think about that![1]

Just four days later, however, the White House (2020) issued a proclamation declaring COVID-19 a national emergency, authorizing state and local governments to take preventive quarantine measures to address the pandemic.

Initially, nine states issued quarantine and shelter-in-place orders to slow the spread of COVID-19: Ohio, Illinois, Washington, Oregon, California, Louisiana,

New York, Connecticut, and New Jersey. By the end of March a total of 30 states were under stay-at-home orders (Mervosh, Lu, and Swales 2020). While the specific orders varied state by state, social distancing guidelines advised persons to avoid congregations of people, to wear protective masks while in public, to remain at home except for essential tasks such as grocery shopping, the closure of public facilities such as restaurants and bars, and the temporary closure of all nonessential businesses. The anticipated shock to the United States economy due to quarantine measures was predicted to have catastrophic short- and long-term impact, so much so that Trump stated that he would "love" to have the economy restarted within a month, "by Easter" (Forgey et al. 2020).

In order to address the economic impact of quarantine orders, on March 27, 2020, the CARES Act (Senate Bill 3548) was signed into law providing immediate and short-term economic relief, expanded unemployment benefits, and relief for businesses and corporations, as well as appropriating funding to hospitals and healthcare facilities. Although criticized for its focus on protecting shareholder wealth rather than preserving jobs, the expanded unemployment provisions within the CARES Act has prevented nearly 12 million families from sinking into poverty due to job loss or underemployment (Parolin, Curran, and Wimer 2020). Relief provided by the CARES Act has been more problematic, however, for small businesses required to close due to quarantine orders, as many owners are without a source of income until their federal assistance is disbursed, a process that has been, unfortunately, delayed by several months (Pofeldt 2020).

The anti-quarantine protest begins

While measures had been taken under the CARES Act to address the economic uncertainty and hardship faced by the public due to COVID-19, national protests against quarantine orders began almost immediately for the purpose of "liberating" their states (Burnett and Slodysko 2020). In contrast to the earlier declaration of national emergency authorizing quarantine provisions, President Trump agreed with the protesters, tweeting on April 17 that his supporters must "LIBERATE MICHIGAN!2" and "LIBERATE VIRGINIA!3" In Texas, the *You Can't Close America* rally was held to "protest the authoritarian lockdown orders being imposed by petty tyrants at the local level" (Jenney 2020). The Michigan state capitol was surrounded by hundreds of anti-quarantine protesters, as were the capitols of North Carolina, Kentucky, Ohio, Oregon, New York, and California (Bogel-Burroughs and Peters 2020). In Washington, an early epicenter of COVID-19, more than 2,500 protesters rallied at the capitol in Olympia decrying the restrictions; in Arizona and Colorado protesters created traffic gridlocks surrounding government buildings; and in Illinois one protester, armed with a semi-automatic rifle, ominously stated that Governor Pritzker must "Re-open the state or we will re-open it ourselves" (BBC News 2020).

Groups protesting the quarantine are varied but tend to be aligned with political conservatism or anti-science movements. Based on attendance, individuals joining the protests are an eclectic mix of anti-government extremists, White supremacists, guns rights advocates, New World Order conspiracy theorists, QAnon followers, Trump supporters, evangelical Christians, alternative medicine gurus and anti-vaccination advocacy groups, anti-globalists, and anti-government militias (BBC News 2020; Bogel-Burroughs and Peters 2020; Burnett and Slodysko 2020; Jenney 2020). A number of anti-science groups, ranging from climate shift denial to anti-vaccination, have also joined the protests (Conrow 2020). Much of the organization and funding for these groups has originated from a network of conservative political action groups such as FreedomWorks, the Tea Party Patriots, the right-wing Save Our Country coalition, and the newly formed, Trump-aligned Reopen America Political Action Committee (Vogel, Rutenberg, and Lerer 2020). Online organization for these protests were largely arranged by far-right extremists who set up Facebook pages for dozens of individual states and amassed more than 200,000 followers within a few weeks (Zadrozny and Collins 2020).

Rationales provided by the anti-quarantine protesters range from denying the existence of the disease – that COVID-19 is actually the more common strain of influenza, minimizing the danger of the virus, to resisting governmental authority to issue quarantine orders, to saying that social distancing guidelines and mask requirements infringe upon their individual choice and civil liberties (BBC News 2020; Jenney 2020). A majority of protesters espoused conspiratorial beliefs about COVID-19 such as that the disease was caused, or amplified, by 5G wireless networks (Duffy 2020), the virus was a human-made biological weapon (Brewster 2020), the disease is a result of consuming genetically modified crops (GMOs), the virus is a hoax perpetuated by pharmaceutical companies, or the pandemic was created by the so-called deep state to undermine President Trump's administration (Lynas 2020). Despite differences in the degree of their beliefs, there is a general agreement among protesters defining quarantine measures as a new, coercive abuse of government power that infringes civil liberties, lacks scientific basis, needlessly damages the economy, and, worrisomely, may be connected to a larger, conspiratorial plot.

Quarantine, governmentality, and the formation of the modern state

Despite protesters' claims, the use of quarantine to contain disease is not an unprecedented or new development. In the United States, quarantine measures were employed in response to the 1918 Spanish influenza outbreak with varying degrees of success. Based on examination of that pandemic, researchers at the National Institutes of Health (2007) concluded that rapid, early quarantine restrictions were vital for containing the disease. Quantitative analysis of mortality rates during the Spanish influenza pandemic indicated that quarantine measures, such as closing nonessential businesses, limiting public gatherings, restricting travel, and mandating mask wearing was linked to a 50% decrease in mortality (Hatchett, Mecher, and Lipsitch 2007). Quarantines have been the standard state response to disease throughout the history of the United States, from 17th-century enforcements of bills of health to prevent diseases coming from overseas, the forced isolation of tuberculosis patients to combat the "Great White Plague" of the 18th century, to containment measures employed to limit the spread of the 2003 SARS outbreak (Gensini, Yacoub, and Conti 2004).

Historically, given the degree of social complexity and adaption required to implement and manage quarantines, authorities' responses to plagues may have assisted in creating the modern state. To illustrate this point, Foucault (1975) observes that quarantine measures were employed to contain the plagues in the 14th through 18th centuries, creating intricate networks of social controls and observations to manage the population. Travel was restricted during the plague years and persons were confined to their residences, only being allowed to move individually under the direction of specially appointed guards known as syndics (Foucault 1975). Inspection of persons, looking for signs of the plague, became commonplace. Individuals exhibiting symptoms of the plague were socially isolated, restricted to remain in their residence and not to come into contact with others. Complex systems to safely allocate food and water, provide medical care, dispose of infected bodies, and maintain commerce were developed. These quarantine methods, directed by the state and sovereign, were successful at slowing, containing, and stopping the plague.

While quarantine methods ultimately proved successful for ending the plague, the new techniques of population management and control innovated during this time period forever altered the relationship between social organization and power in European governance. Foucault (1975, 198) argues the development of quarantine measures gave birth to the "political dream" of the plague, consisting of state-administered populations that are "traversed throughout with hierarchy, surveillance, observation, writing" resulting in the "utopia of the perfectly governed city." In other words, the methods used to combat the plague revealed a previously unimagined way to administer society based on judicious use of state agents, efficient rationality, precise calculability, and constant surveillance and measurement of its population. Foucault (1975, 1978) observes this new *governmentality* (literally a portmanteau of *government* and *rationality*), based on efficiency, calculability, predictability, and surveillance, emerged as the preeminent practice and end-in-itself of modern statecraft for managing its population. In other words, Foucault (1975) argues, plagues represented a challenge that had to be overcome by government-directed measures, fostering the development of the rational techniques ultimately leading to the creation of the modern democratic state.

Complementing its rational foundations, governmentality requires public recognition of state authority to manage the population. Individuals are responsible for regulating their own behavior in compliance with the rational policies of the state (Foucault 1978). In simple terms, governmentality is a social contract between the state and citizens to participate in the management of society for the mutual benefit of both parties. As a rational process, governmentality utilizes clearly defined rules and systematic procedures and employs qualified experts in order to identify, classify, order, and control aspects of the population to maximize the prosperity, health, and happiness of the citizenry. As rational actors, the population is expected to exercise self-discipline by adhering to state policies, as those decrees are ideally designed to increase their prosperity and well-being. In keeping with the principles of governmentality, in instances where there is disagreement between segments of the population and the state, there are prescribed procedures for challenging, altering, or changing the rules such as the right to protest, town hall meetings, lobbying, and other democratic processes.

Since the Industrial Revolution and the emergence of democracy, the principles of governmentality became normal practices for population management, edging out all other types of governance. It makes sense that governmentality would become the dominant form of state management in the modern age. First, governmentality, with its focus on using rational means to maximize gains and minimize losses, is efficacious in achieving societal goals. Second, the participatory nature of governmentality reflects the rights-based values that have spread globally during the modern age. Due to its rational foundation, governmentality has been critiqued for its hyper-focus on efficiency, placing means and ends above persons (Foucault 1978), its tendency towards obsessive bureaucratization (Weber 1922), its potentially depersonalizing and dehumanizing features (Fromm 1973), and the creation of an environment of risk aversion and anxiety (Beck 1992). Despite these critiques, governmentality and its rational, empirical, and scientific underpinnings remain the dominant form of state management, particularly among Western democracies such as the United States.

The motivation of quarantine protesters: anti-governance and anti-rationality

Given the rational basis of governmentality, it is unsurprising that the response to the initial outbreaks of COVID-19 in the United States was to implement quarantine measures to reduce the impact of the disease. In spite of the overwhelming scientific evidence supporting quarantine to combat the spread of COVID-19, quarantine protesters resist any effort to maintain social distance, reduce public contact, restrict nonessential travel, temporarily close nonessential businesses, and require the wearing of protective masks. Although quarantine orders have always been resisted or defied by a small minority of the population due to their inconvenience (National Institutes of Health 2007), contemporary resistance to COVID-19 quarantine measures is unique in the annals of modern public health.

The current protests are unique because, unlike past resistance to quarantine efforts, they are driven by a mass rejection of the principles of modern, democratic governance. When examined thematically, the reasons provided by anti-quarantine protesters represent a total rebuke of the two core tenets of governmentality: (a) recognition of the authority of the state to govern and (b) the use of rational processes to manage populations. First, protesters resist the authority of the state to govern as well as refuse their responsibility to self-discipline their behavior according to quarantine mandates. Second, the protesters refute the medical and scientific rationality underlying the mandate to quarantine to halt the spread of disease. Ultimately, anti-quarantine protesters issue a challenge to the authority of the state, whose role of managing populations includes public health crises such as COVID-19. These protests additionally discount the legitimacy of scientific rationality, whose role is to guide the state in implementing healthcare policy and responses that are empirical, logical, and efficient.

There is ample evidence of anti-governance themes present among these protesters. An anti-quarantine organization, Operation Gridlock Tennessee, issued the following statement: "the pandemic should not give any government body the right to mandate that we close our businesses and order us to 'shelter in place'" (Hernandez 2020). A spokesperson for Reopen Maryland stated, "the government mandating healthy citizens to stay home, forcing businesses and churches to close, is called tyranny!" (Gabbatt 2020). Representatives of Pennsylvanians Against Excessive Quarantine claim, "Politicians are on a power trip, controlling our lives, destroying our businesses, passing laws behind the cover of darkness and forcing us to hand over our freedoms" (Hernandez 2020). When asked about the stay-at-home orders issued by Ohio's Governor Mike DeWine, Melissa Ackison complains that quarantine measures are a government overreach that "enrages something inside of you" (Burnett and Slodysko 2020). At the You Can't Close America Rally in Texas, one protester stated, "By the blood of Jesus may we break every deception of the government that is trying to stop us from our freedom" (Tilove 2020). Protests at the Michigan capitol in Lansing included cries of "lock her [Governor Whitmer] up!" and "Heil Witmer [sic]," referring to the governor's decision to enact stay-at-home orders (Allsop 2020). One Florida protester, screaming at a public health board of physicians for requiring masks to be worn in public, openly stated that the doctors would be "arrested and tried for crimes against humanity" (CNN 2020).

Anti-scientific themes are as common as anti-government messages among protesters, prompting Dr. Anthony Fauci, director of the National Institute of Allergy and Infectious Diseases, to declare that there is "a general anti-science, anti-authority, anti-vaccine" attitude among "an alarming percentage" of Americans (Cohen 2020). Anti-vaccine groups, displaying signs stating: "I do not consent [to being vaccinated]" are commonplace at anti-quarantine protests nationwide (Conrow 2020). At the You Can't Close America protest, crowds of supporters chanted "Fire Fauci," referring to the United States' most visible public health official (Relman 2020). Protest signs, promoting a new conspiracy theory claiming COVID-19 vaccines are being developed to introduce biological surveillance technologies secretly among the public, read, "Bill Gates can keep his poison – I'm homeschooled! No mandatory vaccines!" (Relman 2020). In a Florida town hall meeting discussing quarantine measures, protesters read prepared statements with comments that included claims that wearing masks is "literally killing people" (CNN 2020). Another protester questioned the expertise of the physicians and public health officials, saying that she has: "many question marks about your degrees and what you really know. I'm sorry, but I don't think you are worthy of your credentials and I would ask suggestively that you go back to school and get educated" (CNN 2020).

The rise of postmodernism and anti-rationality

While it is relatively easy to locate examples of anti-rationality and anti-governance among quarantine protesters, explaining *how* these beliefs emerged within modern society presents more of a challenge. Compared to a modernist epistemology, anti-quarantine protesters inhabit a different intellectual culture with their own brand of facts and logic *not* based on empiricism, rationalism, or evidence, instead investing in a type of "post-truth" reality. Clearly, given the recent attention to the problems of the so-called post-truth era, *something* in society has changed regarding the manner in which truth or falsehood, fact or fiction, and real or unreal are established. These new epistemological processes are markedly different from the rational processes underlying governmentality that previously monopolized social discourse as recently as a decade ago.

Although the ramifications of the post-truth age are currently being identified, scholars studying culture and society had anticipated that establishing meaning, and therefore truth, would become increasingly fractured due to technological progress. Jean-François Lyotard, in his influential work *The Postmodern Condition* (1979), argued the increase in communications and information technology posed a threat to the epistemological process modern society used to construct meaning, knowledge, and understanding. This meta-narrative, Lyotard (1979) explained, was built on an epistemological basis of rationality and science, forming the basis of modern society and underlying its increasingly sophisticated technological growth. Once these technologies, particularly in media creation and distribution, became sufficiently widespread, it would prove difficult to maintain a consensual societal narrative.

Lyotard predicted these new, postmodern societies would be fundamentally dissimilar to modernism. Unlike modern societies with its singular meta-narrative of scientific rationalism, future societies would be atomized into *many* smaller, competing narratives, each with its own standards and practices for constructing meaning and truth. These emerging *postmodern* societies would, as a matter of practice, dispense with rationality in varying degrees. Although Lyotard (1979) critiqued scientific rationality for overstating its own objectivity, it still served as a central organizing principle, enabling actors within the modern age to reach consensus, or to at least agree upon a reasonable process in which discussion could be established. In contrast, the postmodern era will lack any epistemological center owing to the constellation of competing worldviews, meanings, histories, and discourse. Consequently, in the postmodern world there is disagreement about facts and meaning, but also entirely contradictory ways to establish what is factual as well as what those facts mean.

These epistemological divisions are a source of concern, but perhaps more worrisome is the rejection of the previously established meta-narrative that defined modernism. Lyotard (1979) warned the postmodern age would be characterized by an innate distrust of meta-narratives. Prior meta-narratives governing the modern world, such as the ideals of capitalism, socialism, science, and reason, are now viewed with doubt and disbelief. On one hand, the rejection of meta-narratives is understandable: Neither capitalism nor socialism has fulfilled their utopian promises of material security; rationality, when pushed to its extremes, becomes dehumanizing; and the technological progress of science has resulted in devastating environmental and social consequences (Best 1994; Jameson 1991). On the other hand, the loss of an agreed upon way to construct meaning and engage in discourse suggests a permanent loss of social consensus, and therefore solidarity, in the coming postmodern world (Giddens 1991; Harvey 1990).

Today, the wholesale repudiation of meta-narratives is evident. Generally, attempts to refer to meta-narratives, particularly ones grounded in rationality, are being met with increasing resistance. This phenomenon is unmistakable when interacting with groups who have abandoned modernist meta-narratives in lieu of a postmodern narrative of their own construction. It is through this process that media becomes "fake news" as it presents a mainstream presentation of events, expertise is viewed with skepticism as it represents the consensus of the scientific community, and government officials are treated with mistrust if they are understood as an "establishment" candidate because they use rational policies (Best 1994; Keen 2007). Outside of the institutions founded on rationality, such as the university, medical, and scientific community, reference to the rational scientific meta-narrative are met with incredulity, animus, and suspicion. Overwhelmingly, the meta-narrative of scientific rationality has been abandoned, forming an essential foundation for the spread of anti-rationality among the general public.

Opposing rationality: plague and the rise of postmodern politics

While postmodern epistemologies have increased overall, it is perhaps most apparent in the differing societal and ideological reactions to COVID-19, of which quarantine protests are merely the most visible. A recent Pew Research poll suggests that 30% of Americans believe that COVID-19 was created in a laboratory, despite scientific experts at the Centers for Disease Control and World Health Organization indicating otherwise (Schaeffer 2020). On social media, new conspiracy theories are developing at such an alarming rate that both Facebook and Twitter have developed new policies to label or remove false and misleading user posts (Wong 2020). Perhaps most worrisome is a report suggesting that fewer than half of Americans intend to become vaccinated against COVID-19 when treatments become available (Cornwall 2020).

While postmodern frames have become prevalent in the general population, political ideology is suggested to be a salient factor for their increase. A recent Quinnipiac (2020) poll indicated that nearly 60% of Republican voters were not concerned about personally contracting COVID-19 versus two-thirds of Democratic voters who worried that they or someone they knew would be infected. Only 55% of Republicans agreed that people should shelter in place until doctors and health officials declared it safe, versus 88% of Democrats (Smith and Kahn 2020). Concerning wearing personal protective equipment such as masks, only 52% of Republicans support wearing masks in public versus 86% of Democrats (Pew Research Center 2020). On June 25, 2020, while COVID-19 cases were increasing nationally, 61% of Republicans believed that the worst of the pandemic was over, whereas only 23% of Democrats agreed (Pew Research Center 2020). Clearly, given the content and themes of anti-quarantine protesters, there is an association between postmodern rejections of governance and rationality and conservative politics. This makes sense given the importance of climate denial movements, anti-vaccination activism, and anti-government organizations to contemporary conservative politics.

While there is a partisan lean towards believing in COVID-19 conspiracy theories, specifically that political conservatism is associated with increased skepticism towards scientific consensus on the disease, perhaps more troubling is that anti-science attitudes were more prevalent among young persons than older (Schaeffer 2020). This makes sense if there is any truth to the Lyotard's critique of technology, as younger persons are more likely to use social media and technology in general. Preliminary investigations suggest there is a link between levels of social media usage and belief in conspiracy theories, providing evidence that the growth of communications and media technologies contributes to the post-truth, postmodern fracturing of social reality, particularly among conservatives (Easton 2020). These findings are consistent with studies linking consumption of new media with irrational, postmodern perspectives (Rotaru, Nitulescu, and Cristian 2020). This trend suggests, regardless of ideology, that postmodern and anti-rational beliefs will continue to rise, forming the epistemological basis of a new type of society hitherto unrealized. These developments imply the formation of a new model of governance, an epistemological anti-rationality, built upon ideology and authoritarian will, as a potential rival against modern rationalized systems of governance.

The political nightmare of the plague

The postmodern framework undergirding quarantine protests implies increasing challenges for managing public healthcare systems. Given the growth of anti-rational and anti-governmental frameworks in recent decades, these difficulties are likely to increase in frequency and strength of resistance. As a consequence of these developments, a disturbing series of questions emerge: *How do officials efficiently and effectively manage public health care in a climate of increasing anti-rationality and political resistance to governmentality?* What would a postmodern healthcare system look like? How does a healthcare system built on whatever narrative happens to be in power, rather than empirical, scientific, and medical rationality, work? What will be the effect on the health and welfare of the population under regimes that are hostile to rationality, knowledge, and expertise? Can rationality and anti-rationality be balanced within a single system, or will public health care simply vanish along with other social programs like entitlements that once defined the modern state? Sadly, there are no immediate answers to these questions.

Based on the nature of disease, however, some possible answers can be surmised. Disease, as a natural process, is unconcerned with the beliefs or politics of its hosts. Pathogens require neither acknowledgement nor consent from their hosts in order to do their damage. Its only motivation is to infect, to debilitate, and, in the case of COVID-19, to kill. The pitiless reality of disease is, oddly, the greatest admonition to the anti-rationality of quarantine protesters.

This is further compounded by the recognition that the purpose of the state is to manage a population, regardless of its fundamental epistemological beliefs. A state that ignores the ravages of a pandemic is, in time, doomed to failure. Accordingly, it seems fair to assume that, at some point, even the most anti-rational state actors will have to implement quarantine measures in order to preserve their own power. In this fashion, quarantine protesters motivated by anti-governance beliefs, by ignoring social distancing recommendations and gathering en masse in protest, risk being *ironically* undermined by their own practices that are assured to increase the spread of COVID-19 and, eventually, require stricter government-mandated quarantine measures. Considering the reversal Vice President Pence and leading members of the Republican Party have undergone regarding mask usage, now advising the public to take precautionary measures against COVID-19, it seems there are limits to the extent reality can be ignored by those entrusted with managing the population of the United States (Bosman 2020). The current administration, however, will certainly face difficulty if they choose to enforce new quarantine measures, as those restrictions will contradict the informal, yet significant, support from Trump for protesters to violate stay-at-home and social distancing orders.

Whether protesters will accept quarantine measures or not, even by a conservative administration with their support, is unknown. Given the anti-rational and anti-governance motivations of the protesters, it is unlikely they will comply with quarantine orders, even if endorsed by President Trump. The most likely outcome is that quarantine protesters would look for more extreme political candidates or movements that share their postmodern beliefs. Given the reluctance of political regimes to simply surrender their supporters, and thus power, it is uncertain how the Trump administration would simultaneously implement quarantine measures *and* retain their following.

While it is evident that society is inexorably moving towards postmodern frames of reference, the transition from modernism is incomplete. A majority of Americans support quarantine measures and the scientific consensus concerning COVID-19 (Pew Research Center 2020; Quinnipiac 2020). With that being said, the quarantine protests are still indicative of a worrisome political development. It is tempting to consider the rejection of modernity to be a product of American conservatism that began with the election of Donald Trump. It is also easy to attribute the rejection of science and quarantine among protesters as being a result of President Trump's dismissive attitude towards COVID-19. These thoughts, while comforting, fail to acknowledge the decades-long trends in global society towards anti-governmentality in general. Furthermore, these observations ignore the COVID-19 quarantine protest movements in the United Kingdom, Canada, France, Germany, Italy, Poland, Russia, and China. In short, postmodernity has truly become international.

Ultimately, the true political nightmare of the plague is the likelihood that modernism will fall victim to COVID-19. Nearly half a century ago, Foucault theorized that the modern state was born from the need to control disease through rational means, using a combination of science, participatory governance, and self-regulation of behavior to serve the common good. That system, even with its contradictions, faults, and omissions, built the modern world. Science, medicine, public health, and the democratic secular state are all products of modernism. It seems sadly poetic that modernism, built from the need to contain disease, is in danger of being eclipsed by a postmodernist system incapable and unwilling to do the same. Clearly, if there is anything to be learned from this pandemic, it is that rational civil society must be defended against the coming storm of anti-governmentality.

Notes

1 Donald Trump, Twitter post, March 9, 2020, 10:47 a.m.
2 Donald Trump, Twitter post, April 17, 2020, 11:22 a.m.
3 Donald Trump, Twitter post, April 17, 2020, 11:25 a.m.

References

Allsop, Jon. 2020. "The Right-Wing Media's Rallying Cry: Anti-Lockdown Edition." *Columbia Journalism Review*, April 17.
Badr, Hamada, Hongru Du, Maximillian Marshall, Ensheng Dong, Marietta Squire, and Lauren Gardner. 2020. "Association Between Mobility Patterns and COVID-19 Transmission in the USA: A Mathematical Modeling Study." *The Lancet: Infectious Diseases*. https://doi.org/10.1016/S1473-3099(20)30553-3.
BBC News. 2020. "Coronavirus Lockdown Protest: What's Behind the US Demonstrations?" *BBC News: US & Canada*, April 21.
Beck, Ulrich. 1992. *Risk Society: Towards a New Modernity*. London, Thousand Oaks, CA and New Delhi: Sage.
Best, Steven. 1994. "The Commodification of Reality and the Reality of Commodification: Baudrillard, Debord, and Postmodern Theory." In *Baudrillard: A Critical Reader*, edited by David Kellner, 41–67. Cambridge, MA: Blackwell Publishers.
Bogel-Burroughs, Nicholas, and Jeremy Peters. 2020. "'You Have to Disobey': Protesters Gather to Defy Stay-At-Home Orders." *The New York Times*, April 20.

Bosman, Julie. 2020. "Amid Virus Surge, Republicans Abruptly Urge Masks Despite Trump's Resistance." *The New York Times*, July 1.

Brewster, Jack. 2020. "A Timeline of the COVID-19 Wuhan Lab Origin Theory." *Forbes*, May 24.

Burnett, Sarah, and Brian Slodysko. 2020. "'Liberate Michigan!' Right-Wing Coalitions Rallying to End Lockdown Restrictions Amid Coronavirus Pandemic." *Chicago Tribune*, April 17.

CNN. 2020. "Angry Residents Erupt at Meeting Over new Mask Rule." *Cable News Network*, June 24.

Cohen, Elizabeth. 2020. "Fauci Says Covid-19 Vaccine May Not Get US to Herd Immunity of Too Many People Refuse to Get It." *CNN Health*, June 28.

Conrow, Joan. 2020. "Anti-Science Groups Drive US Protests Against Lockdowns." *Cornell Alliance for Science*, April 24.

Cornwall, Warren. 2020. "Just 50% of Americans Plan to Get a COVID-19 Vaccine. Here's How to Win Over the Rest." *Science*, June 30.

Duffy, Clare. 2020. "Why Conspiracy Theorists Think 5G is Bad for Your Health and Why Experts Say Not to Worry." *CNN Business*, June 14.

Easton, Mark. 2020. "Coronavirus: Social Media 'Spreading Virus Conspiracy Theories.'" *BBC*, June 18.

Forgey, Quint, Gabby Orr, Nancy Cook, and Caitlin Oprysko. 2020. "'I'd Love to Have it Open by Easter': Trump Says He Wants to Restart Economy by Mid-April." *Politico*, March 3.

Foucault, Michel. 1975. *Discipline and Punish: The Birth of the Prison*. New York and Canada: Random House Incorporated.

———.1978. *Security, Territory, Population*. New York: St. Martin's Press.

Fromm, Erich. 1973. *The Anatomy of Human Destructiveness*. New York: Holt, Rinehart and Winston.

Gabbatt, Adam. 2020. "Thousands of Americans Backed by Rightwing Donors Gear Up for Protests." *The Guardian*, April 18.

Gensini, Gian, Magdi Yacoub, and Andrea Conti. 2004. "The Concept of Quarantine in History: From Plague to SARS." *Journal of Infection* 49 (4): 257–61.

Giddens, Anthony. 1991. *The Consequences of Modernity*. Cambridge: Polity Press.

Harvey, David. 1990. *The Condition of Postmodernity. An Enquiry into the Origins of Cultural Change*. Oxford: Blackwell Publishers.

Hatchett, Richard, Carter Mecher, and Marc Lipsitch. 2007. "Public Health Interventions and Epidemic Intensity During the 1918 Influenza Pandemic." *PNAS* 104 (18): 7582–587.

Hernandez, Salvador. 2020. "This Is How a Group Linked to Betsy DeVos Is Organizing Protests to End Social Distancing, Now With Trump Support." *Buzzfeed*, April 17.

Jameson, Frederic. 1991. *Postmodernism: Or, the Cultural Logic of Late Capitalism*. Durham: Duke University Press.

Jenney, Elizabeth. 2020. "Austin Coronavirus: 'You Can't Close America Rally Draws Crowds." *Patch*, April 18.

Keen, Andrew. 2007. *The Cult of the Amateur: How Blogs, MySpace, YouTube, and the Rest of Today's User-Generated Media are Destroying Our Economy, Our Culture, and Our Values*. New York: Doubleday Press.

Lynas, Mark. 2020. "COVID: Top 10 Current Conspiracy Theories." *Cornell Alliance for Science*, April 20.

Lyotard, Jean-François. 1979. *The Postmodern Condition: A Report on Knowledge*. Minneapolis: University of Minnesota Press.

Mervosh, Sarah, Denise Lu, and Vanessa Swales. 2020. "See Which States and Cities Have Told Residents to Stay at Home." *The New York Times*, April 20. New York: The New York Times Company.

National Institutes of Health. 2007. "Rapid Response was Crucial to Containing the 1918 Flu Pandemic." *NIH*, April 2.

Parolin, Zachary, Megan Curran, and Christopher Wimer. 2020. "The CARES ACT and Poverty in the COVID-19 Crisis: Promises and Pitfalls of the Recovery Rebates and Expanded Unemployment Benefits." *Poverty & Social Policy Brief* 4 (8).

Pew Research Center. 2020. "Republicans, Democrats Move Even Further Apart in Coronavirus Concerns." *Pew Research Center*, June 25.

Pofeldt, Elaine. 2020. "COVID-19 Aid to Small Business Owners Trickles Out as SBA Clarifies CARES Act Rules for Sole Proprietors." *Forbes*, April 15.

Quinnipiac. 2020. "Biden Crushes Sanders in Democratic Race, Quinnipiac University National Poll Finds, More Disapprove of Trump's Response to Coronavirus." *Quinnipiac University*, March 9.

Relman, Eliza. 2020. "An Anti-Lockdown Protest in Austin, Texas, Drew Anti-Vaxxer and Trump Supporters Changing 'Fire Fauci.'" *Business Insider*, April 18.

Rotaru, Ileana, Lavinia Nitulescu, and Cristian Rudolf. 2020. "The Post-Modern Paradigm – A Framework of Today's Media Impact in Cultural Space." *Procedia-Social and Behavioral Sciences* 5 (2010).

Schaeffer, Katherine. 2020. "Nearly Three-In-Ten Americans Believe COVID-19 Was Made in a Lab." *Pew Research Center*, April 8.

Senate Bill 3548. *Coronavirus Aid, Relief, and Economic Security Act: CARES ACT.*

Shear, Michael, Abby Goodnough, Sheila Kaplan, Sheri Fink, Katie Thomas, and Noah Weiland. 2020. "The Lost Month: How a Failure to Test Blinded the U.S. to Covid-19." *The New York Times*, March 28.

Smith, Grant, and Chris Kahn. 2020. "Despite Scattered Protests, Most Americans Support Shelter-in-Place, Reuters/Ipsos Poll Shows." *Reuters*, April 21.

Tilove, Jonathan. 2020. "Chanting 'Let Us Work!', 'Fire Fauci!', Protesters at Capital Decry Virus Restrictions." *Statesman*, April 18.

Vogel, Kenneth, Jim Rutenberg, and Lisa Lerer. 2020. "The Quiet Hand of Conservative Groups in the Anti-Lockdown Protests." *The New York Times*, April 21.

Wallach, Phillip, and Justin Myers. 2020. "The Federal Government's Coronavirus Response – Public Health Timeline." *The Brookings Institute*, March 31.

Weber, Max. 1922. *Economy and Society*. Berkeley: University of California Press.

White House, The. 2020. *Proclamation on Declaring a National Emergency Concerning the Novel Coronavirus Disease (COVID-19) Outbreak*. Washington, DC: The White House.

Wong, Queenie. 2020. "Coronavirus, BLM Conspiracy Theories Collide on Facebook and Twitter." *CNET*, June 28.

World Health Organization. 2020a. "Pneumonia of Unknown Cause – China." *World Health Organization*, January 5.

———. 2020b. *Naming the Coronavirus Disease (COVID-19) and the Virus that Causes It*. Geneva, Switzerland: World Health Organization.

Zadrozny, Brandy, and Ben Collins. 2020. "Conservative Activist Family Behind 'Grassroots" Anti-Quarantine Facebook Events." *NBC News*, April 11.

11

TOXIC WILD WEST SYNDROME

Individual rights vs. community needs

Dinur Blum, Stacy L. Smith, and Adam G. Sanford

May 9, 2020. A tall, broad-shouldered White man with a military-style haircut under his ball cap pulls cash from his pocket to pay for his Subway sandwich during a protest in Raleigh, North Carolina. He wears dark colored cargo pants, a sleeveless red-and-white striped shirt with blue trim, and an AT4 rocket launcher slung across his back. At his sides: dual western-style leather shoulder holsters, one of which holds a revolver. A tattoo on the back of his arm reads "Eagle Scout Dad." Like any good Scout, he comes prepared – to shoot 'em up and blow 'em up.

On the sidewalk outside, a 60-something White man with a receding hairline and long, salt-and-pepper hair tied back in a bun, pauses, unsmiling, to take a selfie. He appears to be standing with an 84-lb M2 Browning .50 caliber machine gun slung casually over his right shoulder. An American flag waves colorfully from the barrel. The "gun," however, is fake, a poorly fashioned wooden replica. At his hip, he carries what one may assume are real weapons: a pistol, and across his back, an AR-15.

(Long 2020)

Across the United States in the spring of 2020, Americans watched in a mixture of horror and skepticism as the novel coronavirus traversed the ocean and landed on the east and west coasts. In the following weeks, skepticism slowly faded and states began implementing social controls: closing nonessential businesses and facilities and asking the population to self-isolate, wear masks when outside their homes, and observe social distancing. Unemployment rates skyrocketed to record levels and the economy slowed as businesses shuttered (Cohen and Hsu 2020). Stimulus checks and increased unemployment benefits from the federal government did little to calm the public's fears and inflamed others who prize free trade and small government as core American values. Public response to the health crisis, therefore, was mixed. For example, the Lake of the Ozarks area in Missouri achieved national notoriety as images of partiers flocking to a crowded swimming pool/bar went viral (Vera 2020). In just over three weeks, 37 partygoers tested positive for coronavirus, with one dead (Hiles 2020).

Public reactions to the public health restrictions imposed due to the COVID-19 pandemic have exposed issues related to social control and how it does, or does not, work in the United States. Social control – the society exerting control over the populace through a system of norms and values – is based on the effect of the community on individual behavior (Durkheim 1951). The community offers people both integration – a sense of belonging – and regulation – a sense of acceptable and unacceptable behavior. Each community has to find an appropriate balance in terms of integration and regulation of its members, or it runs the risk of suicide or other forms of deviant behavior.

Related to social control, Durkheim's (1951) concepts of anomie and egoism help explain the public response to COVID, from fear to recklessness. Anomie refers to a situation in which social regulation has broken down into normlessness, and old ways of acting fail. The unexpected situation means that people struggle to find rules that work in order to maintain some sense of order and control over their lives. The COVID pandemic has made certain prosocial behaviors dangerous, including large gatherings and baring one's face in public due to the way the virus spreads through droplets in the air. Everyday norms of behavior must be suspended and replaced in order to adapt to a rapidly shifting public health situation. Egoism can be an effect of anomie; it refers to a lack of belonging and a heightened sense of isolation. An anomic society lacks community regulation, whereas in an egoistic society, individuals seek independence instead of interdependence, valuing the self over society. If anomie is a lack of regulation by a community, egoism is a lack of integration into a community.

In response to the anomie created by the pandemic, a significant and highly visible and audible minority of American citizens chose the path of egoism, opting to jeopardize public health by gathering in large crowds to protest measures intended to slow the spread of the virus. Typically (though not exclusively) gathering at state capitol buildings in April and May, they loudly protested gubernatorial measures to protect the health of their citizenry, long before health officials recommended weakening those efforts. These protestors appear to demonstrate the rise in nationalism and resurgence of neoconservative ideologies as described by Ryan (2021). Protestors in Michigan and Wisconsin made national news for deliberate and aggressive displays of weaponized strength, verbal aggression, and signage. These protestors presented themselves as local members of a grassroots movement; individuals with a vested interest in their state and local economies, speaking to their elected officials. Significant evidence suggests, however, that these protests are *not* grassroots movements, but Astroturf movements. Astroturf movements are designed to appear organic but are in fact funded by various politically conservative sources (Derysh 2020).[1] Although many of the protestors likely were locals, some of them are not the concerned citizens they portray themselves to be; instead, they are essentially paid crisis actors.[2] A BBC article in April 2020 explains:

> The organizers behind these protests have largely been conservative, pro-Trump and pro-gun activists. Signs calling for freedom over tyranny have also been staples of these protests. Governors have been likened to kings or dictators. "Give me liberty or give me death," a quote harkening back to the American Revolution, has also been a popular mantra.
>
> *(BBC News 2020)*

As Emma Grey Ellis's (2020) *Wired* article notes, although the online support for these movements exceeded a million followers, "in real life, the protests were small, sparse, and few," as well as unpopular, even among conservatives. Ellis (2020) also provides context for how these movements were funded:

> Wealthy funders are absolutely guiding and stoking the frustrations of the people breaking quarantine and turning out in the streets, but those frustrations were pre-existing. . . . The Covid-19 pandemic is nothing if not peculiar, and that has made these demonstrations extra noisy. It is vitally important not to be falsely equivalent here: Most Americans will never shrug off social-distancing guidelines and take to the streets . . . [P]ublic opinion is not the goal, as protesters are laser-focused on moving legislators. [These] events are just a modern permutation of an identity crisis with roots very deep in America's individualist history.
>
> *(Ellis 2020)*

Although the movement appears to be organic, large, and spontaneous, it is a performance, designed to intimidate politicians into easing quarantine restrictions.

Goffman (1956) argues that every interaction between humans constitutes a performance, during which individuals carefully manage their behavior according to specific roles. These roles are governed by scripts that indicate how to speak, costumes or props for how a person presents themselves, and the need for an audience, whether that audience is passive or actively engaged and interactive. Actors manage their self-presentation and alter how they portray themselves, based on their audience and social setting. To ensure the seamless functioning of society, the audience expects, and assumes, that a person's portrayal honestly conveys who they are. The protestors are well aware that their protests grab headlines locally, nationally, and internationally. Those directly funding these protests therefore remain out of sight, and out-of-state protestors mingle, indistinguishable, with local actors. A protest organized by the wealthy elite and spiked with non-local actors does not convey the impression of grassroots outrage to frighten legislators into appeasing local voters.

These protests, which participants assembled during a public health crisis at the risk of their own lives and the lives of their loved ones, do seem to stem from – as Ellis wrote – "an identity crisis with roots very deep in America's individualist history" (Ellis 2020). We submit that these protests can be seen as an example of what we call *Toxic Wild West Syndrome* (TWWS): a combination of (1) a hyper-individualistic emphasis on personal rights and preferences, disguised as the public good, but without any real consideration for the broader community, and (2) toxic masculinity (the combination of aggrieved masculinity with a *conscious, intentional,* and *exaggerated* performance of masculine behaviors with the implied use of violence in order to achieve goals).

TWWS is performative; the empty but overt and aggressive expression of internalized ideals combined with a demand to be heard and deemed important while ignoring or flouting science, including medicine (Howard and Stracqualursi 2020; Meeker 2021). TWWS flourishes in the culture of the United States. Anti-quarantine protestors actively work to portray themselves as champions of freedom while threatening others and showing a wanton, reckless disregard for public health. This chapter combines Goffman's concepts of impression management and framing with Durkheim's anomie to show how Toxic Wild West Syndrome is revealed through the performance of these protestors.

Toxic Wild West Syndrome: origins

We derived the term "Toxic Wild West Syndrome" from the early portrayals of heroes in Classic Western and Spaghetti Western movies and television shows (Kokino 2009). In both genres, the hero is a stoic, unemotional White man, always in control of himself and especially of a chaotic or violent situation. In these movies, there is a clearly defined villain, and the hero of the movie is portrayed as strong when he successfully captures or kills the villain, drawing adulation. The hero does not rely on the help of others, preferring to work alone in his heroic endeavors. Strength is portrayed through violence, a lack of visible emotion, and extreme self-reliance. The main difference between these two types of Western movies lies in the hero's acceptable uses of violence.

The themes of gratuitous violence from Spaghetti Westerns, combined with the intended portrayal of stoic heroism from Classic Westerns, can help us understand the anti-quarantine protestors. However, their threats of violence make them appear more like the protagonists in Spaghetti Westerns, using violence arbitrarily, capriciously, and wantonly, regardless of how appropriate or inappropriate it is for the present situation.

Hyper-individualism

From the Westerns to daily life in the United States, individualism and self-reliance are core to achieving the "American Dream." Individualism is a set of beliefs that economic success comes from one's own hard work (Callero 2017). Individualism holds that private life is more important than public life, with the goal of self-determination; a person can freely choose what they want to do, unencumbered by other people's decisions.

These beliefs, however, are not sustained by reality. A person depends on social groups, such as one's family, friends, classmates, neighbors, and co-workers. Individuals belong to different groups throughout their lifetime, conforming to each group's standards and rules of behavior. Belonging requires at least minimal adherence to these rules, which limits an individual's independence, while enhancing interdependence between members.

Among the protestors, individualism and nationalism have become conflated: Many view public health measures as violations of constitutional rights to assembly and respond by loudly and openly asserting the right to freedom of speech and to bear arms. The quarantine protestors frame quarantine as an unjust power grab by a tyrannical government, rather than an attempt to halt an ongoing health crisis. This framing leads to protesters attempting to convey an image of individual personal strength, bravery, independence, and patriotism. Protestors show these qualities by waving American and other flags, putting these flags on signs and clothes, and brandishing visible weapons, up to and including rocket launchers (Long 2020).

Knowing these weapons attract media attention, protestors keep cameras rolling by answering reporters' questions angrily and carrying signs comparing mask wearing to the Holocaust, abortion, and transatlantic slavery, while simultaneously calling quarantine and mask wearing "governmental overreach" designed to stifle individual freedom. This portrays people in favor of a public health quarantine as weak, as well as indifferent to economic consequences. For example, a protestor in Salt Lake City, Utah, was photographed by KUTV News with a sign saying "I need a haircut," while a protestor in Tennessee held a sign reading "Sacrifice the Weak, Reopen TN" (Serie 2012). Protestors in Michigan held signs reading "Heil Witmer" with the Iron Cross of Nazi Germany, voicing their displeasure with the governor (Stanley-Becker and Romm 2020). Mistakenly claiming, as some have, that they have a "right" to a haircut reveals a desire for normalcy and status: Being consumers allows them to feel like contributing members to society, while simultaneously giving them a sense of status and power (it's someone *else* cutting their hair). They feel like their status and power in society comes not from cooperating with others to suppress the spread of the virus, but from their ability to demand that others work in ways that benefit them.

In addition to being seen as an infringement on citizens' rights, some protestors see mask wearing as a challenge to American values (Mello's chapter in this volume focuses on the change in value in how people broadly view mask wearing, shifting from personal protection to community protection [Mello 2021]). However, for the protesters, the mask is a stigmatizing mark, because it is something "other" (meaning non-American) cultures do (Mello 2021). Mask wearing is unfamiliar: both frightening and an intrusion on the way of life protesters have been accustomed to. Because of the pandemic, mask wearing has shifted from foreign to normalized, and this sudden shift in values (a form of anomie; see discussion of Durkheim) leads to frustration and anger. These protests can in part be understood as a form of "stubborn stability" (Sanford, Blum, and Smith 2021), the need or desire for a stable environment despite rapidly shifting social conditions, and in part what Turner labels "modern theodicies of rage" (Turner 2021).

Rather than recognizing our interdependence, this group understands the idea of "survival of the fittest" as Spencer (1966, 313) did: to mean that only the physically strongest should survive, rather than as Darwin intended: species survival (the collective) is ensured by adapting to environmental changes. Instead, they see hyper-individualism as the only possible outcome (for more information on the isolation this view causes, see MacArthur 2021). These expressions of hyper-individualism leave protestors appearing to onlookers not as heroic, but as loud, selfish, and angrily inconvenienced by a pandemic that, as of mid-August 2020, has resulted in more than 165,0000 confirmed dead in the United States alone, and is approaching three-quarters of a million confirmed deaths worldwide.

Masculinity and violence

While there are women protesting for reopening the economy, most of the highly visible and audible protestors have been men. Gender has long been understood as a set of behaviors individuals are socialized into performing, often unconsciously (West and Zimmerman 1987). Research on masculinity connects it with pride and physical strength, suggesting that humiliation is synonymous with emasculation: "[H]umiliate someone and you take away his manhood. For many men, humiliation must be avenged, or you cease to be a man" (Kalish and Kimmel 2010). For example, in a study conducted by Consalvo (2003), teenage mass shooters felt that their manhood had been compromised due to humiliation or feelings of powerlessness. They reinforced their dominant masculine identity by engaging in violent behavior. Masculinity can also be equated with ego (Consalvo 2003; Kalish and Kimmel 2010). A blow to the ego can be reversed by performing masculinity in a certain manner, usually involving violence. Crime offers a way of performing masculinity because it is considered risky and daring, characteristics that are associated with masculinity.

Aggrieved masculinity (Kimmel 2017) – feeling entitled but not receiving what is expected or wanted – is a recipe for humiliation and sets the foundation for toxic masculinity. However, toxic masculinity is more than gendered entitlement. We argue that toxic masculinity is the combination of aggrieved masculinity with a *conscious*, *intentional*, and *exaggerated* performance of stereotypical masculine behaviors. It is a performance rooted in anger, frustration, and entitlement, designed to restore a person's status as strong and masculine. It is designed to convince the audience that the actor is indeed strong and brave and should be at least feared, if not respected. It is also a way for powerless men to assert a form of power over other people, whether that is physical or symbolic (Levin and Madfis 2009; Rocque 2012).

The examples of violence at the beginning of this chapter are not unique to these protests. Three more examples of implied threatened violence photographed by news outlets include:

> April 15, 2020. Protestors gather in front of the Michigan State capitol building for "Operation Gridlock." Cars full of protestors clog the streets. On the capitol steps, three men in ball caps stand near the photographer, two wearing tactical vests and two carrying rifles. Behind them, a man stands with both hands in the air, holding an American flag modified to have one green and one blue stripe. Others brandish the original American flag, and one carries the Culpeper "don't tread on me" flag – a coiled snake originally representing a group of self-trained militia in Virginia during the Revolutionary War. Others hold hand-lettered signs that read "#RecallWhitmer" (the Michigan governor), "Live Free or Die," and "Stop the Tyranny Open Michigan." The one individual who brought a mask to the protest has pulled it down to dangle, useless, against his chest.
>
> *(Vera 2020)*

> April 30, 2020. On the front lines of the protestors inside the Michigan capitol building, a middle-aged White man leans aggressively forward, his gaping mouth framed by a bristling mustache and beard as he screams, maskless, into the faces of calm and composed Michigan State Police officers. None of the three men in the photo are making eye contact, and in fact, the lack of tension in the man's otherwise aggressive-seeming face suggests that his performance is just that – a performance. In another photo, he can be seen chatting, apparently amicably, with a neighboring woman.
>
> *(Beckett 2020)*

> April 30, 2020. Inside the halls of the Michigan State capitol, a group of six armed and masked individuals pose for a photograph. The caption identifies them as "a militia group stand[ing] in front of the governors [sic] office." All are White and most appear to be male and in their late 20's or 30's. They are clothed in a mixture of denim jeans and sand-colored cargo pants, camouflage, and tactical vests. Each is masked and most wear hats, obscuring their identities. One mask is printed to resemble bared teeth: that fellow also sports a gas mask hanging from an olive drab military pistol belt. Another – also wearing dark sunglasses – sports a faded mask from eyes to sternum, printed with the blue background and white stars and red and white stripes of the American flag. As a group, they are well-armed: from left to right, they carry an AR-15 rifle with a suppressor on the end of the barrel, along with six magazines; an AR-15 rifle, a modified AR-15 rifle, pistol, and hunting

knife; an AR-15 rifle and two-three magazines; an AR-15 rifle, a pistol, three magazines and a knife; and finally, another AR-15, four magazines, and a pistol.

(Beckett 2020)

While the examples used in this chapter are from North Carolina and Michigan, similar protests occurred across the United States; for example, protestors in Wisconsin and Pennsylvania also brought weapons and American flags to their demonstrations. These examples show that protesters are comfortable insinuating that they will use violence against a government they feel has overstepped its boundaries. It does not matter to them that state governments impose restrictions to help preserve public health in the face of a new health problem with a death toll that has far exceeded those of Ebola and swine flu in previous years. To these protestors, any restrictions, regardless of intent, are interpreted as attacks on their specific, individual freedoms. Their weapons suggest that they will fight for their right to assemble in large groups, unmasked, despite the risks of both catching and spreading the virus. They are trying to fight for their right to hurt others by ignoring health experts, because for them, the individual matters more than the community, and the economy is the barometer of how well society functions.

Hyper-individualism + toxic masculinity = consequences

When we combine toxic masculinity with hyper-individualism, the result is Toxic Wild West Syndrome. The components of Westerns (whether Spaghetti or Classic) depict heroes as working alone, using violence to achieve goals, and showing strength through the use of violence. Hyper-individualism demands that heroes be "lone wolves" with few, if any, connections to the community, while toxic masculinity demands that heroes show their strength through violence. Putting these demands together produces people who believe that heroes must be like cowboys to be heroes. This approach does not lend itself to people working together collectively to solve community problems. The cowboy is portrayed as a hero and a leader, whether it is of himself or of a small group of chosen compatriots.

In Classic Western movies (e.g., John Wayne movies such as *True Grit*), the hero only kills when necessary, while in Spaghetti Westerns (e.g., *The Good, the Bad, and the Ugly*), the hero kills at will rather than out of necessity, offering the impression that gratuitous random violence is acceptable and equated with strength as a way to save the day. Modern cinema echoes the values of the Western; in particular, the Spaghetti Western, in which gratuitous violence is the norm (e.g., *The Purge*, the *Kill Bill* series). In both Westerns and many modern action and horror movies, heroes tend to work alone, emphasizing self-reliance in order to achieve their goals and using violence gratuitously, more often than not. In all these cinematic representations, toxic masculinity and hyper-individualism create a dangerous combination: people who fancy themselves as heroic cowboys, despite the risks to others.

The modern versions of these Westerns are seen in action movies (e.g., *Die Hard*) and superhero movies (e.g., the *Avengers* series) where the hero uses violence at least to establish themselves as strong, independent, and in control of a fluid situation.

These beliefs are demonstrated in the COVID-19 anti-quarantine and anti-mask protests. The protesters' view of the hero is centered on individual glory and status, rather than community needs. In a pandemic, this is a dangerous position, as, in the short term, it will increase the chance of community spread, raise the infection rate, and ultimately result in more dead individuals across the planet. The long-term consequences of TWWS may include chronic health issues in survivors, more burdens on an already-struggling health system, and future economic shutdowns. Toxic Wild West Syndrome, therefore, constitutes a public health risk that must be mitigated for the public good.

Concluding thoughts: can we mitigate Toxic Wild West Syndrome?

The immediate problems arising from the sudden COVID-19 pandemic have not been mitigated as of this writing, and the long-term consequences are as yet largely unknown. Although health and economy are linked, a more prudent and prosocial approach to this pandemic prioritizes public health over the economy: Public health is the foundation for a healthy economy and healthy populace. To achieve this state, Toxic Wild West Syndrome must be mitigated or halted.

Just like anything toxic, Toxic Wild West Syndrome can kill – both directly and indirectly, but curtailing TWWS will be difficult. TWWS is cultural, and as Marianne Weber argues, making cultural changes takes time, focused effort, and potentially legislation (Lengermann and Niebrugge-Brantley 1992). Protestors are highly visible and espouse deeply held cultural values (even though many of those values are not conducive to a healthy society). Protesters grab headlines and media attention through their protests, giving their audience an inflated sense of the size of the protests and potentially increasing their impact. It is important to understand the reason we see these protesters so frequently is the same reason news highlights violent crime: It is visible, audible, and shocking, in part because they run counter to how prosocial people are expected to act. Although most Americans appear to be following quarantine guidelines and are not calling for a violent return to a pre-pandemic world, quiet cooperation does not gain media attention.

Because those quarantining have no spotlight on their healthy and prosocial behavior, protestors have had virtually exclusive access to being seen and heard in the mass media, which they use to amplify their messages of economic health over individual and community health. This repeated media attention has the cumulative effect of making the protests seem more widespread and as having more support than reality reflects.

Effectively contending with Toxic Wild West Syndrome will be a long-term goal. Socialization and education, from a young age, must emphasize cooperation and interdependence, rather than rugged individualism. This new approach means we need to teach the values of cooperation and collaboration from childhood through adolescence and into adulthood. As Peter Kropotkin (1902) wrote, "competition may be the law of the jungle, but cooperation is the law of civilization." In order to progress socially, we must work together rather than separately and recognize that violence is not only not the answer, but often one of the problems. While this cultural shift will take time, we should think of anti-quarantine protesters as theatrical or film actors trying to hit their mark, but using a script that fits neither the audience nor the situation. Sheer volume and performative, violent aggression does not change the inappropriateness of their performances, regardless of the attention these performances attract.

Notes

1 It is important to note that while the in-person protests have real people airing their grievances, a *Business Insider* article from May 22, 2020, found that roughly half of the voices on Twitter demanding the economy reopen were bots, or software programs that perform repetitive tasks on the internet (Holmes 2020). These tweets and social media posts are emotionally charged demands to reopen local economies, regardless of the public health implications of doing so.
2 In what may have been an attempt at a joke, a White man toting an AR-15 inside the Michigan State Capitol and shrouded nearly head-to-toe in identity-obscuring clothing, wore a patch or sticker on his tactical vest reading "Crisis Actor" in white lettering on a red background (Beckett 2020).

References

BBC News. 2020. "Coronavirus Lockdown Protest: What's Behind the US Demonstrations?" April 21. Accessed June 24, 2020. www.bbc.com/news/world-us-canada-52359100.

Beckett, Lois. 2020. "Michigan Protests Coronavirus Lockdown at Michigan Capitol." *The Guardian.* www.theguardian.com/us-news/2020/apr/30/michigan-protests-corona virus-lockdown-armed-capitol.

Callero, Peter L. 2017. *The Myth of Individualism: How Social Forces Shape Our Lives.* Lanham, Maryland: Rowman & Littlefield Publishers.

Cohen, Patricia, and Tiffany Hsu. 2020. "'Rolling Shock' as Job Losses Mount Even With Reopenings." *The New York Times,* May 14. Accessed June 24, 2020. www.nytimes. com/2020/05/14/business/economy/coronavirus-unemployment-claims.html.

Consalvo, Mia. 2003. "The Monsters Next Door: Media Constructions of Boys and Masculinity." *Feminist Media Studies* 3 (1): 27–45.

Derysh, Igor. 2020. ""Astroturf": Gun Rights Activists and Prominent GOP Donors Push Protests of Coronavirus Restrictions." *Salon,* April 20. Accessed June 24, 2020. www. salon.com/2020/04/20/astroturf-gun-rights-activists-and-prominent-gop-donors-push-protests-of-coronavirus-restrictions/.

Durkheim, Emile. 1951. *Suicide: A Study in Sociology.* New York: Free Press.

Ellis, Emma Grey. 2020. "The Anti-Quarantine Protests Aren't About Covid-19." *Wired,* April 27. Accessed June 24, 2020. www.wired.com/story/anti-lockdown-protests-online/.

Goffman, Erving. 1956. *The Presentation of Self in Everyday Life.* New York: Doubleday.

Hiles, Sara Shipley. 2020. "Tourism vs. Safety: After Viral Party Pics, It's (Almost) Business as Usual at Lake of the Ozarks." *USA Today*, June 6. www.usatoday.com/story/travel/destinations/2020/06/06/lake-ozarks-covid-cases-community-undeterred-reopening/3156993001/.

Holmes, Aaron. 2020. "Roughly Half the Twitter Accounts Pushing to 'Reopen America' Are Bots, Researchers Found." *Business Insider*, May 22. Accessed June 24, 2020. www.businessinsider.com/nearly-half-of-reopen-america-twitter-accounts-are-bots-report-2020-5.

Howard, Jacqueline, and Veronica Stracqualursi. 2020. "Fauci Warns of Anti-Science Bias Being a Problem in the US." *CNN*, June 18. Accessed June 24, 2020. www.cnn.com/2020/06/18/politics/anthony-fauci-coronavirus-anti-science-bias/index.html.

Kalish, Rachel, and Michael Kimmel. 2010. "Suicide by Mass Murder: Masculinity, Aggrieved Entitlement and Rampage School Shootings." *Health Sociology Review* 19 (4): 451–64.

Kimmel, Michael. 2017. *Angry White Men: American Masculinity at the End of an Era*. New York: Nation Books.

Kokino, Greg. 2009. "The Western and the West." Accessed December 1, 2009. http://exp201014fall09.blogspot.com/2009/12/spaghetti-westerns.html.

Kropotkin, Peter. 1902. *Mutual Aid: A Factor of Evolution*. New York: McClure Phillips and Company.

Lengermann, Patricia Madoo, and Gillian Niebrugge-Brantley. 1992. "Early Women Sociologists and Classical Sociological Theory, 1830–1930." In *Classical Sociological Theory*, edited by George Ritzer, 288–330. New York: McGraw-Hill.

Levin, Jack, and Eric Madfis. 2009. "Mass Murder at School and Cumulative Strain: A Sequential Model." *American Behavioral Scientists* 52 (9): 1227–245.

Long, Travis. 2020. "A Group of About 11 Mostly-Armed Demonstrators Protesting The Stay At Home Order." *Twitter*, May 9. Accessed June 24, 2020. https://twitter.com/vizjourno/status/1259189791150800899.

MacArthur, Kelly Rhea. 2021. "Treating Loneliness in the Aftermath of a Pandemic: Threat or Opportunity?" In *COVID-19: Global Pandemic, Societal Responses, Ideological Solutions*, edited by J. Michael Ryan, 197–208. London: Routledge.

Meeker, James. 2021. "The Political Nightmare of the Plague: The Ironic Resistance of Anti-Quarantine Protesters." In *COVID-19: Social Consequences and Cultural Adaptations*, edited by J. Michael Ryan, 109–21. London: Routledge.

Mello, Heather. 2021. "Innovation Diffusion, Social Capital, and Mask Mobilizations." In *COVID-19: Social Consequences and Cultural Adaptations*, edited by J. Michael Ryan, 134–51. London: Routledge.

Rocque, Michael. 2012. "Exploring School Rampage Shootings: Research, Theory, and Policy." *The Social Science Journal* 49 (3): 304–13.

Ryan, J. Michael. 2021. "The Blessings of COVID-19 for Neoliberalism, Nationalism, and Neoconservative Ideologies." In *COVID-19: Global Pandemic, Societal Responses, Ideological Solutions*, edited by J. Michael Ryan, 80–93. London: Routledge.

Sanford, Adam G., Dinur Blum, and Stacy L. Smith. 2021. "Seeking Stability in Unstable Times: COVID-19 and the Bureaucratic Mindset." In *COVID-19: Social Consequences and Cultural Adaptations*, edited by J. Michael Ryan, 47–60. London: Routledge.

Serie, Kathleen. 2012. "Dozens Rally at TN Capitol, Call for Gov. Lee to Re-Open State Immediately." *WZTV Nashville*, April 20. Accessed June 24, 2020. www.businessinsider.com/wisconsin-supreme-court-overturns-coronavirus-tony-evers-shutdown-packed-bars-2020-5.

Spencer, Herbert. 1966. *The Study of Sociology*. Ann Arbor: University of Michigan Press.

Stanley-Becker, Isaac, and Tony Romm. 2020. "US Lockdown Three Brothers Appear to be Behind Online Network of Far-Right Gun Owners Calling for Protests." *The Independent*, April 20. Accessed June 24, 2020. www.independent.co.uk/news/world/ameri cas/us-coronavirus-lockdown-protests-far-right-guns-facebook-groups-a9473756.html.

Turner, Bryan S. 2021. "Theodicies of the COVID-19 Catastrophe." In *COVID-19: Global Pandemic, Societal Responses, Ideological Solutions*, edited by J. Michael Ryan, 29–42. London: Routledge.

Vera, Amir. 2020. "Another Person Who Attended Lake of the Ozarks on Memorial Day Weekend Tests Positive for Coronavirus." *CNN*, June 13. Accessed June 24, 2020. www.cnn.com/2020/06/12/us/ozarks-missouri-party-coronavirus-positive/index.html.

West, Candace, and Don H. Zimmerman. 1987. "Doing Gender." *Gender and Society* 1 (2): 125–51.

12

INNOVATION DIFFUSION, SOCIAL CAPITAL, AND MASK MOBILIZATION

Culture change during the COVID-19 pandemic

Heather L. Mello

Wearing masks during illness has been rare in the US for over 100 years – since the 1918 flu pandemic, the practice has been considered unnecessary by the general public as a disease preventive measure since that time. Mask-wearing behaviors that had existed were typically only practiced by immigrant and ethnic populations from communities where mask wearing was common practice and, as such, served as a marker of outsider status. With the spread of COVID-19, however, this practice has changed rapidly. From discouragement to adoption and promotion, the rise of mask-wearing behaviors is an unusually rapid cultural practice change.

Reflecting both diffusion from Asian cultures as a method for controlling the pandemic and evolving discourse about mask wearing as both a self- and other-protective behavior, this rapid cultural practice change reflects months of research and discussion concerning masks and their efficacy, back-and-forth messaging by public health and government leaders, and a significant mobilization of mask-making and distribution resources by various levels of social organization across the globe.

Using a "diffusion of innovations" and "social capital" approach applied to recent mask discourse and mobilization, this study hopes to provide insight into the process of diffusion of mask wearing as a pandemic preventive behavior and the role played by formal and informal social networks in the adoption or rejection of masks and mask-wearing behaviors. The current study, in examining the change in mask wearing, will shed light on processes of culture change, generally, and into diffusion of innovation (DOI) and social capital concepts as related to social practices during times of national and even global emergencies.

Diffusion of innovation and social capital in culture change

E. M. Rogers (2010) wrote, "Diffusion is the process by which an innovation is communicated through certain channels over time among the members of a social system" (35). While a pandemic might seem like an urgent, compelling reason to adopt mask wearing across society, according to Rogers (ibid.), the process of diffusion is not always successful, even for life-saving measures – some will adopt the practice and others will not. Furthermore, scientific research, crucial in a pandemic setting, is not always the most compelling factor in adoption. "Near peers" play a key role in this process: individuals who share similarities within a network, have already adopted the innovation, and can report on their experience. Regarding science versus peers,

> Diffusion investigations show that most individuals do not evaluate an innovation on the basis of scientific studies of its consequences, although such objective evaluations are not entirely irrelevant, especially to the very first individuals who adopt. Instead, most people depend mainly upon a subjective evaluation of an innovation that is conveyed to them from other individuals like themselves who have already adopted the innovation.
>
> *(18)*

The term "near" is important here; if the peers are completely similar, especially as regards the innovation and their knowledge and experience of it, then there is nothing new to communicate. In this sense, diffusion is a highly social process requiring some degree of difference between individuals in order to work. This factor highlights the importance of social capital effects within that social system.

Social capital comprises sets of relations between individuals in a society. Beyond simply the number of connections themselves, social capital also concerns the quality of these connections. Applying social capital to health outcomes, Szreter and Woolcock (2004) posit three forms that influence public health in a society: bonding, "trusting and co-operative relations between members of a network who see themselves as being similar in terms of their shared social identity" (654–655); bridging, "relations of respect and mutuality between people who know that they are not alike in some sociodemographic (or social identity) sense (differing by age, ethnic group, class, etc.)" (655); and linking, "norms of respect and networks of trusting relationships between people who are interacting across explicit, formal or institutionalized power or authority gradients in society" (ibid.). The authors note that while material resources are important for public health, "human relationships, effort, and care (or labor) . . . are crucial" (ibid.) and that trust among network members, across networks, and in vertical relationships, such as between society members and institutions of power, will result in compliance with recommended public health behaviors.

Chuang et al. (2015) applied Szreter and Woolcock's social capital concepts in their study of whether social capital influenced respondent likelihood to engage in health protective behaviors during a flu epidemic: wearing masks, getting flu shots, and washing hands frequently. Bonding social capital was defined as relationships and support among neighbors, bridging as association membership, and linking as both trust in government and trust that government had the capacity to handle a pandemic (1). The authors found that intentions to wear a mask during the pandemic were related to higher scores on all three dimensions of social capital. They also found that mask-wearing intentions were lower among men and those older than 65 years (5). Conversely, those with higher education, those who are married, and those with higher susceptibility to a flu were more likely to report intention to engage in the assessed health protective behaviors, to include mask wearing (ibid.).

That mask wearing may legitimately protect the general public during illness may be considered innovative where such ideas and behavior have been uncommon. Masks as material health culture had generally been laid aside in the West in the 100 years since the 1918 Spanish flu pandemic. The rediffusion of this practice during the current COVID-19 pandemic is of special interest as countries across the globe work to contain the spread of the disease, some newly adopting mask wearing as infection prevention measures.

Using Rogers's definition of diffusion, this chapter explores the interrelations between the following concepts: masks as an innovation – not exactly new, but newly rediscovered public health practice; communication channels as patterns of information and resource sharing; over the first seven months of the COVID-19 pandemic; with a focus on the external influence of mass media and public health and political leaders and the internal influence of strong and weak ties and opinion leaders, both within the US social system, generally. The social capital concepts, bonding, bridging, and linking, connect through mask information and resource sharing and through messaging and examples set by external and internal influences.

Methods

This chapter mixes content analysis and corpus analysis methods. Content analysis includes online news articles from December 2019 to mid-July 2020. Although articles from other online US news sites were included, most were taken from CNN and Fox News websites (CNN 2020; Fox News 2020). Two of the biggest online news sources in the US, they typically cover a wide mainstream reader demographic in that country, with CNN on the left of center and Fox News to the right (Farhi 2018; Pasley 2019; Joyella 2020).

Corpus analysis is a digestive approach, using computers to analyze databases of language collected for specific purposes; resulting analyses typically focused on frequency of occurrence for language forms. The NOW Corpus – News on the Web – used for this analysis includes English-language content from online news sites and websites from around the world (Davies 2016–), sourced through Bing News and over 1,000 websites featuring news articles that have appeared within the day of collection. According to the NOW Corpus source website, approximately 10,000 articles are collected for the corpus each day and cleaned to remove non-article content. Data for this chapter includes content from December 2019 to June 2020 originating in the US only. The resulting seven-month corpus contains

645,379,968 words of text with 151,133 instances or hits for "mask" – the central word of analysis. Corpus data were analyzed using the Wordsmith Tools (Scott 2008) corpus analysis program and Microsoft Excel.

Content analysis also supplements corpus analysis techniques, examining concordance lines computed from the original corpus where larger strings of text centered on the word "mask" provided context with final supplementation from online news sites themselves related to corpus analysis topics. The web articles, which may or may not appear within the NOW Corpus data, dated the content and complemented the month-by-month analysis of the corpus. It should be noted that CNN and Fox News content does appear within the NOW Corpus aggregated from Bing News, but due to the structure of the aggregated corpus, extraction of specific whole-article content is not possible.

The results section begins with a content analysis timeline focused on masks and mask-wearing behaviors during COVID-19 (for a more comprehensive timeline of the pandemic, see Ryan 2021, this volume). Search bar queries from the CNN and Fox News websites are supplemented with content from other sites using a Google search. Search terms included "covid," "mask," "need," "hoard," "donate," "sew," "make," "infection," and "surgeon general."

After the timeline, the first corpus analysis examines the word "mask," its frequency and rate. The next three analyses focus on the social capital concepts: bonding, bridging, and linking. Adapting from Chuang et al. (2015), social capital definitions are applied as they relate to masks as pandemic-related material culture and mask wearing as a protective health behavior and as related to the DOI concepts of promoting innovation adoption, behavior commencement and compliance, and trust within and across networks and social systems. Here, bonding social capital is the mobilization of resources to make masks; bridging as the organization and donation of mask supplies; and linking as trust in government and trust that government can handle a pandemic. After having saved each month's concordance into Microsoft Excel, I searched using the "find" function on the varying grammatical forms of "make" (make, makes, making, made) and "sew" (sew, sews, sewing, sewn). Bridging social capital focused on the forms for "donate" (donate, donates, donating, donated) and "organize" (organize, organizes, organizing, organized) and organization types associated with these activities. Linking social capital analysis focused on the timeline content and various mask analyses, with additional corpus results for "mask purposes" and "anti-mask" topics.

Results and discussion

General timeline

Chinese health authorities reported the first cases of a new pneumonia infecting patients in Wuhan, China, to the World Health Organization (WHO) in December 2019. By January 28, 2020, the US had reported its fifth confirmed case of the new coronavirus. Two days later, on January 30, the WHO officially declared the emerging COVID-19 situation a "Public Health Emergency of International Concern" (CNN Editorial Research 2020).

Online news articles reporting out of China starting in January routinely featured photos of Wuhan locals wearing masks on the streets and public transportation. Within this time frame, the US news began reporting runs on medical-grade face masks in stores and online, panic buying, and mask hoarding; this despite suggestions from public health officials not to worry about masks, but to "do what you do every cold and flu season . . . wash your hands, cover your mouth when you cough or sneeze, and stay home from work when you are sick" (Asmelash 2020, para 3–4). Some articles warned that medical-grade masks were not necessary for the general public or the healthy, that general public mask wearing was ineffective as there was a danger of misuse or improper wear that would increase infection rates, and that the lack of masks could be dangerous for healthcare workers and hospitals. The US Centers for Disease Control and Prevention (CDC) began outreach to mask manufacturers to ensure adequate supply.

The prices of masks skyrocketed. Stocks of N-95 and other medical- and surgical-grade mask stocks came up short through February and March as calls were raised to meet surging demand, from healthcare and government sources, as high up as the vice president. Mask supplies typically outsourced globally from China were held back to deal with the pandemic raging there, and authorities in the US reported radically insufficient supply in the US National Strategic Stockpile, an emergency health supply reserve set aside for just such pandemic situations. Efforts arose at all levels to help meet demand; donations came in from Chinese billionaires, rappers, and aid groups. Entrepreneurs outsourced manufacturing for donation, companies like Apple and Facebook donated, and television medical dramas even donated their supplies. Businesses also stepped up, though not for donation, to include a pillow company repurposed to meet demand.

In addition to these larger-scale efforts, individuals and newly formed localized groups stepped in to do their part in making masks – initially for healthcare workers and the ill, to supplement shortfalls, and to strengthen protection during reuse of higher-grade mask materials (Price 2020). A headline from March references a "sewing army" making masks to fill the acute shortage (Enrich, Abrams, and Kurutz 2020):

> They are scrounging for fabric, cutting it up, stitching it together. They are repurposing drapes, dresses, bra straps, shower curtains, even coffee filters. They are building supply chains, organizing workers, managing distribution networks. Most of all, they are sewing. All over the country, homebound Americans are crafting thousands upon thousands of face masks to help shield doctors, nurses and many others from the coronavirus.
>
> *(para 1–3)*

This mask-making army also donated masks to other categories of essential workers: delivery drivers, local police, ambulance workers, firefighters, and grocery store personnel.

As the virus spread globally, scientists learned more about how the virus spread and about the profile of COVID-19 infection.

> From the beginning of the outbreak, which originated in China late last year and rapidly took hold across the globe in recent months, evidence points to the potent influence previous illnesses and underlying conditions have on morbidity rates or rendering a case to be critical.
>
> *(McKay 2020)*

Research further indicated that complications and death rates increased significantly with age, hospitalization was more likely the older the patient, and most deaths occurred in patients over 70. Conversely, the young and the healthy were found to be less likely to suffer COVID-19 complications and death; however, the US surgeon general pointed out that these groups could still spread the virus throughout their communities and to those with health problems (Klein 2020).

As knowledge grew about infection profiles and asymptomatic and potential airborne transmission, messaging between March and April changed from discouraging mask-wear by the general public to tentative encouragement, as long as adequate supply of the higher-grade medical and surgical masks were reserved for the healthcare system and the ill. Global experts, including the WHO, CDC, and researchers from Asian countries with more experience with mask wearing during influenza pandemics, began to advocate for mask wearing among the general public, not only to prevent oneself from contracting the illness, but to protect others as well in cases where the wearer might be infected asymptomatically. The message that virus reproduction rates were lowest when everyone is wearing masks began to proliferate. Consequently, as need for mask supplies grew even further, those cloth-mask-making armies continued their task, turning now to meet the needs of the public doing their part to stop the virus as well. Inspired by those armies, some started anew, sewing masks for friends, family, neighbors, and community in need (BillingsGazette 2020).

In late March, messaging between CNN and Fox News began to diverge: CNN's articles more clearly positive towards masking and Fox News's stance ranging more widely between promotion and skepticism. Pro-mask articles consistently appeared on both sides, including discussing mask how-tos: instructions on crafting your own DIY masks, tips on how to avoid fogged-up glasses during mask-wear, and answers to mask-related questions readers may have. On June 14, both sites reported on the latest from the surgeon general, that "wearing coronavirus masks will give Americans 'more freedom'" (Azad and Cullinane 2020; Moore 2020).

Showing the gap between the sites' orientations, CNN headlines on March 31 and April 1 read, "Masks could be part of the answer" (Lee 2020) and "White

House task force could soon recommend Americans wear masks" (Liptak 2020b); Fox News headlines, dated March 31 and April 2, read "Surgeon general: Data doesn't back up wearing masks in public amid coronavirus pandemic" (Kaplan 2020) and "Should you wear a face mask to prevent COVID-19? Experts disagree" (Geggel 2020). An interesting juxtaposition in mask reference can be seen through reporting on the president's recommendations from a coronavirus briefing in early April: the Fox News headline, "Trump says CDC wants Americans to cover faces with cloth amid coronavirus" (Pappas 2020); CNN, "Trump announces new face mask recommendations after heated internal debate" (Liptak 2020a).

These trends continued through June, revealing political partisanship and deeper divergence on the emerging science. CNN reporting highlighted some Republicans' "defiance" of public health expert guidelines by not wearing masks during meetings (Raju 2020). Additional headlines affirm the site's strong support of mask efficacy: "It's not maskers vs. anti-maskers. It's public safety" (Wolf 2020) and "Want to prevent another shutdown, save 33,000 lives and protect yourself? Wear a face mask, doctors say" (Yan 2020). Meanwhile, Fox News headlines continued representing a wider range of positions: "Former MLB player Aubrey Huff goes on rant about masks amid coronavirus pandemic" (Aaro 2020); "Pence deflects on questions about wearing masks, says White House will 'defer to governors'" (O'Reilly 2020). As late as May 28, 2020, Fox News reported on a *March 2020* WHO report on masks (Casiano 2020),

> The World Health Organization is recommending healthy people, including those who don't exhibit COVID-19 symptoms, only wear masks when taking care of someone infected with the contagion, a sharp contrast from the advice given by American public health officials who recommend everyone wear a mask in public. "If you do not have any respiratory symptoms such as fever, cough or runny nose, you do not need to wear a mask," Dr. April Baller, a public health specialist for the WHO, says in a video on the world health body's website posted in March. "Masks should only be used by health care workers, caretakers or by people who are sick with symptoms of fever and cough." The recommendation has not changed and differs from the Centers for Disease Control and Prevention (CDC), which urges individuals to wear a mask or face-covering in public settings, regardless of infection or not, to limit the spread of the virus.
>
> *(para 1–3)*

As of mid-July, reporting continues on mask needs for healthcare workers, mask-making initiatives for essential workers and community members, DIY mask making, and masks as politics. *The New York Times* reported that seamstresses for the world's top fashion houses had begun their own mask-making network while in quarantine back in March (Testa 2020). Started by a seamstress at Chanel, the ongoing initiative making "haute couture" masks does not sell them for profit, but gives them to frontline workers: bakers, firefighters, and healthcare workers. Back at CNN and Fox News, headlines come back together again on July 12, reporting on the president's visit to a veterans hospital, noting that he wore a mask in public – and on camera – for the first time (Mena and Stracqualursi 2020; McFall 2020).

"Mask"

Corpus analysis methods begin with hits for the word "mask." Figure 12.1 presents the ratio of hits per 1,000 words within each month's corpus. The ratio begins to rise slowly in January and February, hitting a peak in April with a slow descent through June.

Bonding and bridging social capital

From Chuang et al. (2015), bonding social capital works "in epidemic emergencies by mobilizing local institutions for action and by providing information and awareness about the disease through social networks as well as by promoting discussion and problem solving regarding feasible actions" (7). Figure 12.2 counts for lemma for making and sewing masks peak in March and April. Hits begin to rise with the first calls for masks in late January, correlated with spread of the virus, ongoing mask shortages, and public panic buying, reflecting efforts by DOI innovators and early adopters in developing, organizing, planning, and making masks for distribution across the need spectrum, early to healthcare workers, to other essential workers, and then beyond to social networks within the general public.

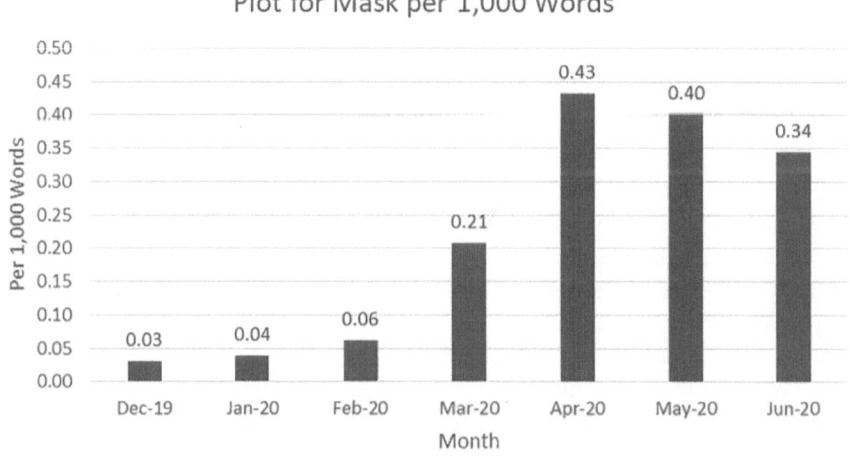

FIGURE 12.1   The Word "Mask" per 1,000 Words by Month

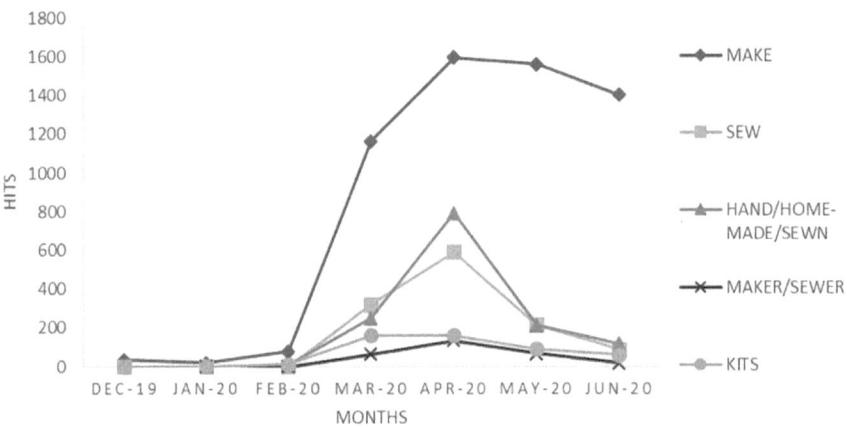

FIGURE 12.2   Bonding Activity Hits by Month

Bonding social capital as social support reflects this mobilization first across networks as calls for help arose and then within both formal and informal social networks as discussed in the timeline. Help arrived in abundance as people from across the country heeded the call. Sewers mentioned in the corpus include a wide range of volunteer types; to name a few: members of sewing circles, seamstresses, city council members, hospital and organization staff members, families, graduate students, sewing shops, classmates, correctional institutes and inmates, homemakers, nursing home residents, soldiers, and lucha libre wrestling mask sewers. Several organizations named include Sew Face Masks Philadelphia, Wisconsin Face Mask Warriors, the Auntie Sewing Squad, Sewing Masks for Area Hospitals, and several different US–Chinese associations.

Bridging social capital lemma hit counts are included in Figures 12.3 and 12.4. From Figure 12.3 we see mask donation and organization among groups referenced that cover the lack of supply of PPE for healthcare workers in the early days of the epidemic and then include community donation and organization beyond the healthcare system. The bonding and bridging analyses here reflect pro-mask actions and processes. Anti-mask topics will be addressed in the linking section.

For Figure 12.4, mobilization terms were searched with the various organizational terms. While companies are the largest organizations involved in the donation of masks, clubs, communities, associations, and various organization members donating, rather than receiving, also comprise noteworthy forces involved in donation. "Interpersonal networks play a crucial role in enhancing communications platforms and augmenting government credibility" (Chuang et al. 2015, 11). Networks organized to ensure and enhance the larger country- and community-wide efforts to provide masks as pandemic preventive material culture and wearing as behavior. Regarding the lower hit count for organizing versus donating, I posit that organizing is an ongoing effort to meet need across the spectrum, led by fewer

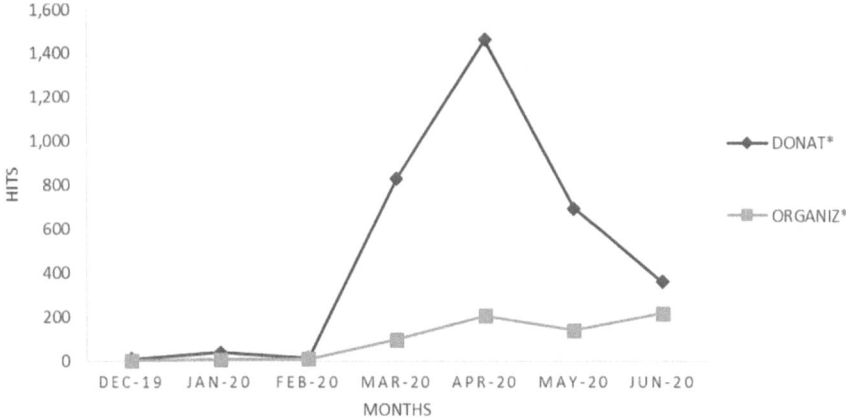

FIGURE 12.3   Bridging Activity Hits by Month

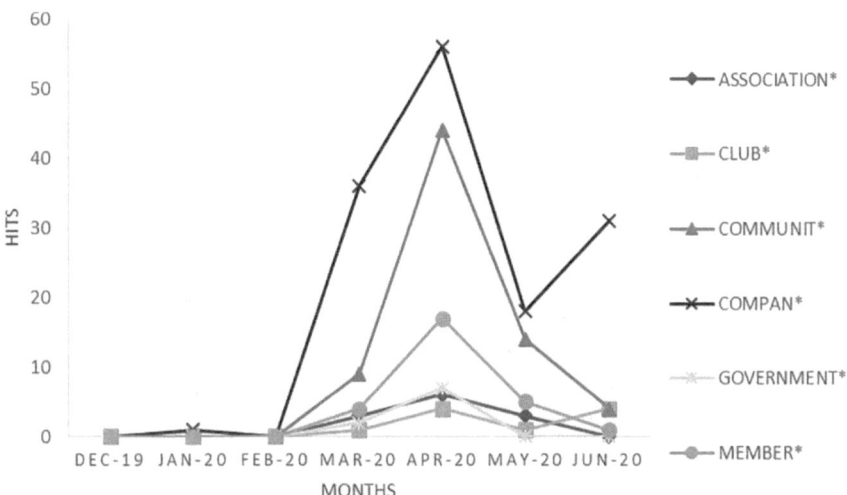

FIGURE 12.4   Bridging Organizational Hits by Month

persons than the initial and ongoing mass donation by companies, celebrities, and governments that enlisted existing processes.

Bridging social capital represents horizontal relations, but between more distant and disparate social networks, those less close than in bonding networks. Relations between mask makers and receivers include connections across boundaries including more formal network relationships as groups interact based on production and need – community groups to hospitals, mask clubs to essential workers, etc. Within the DOI frame, this includes innovators, adopters, and early majority adopters, linked by more similarity; where late majority adopters are concerned, those with higher degrees of mask skepticism, implementation reflects mask mandates and business requirements for workers and customers to wear masks regardless of agreement. Donation eventually also covers connections within informal networks as well.

Linking social capital

Beginning with the question of whether the government has the capacity to handle the pandemic, connected to the DOI concept of external social systems – mass media and health and government authority – messaging from January through March consistently communicated that mask supplies were not going to be enough to meet healthcare workers' needs. Medical and government authorities called for manufacturers to ramp up production and for organizations to donate whatever medical-grade mask supplies they had. Formal and informal network members, from government to companies and the wealthy to groups within communities, started the mask mobilization machine, adapting existing processes and creating new ones to meet this demand and help the government and society to handle the pandemic. In early April, as per the timeline, new research about how COVID-19 spread demonstrated the need for the general public to also wear masks. Ongoing mask-making and distribution processes were extended to the general public and within local informal networks. Later, new networks and individuals joined, further assisting the government in handling the pandemic as it spread.

Moving to the more general concept of trust in government, timeline data provide a much more mixed result. From January through July 12, 2020, the last day of collection for this chapter, we see a 180-degree reversal in the position of the government and medical professionals on whether the public should wear masks to stop the spread of COVID-19. The message careens from one end of the scientific and political spectrum to the other: Masks are only for healthcare workers in January, with the March message from the surgeon general, "Seriously people, stop buying masks!" to June news from the same surgeon general that masks promote freedom, and finally the skeptical, laggard president sporting a mask for public photos for the first time in July. Even before research proliferated that masks might be effective in stopping the spread of the virus among the general public, journalists explicitly discussed the trust lost when health experts communicated that masks were somehow useful for healthcare workers but useless for the general public, even while acknowledging the intent to preserve mask supplies for those same healthcare workers (Tufekci 2020). From Fox News's Tucker Carlson (Creitz 2020): "stop lying to us about why we shouldn't be buying them." Eventually, new science emerged that masks might be good for everyone, not only helping the wearer but also protecting others (see Figure 12.5).

Two other notable points present a challenge to trust for government. As a second challenge, media sources presented different pictures of the science and of differing support for or against changes in preventive knowledge, measures, and

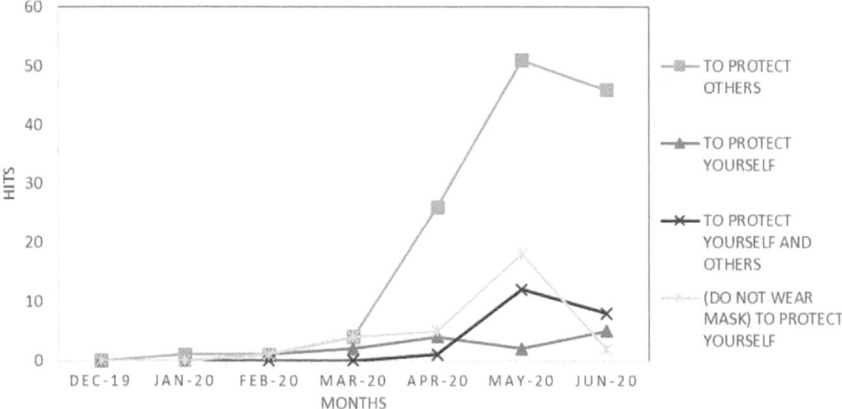

FIGURE 12.5   Mask Purpose Hits by Month

policy. Timely reporting on science as a process and where that science is at any given moment regarding pandemic prevention greatly influence the measures the public may take in response. CNN's positive messaging and persistent reporting on the developing science would engender more consistent mask-wearing behaviors, whereas Fox News ranging between emerging science reporting, celebrity skepticism, and even reporting in May on older public health messaging from March would result in a wider range of attitudes towards masks and their efficacy.

The third challenge to trust for government is exemplified by the highest-ranking potential change agent in the country – the president. During an early April press briefing, as the president discussed new CDC pro-mask guidelines, he emphasized that the practice was "voluntary." From Fox News: "'So it's voluntary. You don't have to do it.' The president added, 'I don't think I'm going to be doing it.' He said he can't imagine himself sitting in the Oval Office of the White House behind 'that beautiful resolute desk' wearing a mask" (Pappas 2020). CNN's quote: "'I don't think I'm going to be doing it,' he said, going on to suggest it was hard to envision such a thing in the Oval Office: 'Wearing a face mask as I greet presidents, prime ministers, dictators, kings, queens – I just don't see it.'" (Liptak 2020a). With this, Trump signals resistance to mask wearing both at the office and among social groups. Trump would go on to appear in public many times without a face mask after this briefing, with his first publicized appearance in a mask on July 12.

Trust in government and its ability to handle a pandemic, centered on the initial no-mask messaging, are less likely when that messaging changes so completely and so rapidly in time. Anti-mask attitudes may be developed at any point and may change for or against the innovation depending on other factors as well, to include emerging information on who is most likely to be infected. In the case of COVID-19, the elderly and chronically less healthy would be assumed to be more likely to wear masks, depending on how much they trust that emerging science. Conversely, lower infection severity among the young and the healthy has led to their lower mask implementation despite the accompanying messaging that community spread is halted best when all those in contact wear masks. The virus's novelty may also contribute to lower trust in government's messaging about the reality and severity of the virus: on April 7, only 14% of Americans reportedly knew someone who had tested positive (Vaidya 2020); by May 26, only 20% of Americans knew someone who had been hospitalized for or died from the virus (Johnson, Ferno, and Keeter 2020). These bases for skepticism may be exacerbated by mass media outlets and prominent public figures who themselves are late adopters, if not laggards or outright rejecters.

Figure 12.6 represents the anti-mask concept found within the corpus. Concordance lines reveal some very interesting findings related to past and current law, reactions to mask mandates during the 1918 Spanish flu pandemic, and as expected, rising anti-mask sentiments in the US.

The January, March, and April 2020 hits constitute prior and recent anti-mask laws aimed at protest groups, KKK, and criminal activity; to prevent identity concealment during both legal and illegal activities. Hits include discussion of New York City reviving old anti-mask laws during the Occupy Wall Street movement in 2011, the earliest dates for enactment of anti-mask laws is the 1840s, with many states enacting such laws between the 1920s and 1950s. Beginning in April, articles discuss repeal of those anti-mask laws in a few states, in the face of the CDC's "pro-mask stance." There is even discussion of anti-mask laws in other countries that contravene current public health measures.

April and May discourse reflects back to the anti-mask movements in the 1918 Spanish influenza pandemic; mask ordinances were considered by some to be "contrary to the desires of the majority." Lines mention a marshal shooting someone

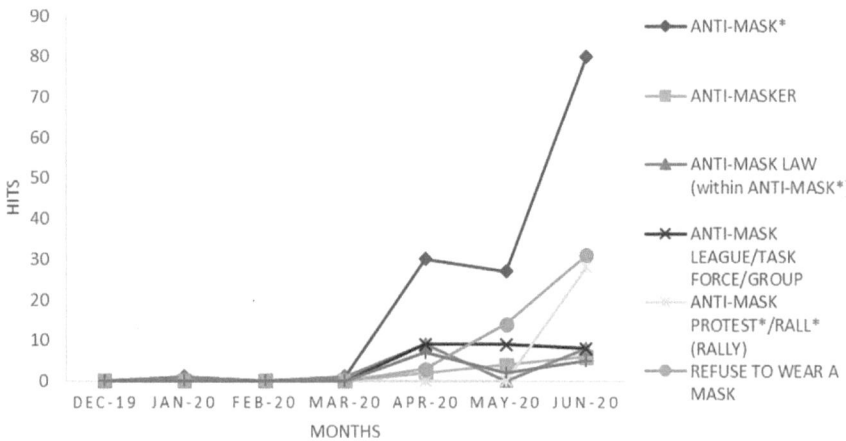

FIGURE 12.6 Anti-Mask/Mask-Refusal Concepts by Month

who refused to put on a mask, which led to anti-mask rallies. The San Francisco Anti-Mask League held rallies of up to 4,500 persons. May to June discourse moves into the present with the anti-mask position held by the sitting US president mentioned as "helping fuel an anti-mask movement across the US." Anti-mask rallies and protests occur in at least six states. Disputes pop up between business owners and customers over the owners' right to refuse service to those refusing to wear a mask. Terms used in reference to mask requirements in the present mirrored those of the 1918 anti-maskers as "ineffective," "tyrannical," and "unconstitutional." Slogans deployed include "My body, my choice" and "I can't breathe," lines borrowed (coopted?!) from the pro-choice movement and the line repeated by George Floyd as he died during an arrest in Minneapolis. An anti-mask "Freedom to Breath Agency" has been formed, with an interesting anti-mask tactic, mentioned several times, of presenting an Americans with Disabilities Act card indicating that the bearer has a disability that prevents mask wearing. Terms for these anti-mask movements include "reckless" and reflecting a "me first" attitude.

I want to comment here on some of the nuances related to mask-wearing behaviors. In this chapter, I am concerned with social capital and diffusion of masks as prosocial behaviors, but I do touch on anti-social, i.e., anti-mask, attitudes and behaviors. Blum, Smith, and Stanford (2021, this volume) talk more in-depth about prosocial versus "hyper-individualist" and "inflexible" attitudes towards mask wearing and the wider range of infection-prevention measures during the recent pandemic. This should be contrasted with reactions to mask behavior and concerns of racism and discrimination among Asian Americans and other persons of color. For Asian Americans, mask wearing has been seen as evidence of "disease status" despite the fact that this was a common community behavior even before the pandemic, sometimes simply to combat the effects of pollution (Yan, Chen, and Naresh 2020; Chiang 2021, this volume). For Blacks and Latinos, specifically, mask wearing has been seen as evidence of criminality and may lead to racial profiling (Fernando III 2020).

Conclusion

Using the diffusion of innovation and social capital perspectives, this research showed how masks, an innovation within the US context, diffused across US society. This innovation spread as information and patterns of action along communication channels during the early days of the coronavirus pandemic under various social system influences. Influence flowed externally from mass media and public health and government authorities and internally through social networks, according to connection to opinion leaders and change agents, from as high up as the sitting president, at the level of organizations creating mobilization networks, to as local as a neighbor sitting in front of a sewing machine.

Masks as material culture and general mask-wearing behavior began in the US with examples from Asia fighting the early pandemic mixed in with panic buying and hoarding and has ended at the time of this writing with a majority of state-level governments mandating general mask wearing in public to combat the virus. This research supports the hypothesis that the mass mobilization of mask making and donating, upon calls from health and government leaders to support essential healthcare and service workers, has been one of the largest and most crucial influences in the adoption of the general public's mask-wearing behaviors. When science shifted to support mask wearing by the general public, these networks were already in place to meet the newer demand and were already predisposed to see masks as beneficial, even if scarce. The enlistment of additional society members to meet the new demand added to positive perceptions of masks as pandemic practice.

Bonding social capital as local social support and bridging social capital as extension of support exemplify investment in masks as crucial in promoting the health of society during the pandemic. This is further supported by the linking social capital concept of trust that government can handle the pandemic, as innovation and change leaders across the country mobilized in support, supplementing efforts by the government. As Chuang et al. (2015) noted, such networks have a key role to play in enhancing the government's credibility.

On the other hand, such mobilization was insufficient to create an atmosphere of overwhelmingly positive trust in government, apart from its ability to handle the pandemic, due to rapidly and radically changing messaging, differing information channels, and systems of influence. At the time of this chapter's final writing, masks and mask wearing have proliferated but have only just reached around 55% health expert guided compliance (Kane 2020). In order to bend the infection rate curve, required compliance rates as high as 95% have been suggested. I argue that the mixed messaging by health experts early on has been a major source of confusion and skepticism of mask science. While some influences have successfully persuaded the implementation and continuation of adoption of masks for pandemic prevention as a country-wide, social support mobilization over time, other influences – mass media and influential members of society communicating on various platforms – continue to question the efficacy and constitutionality of the mask as innovation, frustrating compliance.

Innovations do not always diffuse evenly or completely across a social system. While innovations typically take time to make their way from innovators to early and later stage adopters, it may also be the case that a diffusion fails to reach 100% adoption. That social and cultural change for mask wearing has not (yet?) reached into many layers and communities in the US should not be a surprise. In a country that holds up individualism, freedom, and the maverick spirit as treasured values, resistance and noncompliance should be expected, as seen during the 1918 pandemic. Social media and its proliferation have contributed to the ability of agents on both sides of the debate to raise their voices and have their arguments considered in the marketplace of ideas, sometimes on equal footing.

Science is a process, one that takes time and relies on evidence before making assertions. That mask-related messaging would change over time as new evidence replaced older evidence is the heart of that process. In the face of reliance on older messages or skepticism about new messages, the voices of public health and government experts communicating that new evidence across as many channels and among as many social systems as possible are needed more than ever.

References

Aaro, David. 2020. "Former MLB Player Aubrey Huff Goes on Rant About Masks Amid Coronavirus Pandemic." *Fox News*, June 17. www.foxnews.com/sports/former-mlb-player-aubrey-huff-goes-rant-having-wear-masks.

Asmelash, Leah. 2020. "The Surgeon General Wants Americans to Stop Buying Face Masks." *CNN*, March 2. https://edition.cnn.com/2020/02/29/health/face-masks-coronavirus-surgeon-general-trnd/index.html.

Azad, Arman, and Susannah Cullinane. 2020. "US Surgeon General: Coronavirus Face Masks Promote Freedom." *CNN*, June 14. https://edition.cnn.com/2020/06/14/health/us-surgeon-general-coronavirus-masks/index.html.

BillingsGazette. 2020. "Sew Masks for Friends and Family." *Billings Gazette*, April 22. https://billingsgazette.com/travel/sew-masks-for-friends-and-family/article_81e0e7ba-3d9a-5d8e-8cc2-75710e7149d3.html.

Blum, Dinur, Stacy L. Smith, and Adam G. Stanford. 2021. "Toxic Wild West Syndrome: Individual Rights vs. Community Needs." In *COVID-19: Social Consequences and Cultural Adaptations*, edited by J. Michael Ryan, 122–133. London: Routledge.

Casiano, Louis. 2020. "WHO Guidance: Healthy People Should Wear Masks Only When 'Taking Care of' Coronavirus Patients." *Fox News*, May 28. www.foxnews.com/world/who-guidance-healthy-people-wear-masks-around-coronavirus-patients.

Chiang, Pamela. 2021. "Anti-Asian Racism, Responses, and the Impact on Asian Americans' Lives: A Social-Ecological Perspective." In *COVID-19: Social Consequences and Cultural Adaptations*, edited by J. Michael Ryan, 215–29. London: Routledge.

Chuang, Ying-Chih, Ya-Li Huang, Kuo-Chien Tseng, Chia-Hsin Yen, and Lin-Hui Yang. 2015. "Social Capital and Health-Protective Behavior Intentions in an Influenza Pandemic." *PLoS One*, 1–14.

CNN. 2020. www.cnn.com.

Creitz, Charles. 2020. "Tucker Blasts Feds Over Medical Masks, Says 'Stop Lying to Us' About Why We Shouldn't Buy Them." *Fox News*, March 30. www.foxnews.com/media/tucker-carlson-blasts-feds-medical-masks coronavirus.

Davies, Mark. 2016–. "Corpus of News on the Web (NOW): 10 Billion Words from 20 Countries, Updated Every Day." Accessed June 3, 2020. www.english-corpora.org/now/.

Enrich, David, Rachel Abrams, and Stephen Kurutz. 2020. "A Sewing Army, Making Masks for America." *New York Times*, March 25. www.nytimes.com/2020/03/25/business/coronavirus-masks-sewers.html.

Farhi, Paul. 2018. "CNN vs. Fox: Why These Two Cable Networks Can't Stop Talking about Each Other." *The Washington Post*, February 28. www.washingtonpost.com/lifestyle/style/cnn-vs-fox-why-these-two-cable-networks-cant-stop-talking-about-each-other/2018/02/27/d30ad4ea-1360–11e8–9065-e55346f6de81_story.html.

Fernando, Alfonso III. 2020. "Why Some People of Color Say They Won't Wear Homemade Masks." *CNN*, April 7. https://edition.cnn.com/2020/04/07/us/face-masks-ethnicity-coronavirus-cdc-trnd/index.html.

Fox News. 2020. www.foxnews.com.

Geggel, Laura. 2020. "Should You Wear a Face Mask to Prevent COVID-19? Experts Disagree." *Fox News*, April 2. www.foxnews.com/science/should-you-wear-a-face-mask-to-prevent-covid-19-experts-disagree.

Johnson, Courtney, Joshua Ferno, and Scott Keeter. 2020. "Few U.S. Adults Say They've Been Diagnosed with Coronavirus, But More Than a Quarter Know Someone Who Has." *Pew Research*, May 26. www.pewresearch.org/fact-tank/2020/05/26/few-u-s-adults-say-theyve-been-diagnosed-with-coronavirus-but-more-than-a-quarter-know-someone-who-has/.

Joyella, Mark. 2020. "Fox News Dominates May Ratings, But CNN Prime Time Jumps 117%." *Forbes*, June 2. www.forbes.com/sites/markjoyella/2020/06/02/fox-news-dominates-may-ratings-but-cnn-prime-time-jumps-117/#740f3aa71e6d.

Kane, Andrea. 2020. "There Aren't Enough Americans Wearing Masks, Coronavirus Researcher Says." August 2. https://edition.cnn.com/world/live-news/coronavirus-pandemic-08-01-20-intl/h_23c591930574b017c6357eba45312bd1.

Kaplan, Talia. 2020. "Surgeon General: Data Doesn't Back Up Wearing Masks in Public Amid Coronavirus Pandemic." *Fox News*, March 31. www.foxnews.com/media/surgeon-general-explains-masks-public-coronavirus.

Klein, Betsy. 2020. "The Average Age of Death from Coronavirus is 80, US Surgeon General Says." *CNN*, March 9. https://edition.cnn.com/asia/live-news/coronavirus-outbreak-03-09-20-intl-hnk/index.html.

Lee, Jennifer. 2020. "Face Masks Could Be Part of the Answer." *CNN*, March 31. https://edition.cnn.com/2020/03/31/opinions/face-masks-part-of-the-answer-lee/index.html.

Liptak, Kevin. 2020a. "Trump Announces New Face Mask Recommendations After Heated Internal Debate." *CNN*, April 4. https://edition.cnn.com/2020/04/03/politics/trump-white-house-face-masks/index.html.

———. 2020b. "White House Task Force Could Soon Recommend Americans Wear Masks." *CNN*, April 1. https://edition.cnn.com/2020/04/01/politics/trump-coronavirus-masks/index.html.

McFall, Caitlin. 2020. "Trump Wears Face Mask in Public for First Time During Coronavirus Pandemic." *Fox News*, July 12. www.foxnews.com/politics/trump-wears-face-mask-in-public-first-time-coronavirus.

McKay, Hollie. 2020. "Coronavirus' Frightening Profile: Who Is More Likely to Die from COVID-19?" *Fox News*, March 31. www.foxnews.com/health/coronavirus-who-is-more-likely-to-die.

Mena, Kelly, and Veronica Stracqualursi. 2020. "Trump Wears a Mask During Visit to Wounded Service Members at Walter Reed." *CNN*, July 12. https://edition.cnn.com/2020/07/11/politics/trump-walter-reed-visit-mask/index.html.

Moore, Mark. 2020. "Surgeon General Jerome Adams Says Wearing Coronavirus Masks Will Give Americans 'More Freedom'." *Fox News*, June 14. www.foxnews.com/health/surgeon-general-jerome-adams-coronavirus-masks-freedom.

O'Reilly, Andrew. 2020. "Pence Deflects on Questions About Wearing Masks, Says White House Will 'Defer to Governors'." *Fox News*, June 28. www.foxnews.com/politics/pence-deflects-on-questions-about-wearing-masks-says-wh-will-defer-to-governors.

Pappas, Alex. 2020. "Trump Says CDC Wants Americans to Cover Faces with Cloth Amid Coronavirus." *Fox News*, April 3. www.foxnews.com/politics/trump-cdc-recommending-face-covering-voluntary.

Pasley, James. 2019. "Fox News and CNN are 2 of America's Biggest News Sources – But They Couldn't Be More Different. Here's How They've Changed in the Past

Decade." *Business Insider*, December 19. www.businessinsider.com/fox-news-cnn-change-evolution-2010-2019-11.

Price, Emily. 2020. "In the Face of an N95 Mask Shortage for Coronavirus Healthcare Workers, Sewists Got to Work." *Fortune*, March 24. https://fortune.com/2020/03/23/n95-mask-shortage-coronavirus-sewists-seamstresses/.

Raju, Manu. 2020. "GOP's no-Mask Caucus: 'Can You Smell Through That Mask?'" *CNN*, May 29. https://edition.cnn.com/2020/05/28/politics/house-republicans-masks-debate-covid/index.html.

Rogers, Everett M. 2010. *Diffusion of Innovations*. 4th ed. New York: The Free Press.

Ryan, Michael J. 2021. "Timeline of the COVID-19 Pandemic." In *COVID-19: Social Consequences and Cultural Adaptations*, edited by J. Michael Ryan, xiii–xxxi. London: Routledge.

Scott, Mike. 2008. "Wordsmith Tools Version 8." Accessed June 3, 2020. www.lexically.net/wordsmith/.

Szreter, Simon, and Michael Woolcock. 2004. "Health by Association? Social Capital, Social Theory, and the Political Economy of Public Health." *International Journal of Epidemiology* 33: 650–67.

Testa, Jessica. 2020. "In Paris, Haute Couture Face Masks for All." *New York Times*, July 7. www.nytimes.com/2020/07/07/fashion/in-paris-haute-couture-face-masks-for-all.html.

Tufekci, Zeynep. 2020. "Why Telling People They Don't Need Masks Backfired." *New York Times*, March 14. www.nytimes.com/2020/03/17/opinion/coronavirus-face-masks.html.

Vaidya, Anuja. 2020. "1 in 8 Americans Know Someone with COVID-19." *Beckers Hospital Review*, April 7. www.beckershospitalreview.com/public-health/1-in-8-americans-know-someone-with-covid-19.html.

Wolf, Zachary B. 2020. "It's Not Maskers vs. Anti-Maskers. It's Public Safety." *CNN*, June 16. https://edition.cnn.com/2020/06/16/politics/what-matters-coronavirus-covid-mask-politics/index.html.

Yan, Holly. 2020. "Want to Prevent Another Shutdown, Save 33,000 Lives and Protect Yourself? Wear a Face Mask, Doctors Say." *CNN*, June 29. https://edition.cnn.com/2020/06/25/health/face-mask-guidance-covid-19/index.html.

Yan, Holly, Natasha Chen, and Dushyant Naresh. 2020. "What's Spreading Faster Than Coronavirus in the US? Racist Assaults and Ignorant Attacks Against Asians." *CNN*, February 21. https://edition.cnn.com/2020/02/20/us/coronavirus-racist-attacks-against-asian-americans/index.html.

13

CHANGING TIMES

New sources of parenting stress and the shifting meanings of time with and for children

Melissa A. Milkie

Time during the COVID-19 pandemic passed before us in an unrecognizable pace and form. During lockdown, our schedules from just weeks earlier became cut off abruptly, with new routines, and lack thereof, suddenly thrust in front of us to make sense of. And our time took on new emotional elements. The year 2020 saw uncertainties and fear color how, with whom, and where we spent our time, as days upon days stretched into a murkier future. What is "quality time" and how can we achieve it? Under the "new normal," what will our time be like? These are among the big questions being asked by scholars, as we march forward into the decade that has begun by upending our time use and our perceptions of time.

For those living with children during the COVID-19 pandemic, questions about how they spend their time are further complicated. Parents are tasked with providing optimal conditions for children's health and development. To the extent possible, most parents try to craft their own and their children's time to maximize children's academic and skill growth, as well as their happiness. Yet pandemic conditions exploded both parents' and children's time use – the normal allocations to work, school, and family – deeply upending schedules and locales. Parents watched children's schedules – even those organized meticulously with an eye toward children's futures – quickly crumble away.

This chapter will analyze parents' pandemic time upheavals, time stressors, and the new meanings of quality time when much work and schooling moved to homes and most parents became isolated alone together with their children. It will focus on three forms of parental time: time spent *with* children at home and in activities out in the social world, time spent *for* children – to meet their material, care, and educational needs, and time spent *toward safeguarding* and managing children's futures. The essay shows that parents' roles became more demanding, while rewards shifted. The pandemic's untethering of children's and families' time provoked questions about the benefits and costs of time allocations, exacerbated class and gender inequalities in parenting, and highlighted the sources of institutional (dis)investments in children's lives.

The upending of family time

The *demands-rewards* theoretical perspective on parents' well-being (Nomaguchi and Milkie 2020) frames this essay. This model emphasizes the shifts in factors influencing parents' mental health and well-being in 2020 once the pandemic hit. In examining demands, in line with stress process theories (Pearlin 1999), the focus is on shifting time-based and other *stressors* parents experience, both objective and subjective, and how these influence parents' levels of *distress*. Individual and institutional resources may buffer parents' stress, though these are unequally distributed, especially by social class. In examining the rewards of parenting, emphasis is upon how new sources of meaning and happiness in time with and for children might unfold during the pandemic and beyond.

The demands-rewards perspective underscores the overarching place of social statuses, and thus variations in the stress process across statuses will be emphasized. For example, socioeconomic status (SES) is a paramount influence on parents' experiences, and thus the time stressors of parents with more versus fewer resources are considered. Work investments vary by SES and occupation, and the pandemic created an uneven shock to parents' work time and conditions. Some parents' work intensified, others lost their jobs and security, and still other parents' work put them on the front lines and at risk of disease, potentially pulling them apart from children for safety reasons (J. W. Cox 2020). SES is also relevant to how parents are able to invest in children. Across the socioeconomic spectrum, parents spend time and energy toward *safeguarding* children's futures, but this takes very different forms. Gender is another key status inequality, with mothers' time and parenting stressors more deeply shocked by the pandemic as they face endless tasks, impacts on their paid work, and worse mental health than fathers (Chung et al. 2020; J. Cox 2020; Gerber 2020; Landivar et al. 2020; Manzo and Minello 2020).

In all, the pandemic upended parents' and children's lives – their work, schooling, and play and their schedules, rhythms, and relationships. Just about all those things that made life normal for children and their families before the pandemic shifted abruptly. From parents' perspectives, important changes may have come to the time they spend with children, the time they allocate for children's provision, and the way they approach safeguarding children's futures. Next, I elaborate on these forms of time and how they have been dramatically altered, making the balance of demands and rewards less favorable for parents, though divergent based on parents' social statuses. I discuss how some time patterns for parents and families may stick across the coming years.

Time with children

In "normal times," many parents felt they had too little time with children, with about half in the US, Canada, and many European countries expressing this sentiment (Milkie, Nomaguchi, and Schieman 2019; Berghammer and Milkie 2020). Suddenly, once the pandemic hit, most parents whose minor children lived with them had nothing *but* time with children. The children's school became home, friends were out of reach for the most part, and for many children, their only young companions were siblings, if they had them. Kids' activities were cancelled, as well as parents' outside leisure time and ways to take breaks away from the unending day-to-day responsibilities they face as parents. Many parents' paid work came home to couches, desks, makeshift spaces across cramped spaces, or more luxurious home offices. Some parents lost jobs, making their at-home time with children more complex, as the future looked less secure. No matter the size of the home, the makeup of the household, the amount of outdoor space, the weather, or the neighborhood, parents' time with children radically changed during the lockdown months – there was more of it – and its qualities may have shifted. Such a sudden transition may have juxtaposed the experiences in a way that made parents especially reflective of the meaning of time with children. While about half of parents had longed for more time with children in the recent past (Berghammer and Milkie 2020; Milkie, Nomaguchi, and Schieman 2019), the kind of time that they suddenly had with children was likely not what they had been envisioning. Indeed, stuck in a "bubble" with children meant high care needs within the household, with limited ability for parents to tap into even those in nearby "bubbles" (Trnka and Davies 2021, this volume) who could help parents out with high demands.

Time spent in the company of children has at least three central qualities under normal times: compared to time apart from children, it is especially enjoyable and it is meaningful, but it can also be stressful and demanding (Negraia and Augustine 2020; Nomaguchi and Milkie 2020; Musick, Meier, and Flood 2016). In the pandemic, each of these became magnified. Taken together, given that parents were stressed from work – either due to overwork and the blurring of work-family boundaries or because jobs themselves were lost or upended, the overall quality of time in the pandemic could be characterized as off and unbalanced. And for single parents with few or perhaps no other adults to pull into children's lives directly due to the pandemic, maintaining quality time with children became even more challenging (Rogers 2020). As the pandemic worsened, with more virus cases in the community and tighter lockdown conditions, the stressful part of time spent with children became more prominent, and the normal feelings of happiness at being together on the part of both parents and children may have felt dampened (Galinsky 1999). How time with children was experienced in terms of its quality for parents and family life became more glaringly obvious as life slowed way, way down, and paradoxically for some, accelerated in terms of time demands.

The pandemic likely made each of these qualities of time with children – stress, enjoyment, and meaningfulness – more deeply felt. In terms of stress, time parents spent for children became fraught as it conflicted with parents' work – spilling directly into the day-to-day interactions parents have with kids. Moreover, the time parents spent with children could easily become conflictual, given the host of new restrictions and guiding behavior that parents needed to enforce with their children. For school-aged kids and teenagers, this meant parents sometimes had to create, maintain, and/or encourage educational connections and activities – really an entirely new ballgame that parents and children had not negotiated in modern times. For the most part, children did not like online schooling, as they felt the deprivation of the richness of in-person lessons and greatly missed their friends and teachers (CBC 2020). Heavily dependent on the quality of the educational experience to begin with, those parents, typically of higher SES, whose kids attended schools that were able to quickly adjust and provide high-quality experiences in real time, were going to experience less stress. In all, for many reasons, then, due to parents' work stresses and overload (Galinsky 1999; Tubbs, Roy, and Burton 2005), the enforcing of educational work for kids that might cause conflicts, and the great amounts of time families spent together with few "real" connections to others outside their household, time with children likely became more stressful – crowding out quality time.

Though time with children had great potential to become more stressful, it also had a potential upside. The new forms and amounts of time could also be quite positive. In terms of feelings of enjoyment and happiness with children, there were fresh possibilities. As the outside social sphere became restricted and some parents found their job pressures were at least temporarily lessened or had commutes evaporate, parents tried new things. Time with children became conducive to sustained blocks of focused or creative time together – like hiking, biking, board games, baking, and the like, if resources allowed. For some, cooking together may have become a high-quality activity to enjoy.[1] Some parents were even able to experience new joys with their children through adopting pets into the family (Kavin 2020). In all, since many of the normal ways of life were suddenly gone – including all the normal extracurriculars like sports and lessons that children participated in, parents were able to (or were forced to) get creative and try new things, thus affecting the quality of time in everyday family life. Quality time often is more of an ideal than a reality, though, even in normal times (Christensen 2002; Daly 2001). To the extent that fears of the virus, stresses from economic fallout, and demands and conflicts parents experienced during their long days at home with children, these joys could get crowded out.

Parents' social class mattered in that lockdowns varied by the resources parents had going into "lockdown." The types of new activities that parents could do with children might have varied based on space – and so how happy versus stressful the time parents experienced with children might follow (Carmona 2020). There were fewer escapes for parents who are in urban areas or small dwellings, as even outside space became extremely difficult to navigate when basic but treasured city playgrounds were off limits. Without vehicles like cars or bikes to get to parks or trails that were conducive to quality time out in nature, some low-resourced urban parents may have been stuck in small places where, over time, it would become more and more difficult to enjoy time together. The quality of time with children was also conditioned by the severity of the outbreak across societies. Extreme examples occurred in regions of China, Italy, and Spain, when parents were completely locked inside with children by government mandates for weeks on end, without the ability to even move outside their apartment or house for fresh air or exercise (Carmona 2020).

Time with children not only might have become, paradoxically, both more stressful and potentially more enjoyable, it may have become more meaningful. Some parents, no doubt, found the extra and different time at home with children a gift – to more fully appreciate their presence and to discuss the world in new ways with their children. This might have been especially true for those with older children and teenagers, wherein parents could have potentially taken advantage of an awareness that they may have just a little time left before offspring move into futures outside the household. Moreover, these teenagers also had their social lives drastically curtailed for a time, allowing them to potentially be fully more available. At the same time, parents may have had more reason for discussion of values, given the major social movements like Black Lives Matter that co-occurred during the pandemic. Moral issues surrounding family, the economy, health care, policing, anti-Black and anti-Asian discrimination (Chiang 2021, this volume), and multiple urgent social problems became central in many families' conversations during these times. Moreover, the value of work, and working from home, became more clear, with many parents expressing hopes of continuing remote work into the future, in part to spend more time with children (Chung et al. 2020). Parents, like other adults, became confronted with what matters in life, the world, and the future – and had new opportunities to share important life lessons with their children – potentially making time with children especially meaningful.

The quality of time *with* children surely changed. Perhaps there was more stressful time with children, but also there may have been more opportunities for unique or new ways to enjoy spending days together. Parents and children alike surely learned lessons about what they value and how they want to spend their time. How "quality" the time with children became depended a great deal on parents' resources – money, work conditions, education level, health, space, and so on. In order to make room for quality time, stressors need to be held at bay (Tubbs, Roy, and Burton 2005). In essence, for the time with children to be high quality during the pandemic, many resources would have had to be already in place, and supports from the larger community, workplace, and government able to be leveraged.

Time for children

The pandemic altered *time for* children, that is the labor it takes to provide the very basics of income and care as parents.[2] Thinking about this within the framework of the demands-rewards perspective, the pandemic tipped the balance, creating more distress among parents. Under normal circumstances, most parents' workloads are very high in total – that is paid and unpaid work hours – because a large part of their lives are given to time for children's provision in the form of direct child care. For most fathers this is typically in the form of many hours on the job, or even taking two jobs to make ends meet given the expenses of children. Mothers do more housework than fathers do, but are also employed at quite high levels, with about two-thirds in the labor force, though this varies across countries (Berghammer and Milkie 2020).

When the pandemic hit, many parents' investments of time for children became greater and more difficult. Most fundamentally, work and care time dedicated to provide for children became a bigger stressor, creating greater distress in the form of work-family conflicts (Chung et al. 2020; Craig and Churchill 2020). For some, work-family conflicts arose as duties from the job, often done remotely from home, directly confronted (new and extra) parental duties (Schieman et al. 2020). Other parents lost jobs, and thus the uncertainties hit hard, given the responsibilities of providing for children and the deep ache of potentially becoming evicted from their home in some countries where social protections were weak. Still other parents were essential workers – and their work became more difficult and exhausting, with added concerns about their own health and their family's health as the possibility of catching the virus was heighted (J. W. Cox 2020).

For one group of parents, typically professionals in more developed countries, the time that they spent for children in paid and unpaid labor was dramatically altered in that paid work moved into telecommuting from home. This then faced direct competition with child care or guided schoolwork that parents become suddenly charged with. A unique feature of the pandemic for parents was the fact that child care and the education of children became fully under their roof. And with few other adults to assist – including teachers who were newly attempting to reach students remotely – this was a complex situation. For a multitude of reasons – technologies, uninterested children, material that did not translate well to online work, parents ended up in the drivers' seats of children's educations – on top of their paid work, if they still had it, resulting in more work-family conflict. This meant to take on the new load of work, parents' mental and physical health could suffer (Chung et al. 2020).

Time parents spent for children during the pandemic also includes another form of labor – that of housework. Here, demands also increased and became more stressful for parents, especially mothers (Chung et al. 2020). During the pandemic, more dishes piled up, shopping became especially fraught and time consuming, and households experienced new levels of use. Perhaps some older children became more involved in helping with household tasks – although for many parents, this may have been offset by difficulties in creating and enforcing new rules for kids, in the midst of the children having to adjust to their own new worlds of the pandemic.

A final key component of parents' time invested for children – what sociologists count as hours of child care in the direct service of children's needs – also increased, sometimes dramatically. Where young children are concerned, this came in the form of direct care that children would have otherwise received from daycares and elementary schools. Babysitters were typically off limits. Parents thus spent countless extra hours in direct care and supervision for especially young children – something that those without children in the home clearly did not have as part of their portfolio – and as noted, a key feature of this extra child time is that it became in direct conflict with paid work. The hours added up – and piled on top of the housework, and alongside the paid work. The collisions across the forms of work undoubtedly formed new types of work-home conflicts for parents (Schieman et al. 2020).

To underscore the severity of how parents' time *for* children was affected by the pandemic, it is important to note that an entire societal institution – that of education – was cut off from the children (and others) it was supposed to serve – and though this was uneven between and within countries, its effects on parents' lives cannot be overstated. Instructional time by schools dropped dramatically and the content often did not include new material. In some countries, after a period of lockdown, they reopened, though with many uncertainties. However, in many other countries, the vast majority of schools did not reopen in spring 2020, or beyond, creating a chasm of months of unstructured time when the educational content provided by schools was minimally engaging to children. Summer camps, which some privileged parents count on for supporting both care and education for children, were also cancelled or went online from home, across the United States, Canada, and other places. Even into the new academic year, for example in the United States, parents' demands stayed high as they had to supervise and supplement time that children normally spent in educational institutions, when many school districts declared school would be online for the new school year. This effectively places the huge educational workload onto parents for months upon months. This was not just a matter of extra hours that exhausted parents faced in educating children – but as will be discussed later, it placed undue strain on how parents across the class spectrum felt able to safeguard children's futures (Milkie and Warner 2014).

In all, the pandemic created a new world in terms of parents' time *for* children – by increasing time demands on parents in terms of child care and especially creating and overseeing the education of their children (Shafer, Scheibling, and Milkie 2020). For mothers more so than fathers, this pushed some of them to reduce hours or leave jobs and careers when things reached a breaking point (Landivar et al. 2020; Qian and Fuller 2020). For single mothers and fathers, often providing the main income for their children, leaving jobs might have been extremely difficult, even when demands became very high (Rogers 2020), and they likely experienced high levels of distress. The pandemic created more stress linked to the provider role too, as some parents had to work from home when children were present, some became laid off, and others had to work in essential jobs, putting themselves and their families at risk. A small portion of parents, though, may have had steady income even with reduced job demands, and short or no commutes such that the amount of time they spent for children's provision stayed similar or possibly was reduced.

Safeguarding: time toward children's futures

Guiding children is much more than the time parents spend directly with them and for them. Raising kids involves a great deal of anticipatory planning work to attempt to assure that children's pathways are smooth as they grow. Children's successes are often marked and celebrated along the way – which they likely enjoy – but these are also a vastly underappreciated form of rewards from the society for parents. In short, the pandemic may have altered this third form of time for some parents – from hopeful to fearful, and from joyous to filled with loss. This parental *time toward* children's futures became emotionally fraught during the pandemic as rewards lessened and uncertainties rose.

Parenting requires great efforts across many years – through infancy, toddlerhood, childhood and adolescence – and toward an imagined future in adulthood. The markers and rituals that a child moves through are normally multifaceted and meaningful. These are both greatly anticipated and marked socially in dramatic and profoundly felt ways, including through organized religions (e.g., bar and bat mitzvahs, confirmations and first communions), through the education system in the form of graduations, awards ceremonies, musical events, and so on – in high school but also middle and elementary school, and even in pre-K. In extracurricular activities, these are capped by playoffs, tournaments, competitions, awards banquets, and the like, with kids from working-class families typically enjoying at least one team or club, and middle- and upper-class children more regularly participating (Lareau 2003). These events serve as markers of a job well done for parents and a time when they are sometimes formally recognized by schools, community organizations, and the like for contributing time toward children's futures.

The anticipation phase related to these markers are vitally important – in essence it helps parents and children persevere and work hard through the many hours of learning that it takes to achieve. These markers are of the work called *status safeguarding* (Milkie and Warner 2014) – the efforts of parents, most often especially mothers, to maintain their child's move toward success and well-being into the child's future. The pandemic cancellations of children's ceremonies and ritual markers were vast – although many moved online or were attempted in unique ways, parents were prevented from observing key, long-anticipated events with their communities – for example, graduations – in the normal, expected, and highly anticipated ways. Instead of the expected community-level joys at a high school graduation, there was sadness and loss associated with distanced or online ceremonies, if they were conducted at all. Instead of hope about the future of the child's next steps, there may have been apprehension or fear (Null 2020).

The work of safeguarding children's futures became harder for parents, as the rest of the world shrunk away and each household was on its own. Relentless days and weeks of feeling alone in their work of guiding children turned to months of parents feeling relatively isolated in their raising of the next generation. Moreover, fears related to children's futures likely increased a great deal, making the time parents spent monitoring, planning, and organizing for children's daily lives and building toward their futures more fraught with questions about whether the future they once expected would look the same. An expected pathway (at least for the globally privileged) – a quality education leading to a college degree and a decent job – appeared increasingly precarious, as education became upended and good jobs – already precarious – became even more so.

Unevenness across social statuses: time inequality and parents' lives

Parents' time with and for children, and their time in working toward children's futures, absolutely and dramatically shifted during the pandemic. But the differences among parents are many, across a number of parents' central statuses. For one – were parents comfortable, income-wise, with a great deal of wealth to support their lifestyle? Or were they just getting by, and perhaps experiencing a loss of income due to a temporary or permanent job loss, to add stress to their provider role? Parents' economic status sharply determined how they experienced time with and for children during the pandemic. Those with large homes, multiple technologies, adequate transportation, and money to buy new things during otherwise economically constrained times would be more easily able to weather the time shifts with their children. Those at the other end of the SES spectrum became at further disadvantage during pandemic times, with lost work or more stressful situations regarding their children's educations evident. Single parents may have been at great risk of both economic precarity and overload from extra time spent on children's provision. In terms of children's futures, wealthier families may have gained even more of an edge as they scrambled to safeguard their children's academic distinctions, talents, and happiness (Milkie and Warner 2014) when pre-pandemic education and extracurricular systems were upended. Thus, parenting inequalities prior to 2020 became exacerbated as the pandemic wore on.

The parental roles of mothers and fathers also mattered a great deal as to how they experienced the work of childrearing in the pandemic. Fathers stepped up their work in the home during the early months, in both housework and child care (Carlson, Petts and Pepin 2020; Craig and Churchill 2020; Shafer, Scheibling, and Milkie 2020). But more so than mothers, fathers might feel the pressures of time *for* children through paid work and how it changed. Mothers also experienced more work occurring through housework, child care, and the education of children (Shafer, Scheibling, and Milkie 2020). As the pandemic continued, and some changes to time with children became entrenched, the direct conflicts with paid work became more glaring. Some parents, but most often mothers, had to reduce their paid work hours or leave the workforce, exacerbating gender inequalities between mothers and fathers (Landivar et al. 2020). Mothers did so in order to manage family life during pandemic times (Qian and Fuller 2020), helping "solve" the problem of demands from children's care and education in the short term, but at potential cost to mothers' own career and future well-being. Will the pandemic mean that it is mothers whose careers become sacrificed, where governments and workplaces cannot prioritize children's care and education? Research from early in the pandemic, such as that by Qian and Fuller (2020), shows that because mothers' work was devalued prior to the pandemic, and due to the wage gap that in part exists because of the care work mothers are pushed to take on, mothers did reduce hours or leave paid work more than fathers did. The pandemic will likely have long-term effects on mothers' care time and in exacerbating gender inequalities (Chung et al. 2020; Craig and Churchill 2020; Landivar et al. 2020).

Changing values: parents' and society's

As the pandemic became enduring over many months, the possibility of redistributions of how, with whom, and where parents spent their time potentially shifted more permanently. As parents weathered the storm of the pandemic, and as they led their children through this difficult time, values related to health, education, and inequalities and how parents spend time became clearer. How does parents' time for children and their futures matter in a society? What is the social response (Ryan 2021, this volume) to the way that the virus has upended children's education and care and parents' lives? It is an underappreciated question – but one that could, and should, be asked more often. How parents' time is important became more obvious during the pandemic as parents scrambled to do it all, including working for pay (if they could maintain their employment) alongside also caring for and guiding, supplementing, and even creating children's education from home. Parents' new stressors in the form of big workloads and exhaustion became glaringly clear. The need for prioritizing education and child care so that parents can distribute their time allocations in a healthy way across paid work and care became more dire in places where parents were most disadvantaged prior to 2020 (Collins 2019; Glass, Simon, and Andersson 2016). A lack of investments in children, and thus in their parents, must be recognized as a structural problem to be addressed (Folbre 2008; Manzo and Minello 2020). How do, and how will, local, state, and federal governments prioritize children and parents, particularly those with fewer means? Will governments invest in supporting high-quality care and educational systems that not only help children but also ease time burdens on parents (Folbre 2008)? Do they recognize the great investments many parents make in terms of time for and with children – both of which have become more stressful and burdensome during the pandemic? Will they support parents, especially those with fewer resources, in investing in children's futures? How do governments help the well-being of this vitally important group raising the next generation?

Conclusion

In all, the unpaid work of parenting has been put into shock, as the juggling of the roles of parent and worker became upended in the pandemic, and normal time schedules and timelines exploded. What were taken-for-granted ways of parenting in many societies at the turn of the decade – parenting that was described as "intensive" (Nomaguchi and Milkie 2020) due to the deep financial and time investments parents made into children – is now even more so. Time spent with and for children took on, and will continue to take on, new forms and meanings. Given parents' time allocations and well-being are relevant not only for themselves but also for the next generation of citizens, assessing the pandemic's shock on parents' time strains and mental health is vital. How societies support parents through the pandemic will have a lasting impact on those currently raising children during this era. More importantly, these supports will also be manifest now and for generations to come through how the children and youth of 2020, and potentially beyond, weather this storm.

Notes

1 However, for parents with few resources, ingredients and time needed to try new recipes may have been scarce. Indeed, for many parents with lower incomes, even feeding their families had to be renegotiated during pandemic times. Given that children's meals had been delivered at school through government or other programs, new routines to obtain regular meals became necessary with school closures (Dunn et al. 2020).
2 There are clearly overlaps between what I distinguish as time *with* and *for* children. I count the basic physical care of young children, which takes large amounts of time, as being part of time provided for children in unpaid care work. Beyond physical care, childcare in the time diary literature (e.g., Musick, Meier, and Flood 2016) also includes teaching, educational activities, and helping children, which became heavy during the pandemic, and I include in this category of time spent for children. Time spent with children includes more of the interactive leisure-like activities, discussed earlier. The lines of time *with* versus *for* children, though, are drawn here only for analytical purposes.

References

Berghammer, Caroline, and Melissa A. Milkie. 2020. "How Much Time with Children Is Enough? Actual Childcare Time and Subjective Perceptions across European Countries." Paper Prepared for the Population Association of America (PAA) Annual Meeting, Washington, DC, April.

Carlson, Daniel L., Richard Petts, and Joanna R. Pepin. 2020. "Changes in Parents' Domestic Labor During the COVID-19 Pandemic." https://doi.org/10.31235/osf.io/jy8fn.

Carmona, Rocio. 2020. "What if They Confine Us Again? Coping with Fear of New Restrictions." *La Vanguardia.* www.lavanguardia.com/vivo/psicologia/20200802/482575966265/confinamiento-afrontar-covid-19.html.

CBC. 2020. "Canadian Kids Bored and Missing Friends in Isolation, New Poll Suggests." www.cbc.ca/news/canada/toronto/canada-covid-children-poll-1.5564425.

Chiang, Pamela P. 2021. "Anti-Asian Racism, Responses, and the Impact on Asian Americans' Lives: A Social-Ecological Perspective." In *COVID-19: Social Consequences and Cultural Adaptations,* edited by J. Michael Ryan, 215–29. London: Routledge.

Christensen, Pia Haudrup. 2002. "Why More 'Quality Time' is Not on the Top of Children's Lists: The 'Qualities of Time' for Children." *Children & Society* 16: 77–88.

Chung, Heejung, Hyojin Seo, Sarah Forbes, and Holly Birkett. 2020. "Working from Home During the COVID-19 Lockdown: Changing Preferences and the Future of Work." https://drive.google.com/file/d/1OoyxkO__fCKzMCnG2Ld14fVI8Hl7xRGe/view.

Collins, Caitlyn. 2019. *Making Motherhood Work: How Women Manage Careers and Caregiving.* Princeton: Princeton University Press.

Cox, John Woodrow. 2020. "What Happens if You and Daddy Die?" *The Washington Post.* www.washingtonpost.com/graphics/2020/local/children-doctors-nurses-coronavirus-death/?tid=graphics-story.

Cox, Josie. 2020. "New Research Shows Covid-19's Impact on Gender Inequality and Mothers' Mental Health." *Forbes.* www.forbes.com/sites/josiecox/2020/07/30/covid-19-gender-equality-mental-health-working-mothers-flexible-working/#7f600251e4a5.

Craig, Lyn, and Brendan Churchill. 2020. "Dual-Earner Parent Couples' Work and Care during Covid-19." *Gender, Work and Organization.* https://doi.org/10.1111/gwao.12497.

Daly, Kerry J. 2001. "Deconstructing Family Time: From Ideology to Lived Experience." *Journal of Marriage and Family* 63: 283–94.

Dunn, Caroline G., Erica Kenney, Sheila E. Fleischhacker, and Sara N. Bleich. 2020. "Feeding Children During the COVID-19 Pandemic." *New England Journal of Medicine.* www.nejm.org/doi/full/10.1056/NEJMp2005638.

Folbre, Nancy. 2008. *Valuing Children: Rethinking the Economics of the Family.* Cambridge: Harvard University Press.

Galinsky, Ellen. 1999. *Ask the Children: What America's Children Really Think About Working Parents.* New York: William Morrow and Company.

Gerber, Cassie. 2020. "The Lockdown is Damaging Mental Health but Only for Women." *Quartz.* https://qz.com/1853394/lockdown-is-damaging-mental-health-but-only-for-women/.

Glass, Jennifer, Robin W. Simon, and Matthew A. Andersson. 2016. "Parenthood and Happiness: Effects of Work-Family Reconciliation Policies in 22 OECD Countries." *American Journal of Sociology* 122 (3): 886–929.

Kavin, Kim. 2020. "Dog Adoptions and Sales Soar During the Pandemic." *The Washington Post* www.washingtonpost.com/nation/2020/08/12/adoptions-dogs-coronavirus/.

Landivar, Liana Christin, Leah Ruppanner, William J. Scarborough, and Caitlyn Collins. 2020. "Early Signs Indicate That COVID-19 Is Exacerbating Gender Inequality in the Labor Force." *Socius: Sociological Research for a Dynamic World.* https://journals.sagepub.com/doi/10.1177/2378023120947997.

Lareau, Annette. 2003. *Unequal Childhoods: Class, Race, and Family Life.* Berkeley: University of California Press.

Manzo, Lidia Katia C., and Alessandra Minello. 2020. "Mothers, Childcare Duties, and Remote Working under COVID-19 Lockdown in Italy: Cultivating Communities of Care." *Dialogues in Human Geography* https://journals.sagepub.com/doi/full/10.1177/2043820620934268.

Milkie, Melissa A., and Catharine H. Warner. 2014. "Status Safeguarding: Mothers' Work to Secure Children's Place in the Status Hierarchy." In *Intensive Mothering: The Cultural Contradictions of Modern Motherhood*, edited by Linda Ennis, 66–85. Bradford, ON: Demeter Press.

Milkie, Melissa A., Kei Nomaguchi, and Scott Schieman. 2019. "Time Deficits with Children: The Link to Parents' Mental and Physical Health." *Society and Mental Health* 9: 277–95.

Musick, Kelly, Ann Meier, and Sarah Flood. 2016. "How Parents Fare: Mothers' and Fathers' Subjective Well-being in Time with Children." *American Sociological Review* 81 (5): 1069–95.

Negraia, Daniela Veronica, and Jennifer March Augustine. 2020. "Unpacking the Parenting Well-Being Gap: The Role of Dynamic Features of Daily Life across Broader Social Contexts." *Social Psychology Quarterly*. doi.org/10.1177/0190272520902453.

Nomaguchi, Kei, and Melissa A. Milkie. 2020. "Parenthood and Well-Being: A Decade in Review." *Journal of Marriage and Family* 82: 198–223.

Null, Christopher. 2020. "The Reality of Covid-19 is Hitting Teens Especially Hard." *Wired*. www.wired.com/story/covid-19-is-hitting-teens-especially-hard/.

Pearlin, Leonard I. 1999. "The Stress Process Revisited." In *Handbook of the Sociology of Mental Health*, edited by C. S. Aneshensel and J. C. Phelan, 395–415. Boston, MA: Springer.

Qian, Yue, and Sylvia Fuller. 2020. "COVID-19 and the Gender Employment Gap Among Parents of Young Children." *Canadian Public Policy*. DOI: 10.3138/cpp.2020-077.

Rogers, Kristen. 2020. "Frosted Flakes for Dinner. Hiding in the Laundry Room. This is Life for Single Moms Right Now." *CNN*. www.cnn.com/2020/05/08/health/single-mom-challenges-mothers-day-coronavirus-wellness/index.html.

Ryan, J. Michael. 2021. "The SARS-CoV-2 Virus and the COVID-19 Pandemic." In *COVID-19: Social Consequences and Cultural Adaptations*, edited by J. Michael Ryan, 9–19. London: Routledge.

Schieman, Scott, Philip J. Badawy, Melissa A. Milkie, and Alex Bierman. 2020. "Work-Life Conflict During the Covid-19 Pandemic." http://dx.doi.org/10.13140/RG.2.2.32315.44329.

Shafer, Kevin, Casey Scheibling, and Melissa A. Milkie. 2020. "The Division of Domestic Labour Before & During the COVID-19 Pandemic in Canada: Stagnation vs. Shifts in Fathers' Contributions." *Canadian Review of Sociology* 57 (4).

Trnka, Susanna, and Sharyn Graham Davies. 2021. "Blowing Bubbles: Covid-19, New Zealand's Bubble Metaphor, and the Limits of Households as Sites of Responsibility and Care." In *COVID-19: Global Pandemic, Social Responses, Ideological Solutions*, edited by J. Michael Ryan, 167–83. London: Routledge.

Tubbs, Carolyn Y., Kevin M. Roy, and Linda M. Burton. 2005. "Family Ties: Constructing Family Time in Low-Income Families." *Family Process* 44: 77–91.

14

SITES OF SILENCE

Deaf online communication in the time of corona

Marilyn Plumlee

As the COVID-19 virus spread around the globe in the spring of 2020, confinement protocols dramatically reduced face-to-face interaction opportunities for the majority of the world's population. The resulting social isolation led to a surge in use of the internet as it became a lifeline for people searching for virus-related medical information and for sources of financial support, food, and essential supplies, along with entertainment and leisure-time distractions. It also became the lifeline for those seeking to stay socially connected to their network of friends and family. For one group of people – the Deaf[1] – the opportunities afforded by the internet to communicate with other Deaf people during this crisis became even more significant. Under the best of circumstances, due to communication barriers resulting from the inaccessibility of audio input, Deaf people have less access to information than hearing people have. Under imposed COVID-19 quarantine regimes, movement restrictions created additional barriers to accessible information sources and reduced opportunities to meet with people sharing the same language who could provide missing information as well as social support. The increasingly strict restrictions on normal modes of interaction as news of the severity of the pandemic's spread threatened to lead to a heightened sense of isolation. These circumstances motivated tech-savvy Deaf people to turn to an online platform for support from other Deaf people.

This study thus focuses on the online communication among a group of Deaf adults in Kazakhstan in the spring of 2020 as the spread of coronavirus accelerated. There were nine participants, all friends who interacted socially offline when not under lockdown. After the introduction of confinement regulations in March 2020, they established a support group on the WhatsApp platform, which they called "Antistress." They collectively posted 14,066 messages between March 28 and July 4, 2020, the period of this study, at a rate of sometimes over 500 messages per day during peak periods of concern and stress.

This study analyzes the themes expressed in these messages as well as the social interaction moves engaged in, focusing on two aspects of the group's interactions: what aspects of the COVID-19 crisis were most salient for participants and emerged discursively in their "Antistress" group, and what the "Deaf" *habitus* is in their communicative practices.

Cross-border and international communication

The worldwide pandemic has introduced a sense of shared collective experience among much of the world's population. That same sense pervades Deaf communities. Even prior to the spread of the coronavirus, Deaf people were communicating transnationally both in real spaces where international Deaf events were convened and in cyber spaces. The vocabulary of the national sign languages varies by country, but there are a sufficient number of grammatical features shared in the visual modality that proficient signers can improvise an *ad hoc* form of communication known as International Sign (IS) that leads to extended communication within minutes of first contact. (For further discussion of international Deaf spaces and International Sign, see Supalla and Webb 1995; Moody 1987, 2002; Plumlee 2009; Hiddinga and Crasborn 2011; Green 2014; Crasborn and Hiddinga 2015; Friedner and Kusters, eds. 2015.)

This intelligible cross-linguistic signed code (IS) that fluent signers can generate after a brief exposure and without lengthy formal instruction accounts for the ability of Kazakh Deaf signers, particularly those with prior experience meeting signers who do not use Russian Sign Language (RSL), to largely comprehend signed recordings posted in IS, albeit with gaps in understanding some specific signs.

Theoretical framework

One might reasonably ask the purpose of studying a minority representing just over 6% of the world's population (www.who.int/pbd/deafness/estimates/en/) and whose members struggle to be recognized by the majority culture due to significant linguistic and attitudinal barriers. With so many people suffering worldwide in the era of COVID-19, do the perspectives of Deaf Kazakhs have something to contribute to the worldwide discussion on how to deal with the current or predicted challenges of the post-COVID-19 period? The answer to this question lies in the position one takes on the value of human diversity and human rights for minorities. If we concede that studying the planet's human diversity is an intrinsically worthwhile endeavor and that all minorities have a right to be shown respect and a right to realize their full potential, then yes – the Deaf minority's contribution to an examination of the full spectrum of human diversity has a rightful place at the discussion forum. Note that the estimated number of deaf people in the world in 2020 (466 million) surpasses the total estimated population of the United States (331 million). In an era when the COVID-19 pandemic has revealed stark individual and societal vulnerabilities (see Nanda 2021), there is a growing recognition that more attention needs to be given to equitable treatment of heretofore marginalized citizens. In this era of increased sensitization, the time is certainly right to ensure that the realities of Deaf lives are also portrayed.

Furthermore, as Ryan (2021, this volume) stated, one of the goals of this volume is to unveil individual and social inequalities. This study, then, hopes to shed light on the experiences of members of a Deaf community as they navigate the uncertainties of the coronavirus pandemic from their vantage point of a vibrant but often misunderstood linguistic and cultural minority and to make that community more accessible and more relatable to members of the majority culture.

Underscoring the importance of documenting the Deaf experience during the pandemic, two scholars who conducted an exhaustive review of the research on sign languages and deaf experiences in several countries had this to say about the relevance of studying deaf cultures:

> Anthropological studies show us that deafness impinges on many aspects of human activity. Furthermore, studies involving deaf people reveal issues of general anthropological significance, even to those who may not (yet) have particular interest in issues of deafness. For example, social organization, identity, culture, ideology, and sociolinguistic variation are all issues [of concern]. The social implications of deafness are often counterintuitive and merit more than commonsense assessments. Deafness is, at least in part, a social construction.
>
> *(Senghas and Monaghan 2002, 70)*

To determine the Deaf cultural norms of interaction that the participants oriented to in their postings to the WhatsApp group, two key principles of the ethnography of communication were utilized, i.e., observation of topics raised for discussion by the group members and attitudes toward these topics. An ethnographic approach to the Deaf group's communication was opted for, since, as Saville-Troike (1989, 107–8) has stated, "[o]bserved behavior is now recognized as a manifestation of a deeper set of codes and rules, and the task of ethnography is seen as the discovery and explication of the rules for contextually appropriate behavior in a community or group." In addition to the ethnographic framework that focuses on behavioral moves in established communities, to ascertain the salient aspects of the group's engagement with the COVID-19 pandemic, the study used discourse analysis as a complementary approach, which emphasizes the linguistic component of an interaction.

Design of the study: participants, data, and research methods

The participants

The participants all reside in Kazakhstan and they had all been living in the capital city of Nur-Sultan (formerly known as Astana) prior to the outbreak of the pandemic. During the coronavirus quarantine period, several returned to their hometowns in other regions of Kazakhstan. Other than the author of this study, the participants in the WhatsApp group consisted of nine individuals, eight of whom are deaf: three women and five men. The ninth member of the group is a trilingual hearing woman who has deaf parents, i.e., she is a native RSL signer and speaks both Russian and Kazakh. The hearing woman works as a professional interpreter in the local deaf community but is also a personal friend of the deaf members of the WhatsApp group and socializes with them outside of her professional role as a community interpreter. The nine participants range in age from 22 to 35.

The basis of my relationship to the group is that I am proficient in American Sign Language (ASL) and International Sign (IS) and have an international circle of Deaf friends. I have been learning Russian Sign Language through contact with the local Deaf community in Kazakhstan for approximately one year, which afforded me "guest status" within the group. I functioned primarily as an observer and only occasionally actively participated in group discussions.

In their postings, the Deaf group members use both written Russian, the language in which they were educated, and Russian Sign Language (RSL). Because RSL is also the sign language used by Deaf people in Russia and in other former Soviet Central Asian Republics as well as in several countries of Eastern Europe, the Kazakh Deaf have access not only to their own Kazakhstan-based support group, but also to a large pool of Deaf RSL signers who regularly post on Instagram, YouTube, or other social media platforms. RSL thus serves as a lingua franca across national boundaries and connects Kazakh Deaf people to an international pool of Deaf interlocutors and bloggers.

Seven of the nine group members posted actively to the group, usually on a daily basis. Over the 14 weeks of the study, the group generated a total of 14,066 postings, i.e., the WhatsApp group was intensively used by the members to communicate with each other while under varying stages of lockdown.

The data: general description

The main corpus consists of the 14,066 postings to the WhatsApp group called "Antistress," which was initially launched on March 3, 2020, by one of the members of the Deaf community of Nur-Sultan. On March 28, the founder of the group invited me to join them. Most of the members of the group were already acquainted with me, and we had previously interacted socially several times in offline contexts. I did not initially intend to analyze the postings on the WhatsApp group to which I had been invited, but several days after joining the group, I realized that the conversations presented a unique opportunity to document how the coronavirus pandemic was being experienced by individuals in an underdocumented culture-specific group. After obtaining general consent from the founder of the group to analyze the messages for publication, and after approval from my institutional review board, I then obtained consent from the group members to proceed with the analysis of their postings. The data consist of postings to this group beginning from March 28 through July 4, 2020. Of the 14,066 postings, the majority (8,885) consists of the members' own written text messages, usually written in Russian in a cryptic shorthand style in a bantering, informal conversational register. The remaining 5,181 postings are in various multimedia formats, which can be divided into three categories: (1) still images, consisting of emojis, selfies, forwarded GIFs, or scenes they encountered in their daily lives and recorded on their own phones; (2) filmed scenes of daily life during the pandemic such as flooded streets, dinner gatherings with friends, police raids on noncompliant public gatherings during the confinement period, and forwarded postings from international websites, usually of a humorous nature; and (3) messages in sign language, i.e., "selfie"-style uploaded videos.

The corpus contains 1,101 messages in sign language, which can be further subdivided into two groups: (1) messages in sign language that the members recorded of themselves (486) and (2) forwarded sign language recordings originally posted by Deaf people in other countries (615). Postings from other countries usually originated from within the former Soviet-influenced sphere and were usually signed in RSL, although occasionally the members posted sign language videos recorded in International Sign or other sign languages.

A number of the uploaded media postings contained audio tracks in spoken Russian lacking written titles or captions, which would have rendered them fully accessible to Deaf viewers. However, these uploaded clips were visually humorous and could therefore be enjoyed by a deaf viewer without relying on the audio track. The presence of these Russian language clips with audio soundtrack is a clear indication that the participants were browsing Russian-language websites beyond those created by and for Deaf people.

The research methods

The corpus of 14,066 messages was downloaded and archived. The 8,885 written Russian texts were translated into English using an automatic translation application. The 5,181 multimedia texts, of which 1,101 were in sign language, were preserved in their original format so that they could be consulted for content relevance. Postings mentioning the coronavirus situation or that reflected a Deaf perspective were culled from the corpus. Signed messages were also reviewed to ensure that their thematic content would be included in the categories retained for analysis. The selected texts were then categorized and coded for further analysis, a summary of which is presented in this study.

To determine the norms of Deaf culture appearing in the data, a triangulated method was used: (1) explicit mention of deaf-related experiences in group members' postings, (2) review of the published literature on Deaf culture norms by both hearing and Deaf authors (see, *inter alia*, Lane 1984; Padden and Humphries 1988; Wilcox, ed. 1989; Ladd 2003; Pursglove and Komarova 2003; Bauman, ed. 2008;

Ladd 2003), and (3) reliance on my own familiarity with multigenerational Deaf communities, gained from years-long relationships with Deaf people in several countries.

The next section will present findings of the study, in response to the two main questions the study was designed to answer:

1   What are the responses and reactions to the coronavirus pandemic in this community, and
2   what is "Deaf" about interactions within this group of Deaf people?

Findings: emergent themes

The themes emerging in the data are presented in two sections, with illustrative examples from the corpus: (1) themes related to the pandemic and (2) themes reflective of Deaf perspectives.

The discussion threads related to the pandemic centered on the five following themes:

1   Medical questions and infection rates
2   Government announcements: lockdown measures; procedures for obtaining government subsistence payments
3   Employment
4   Apprehension, frustrations, complaints, suffering, and sorrow
5   Displays of socializing and relaxing despite COVID lockdown or during periods of loosened restrictions

The discussion threads reflecting Deaf-specific concerns fall into the following seven categories:

6   Group solidarity (care, support, and affection)
7   Language and communication: literacy and information gaps; seeking explanations from other Deaf
8   Accessibility issues; misunderstandings with hearing people
9   Seeking or offering pandemic-related help
10 Social responsibility and assistance to others (non-group members)
11 Miscellaneous topics of conversation
12 International network of online resources in sign language

While the research questions are separated into two separate categories (pandemic-related and Deaf-related), the two themes in some cases overlap as when sharing pandemic-related information from international sources in sign language or relying on a trusted hearing person to provide information about how to obtain government subsistence payments.

Pandemic-related themes

Related to theme (1) "Medical questions and infection rates," the group members were active in searching out and sharing information throughout the spring and on into the summer of 2020. This usually took the form of uploaded lists from internet sites detailing the number of daily infections in the world or in regions of Kazakhstan. These basic facts were not readily accessible to all members of the group, particularly in intermittent periods when a local television station cancelled sign language interpretation of the evening newscasts, which led to low viewership by the Deaf. On key dates in the pandemic, when high infection rates due to the virus or death toll counts in Kazakhstan were announced, or when tightening, loosening, or further restricting of the confinement measures were announced, there would be an increase in the postings and comments on this topic.

The comments related to theme (2) "Government announcements: lockdown measures; procedures for obtaining subsistence payments" and theme (3) "Employment" were more frequent at the beginning of the period under study, as these deaf citizens, along with other Kazakhstanis, tried to determine if they qualified for the government support programs being launched. These extracts illustrate the tendency of Deaf people to reach out to and rely on other Deaf people or a trusted hearing person who signs to provide them with accurate information, since communication is often frustratingly incomplete or imprecise with hearing members of their families. One of the key issues during the pandemic was to know the specific amount of subsistence payments that people with disabilities would receive and whether it was based on their employment status.

The postings related to theme (4) "Apprehension, frustrations, complaints, suffering, and sorrow" all document the emotions the group members were experiencing during the period, particularly at the beginning when people in Nur-Sultan were under a strict lockdown order and were not yet accustomed to staying home for long periods of time. Utterances like "it's the end of the world," "I lost my mind bored at home," "we cannot sit at home, going mad," and "as if everyone is sitting under house arrest, it is horrible" indicate the level of frustration experienced. Other statements contain slightly more upbeat and practical attitudes to the restrictions, with members suggesting positive perspectives on the mandated movement restrictions (e.g., "think of your mom and dad," "lucky to walk," "maybe you can call people you know" [to find out if service stations are open]).

For theme (5) "Socializing and relaxing despite COVID lockdown or during periods of loosened restrictions," the corpus contains many examples of jocularity and humor in the group. In one posting, the members are playfully telling each other what they are dreaming of eating or doing whenever the lockdown is lifted. One says he misses going to KFC, another dreams of eating raw fish, and yet another asks when they can all go eat shashlik, to which the joking response is "you'll lie on the sofa like the Sultan of Turkey."

Deaf-related themes

The excerpts illustrating theme (6) "Group solidarity" demonstrate the strong bonds of friendship and affection between the group members. Their feelings are sometimes expressed with great seriousness and solemnity: "I feel like I will die soon" or "Guys, I love you all . . . If I die remember this . . . I forgive everyone, and forgive me, my fav people," when referring to their anxiety and the very real possibility of dying in the context of the coronavirus pandemic. In another posting, group members are telling the hearing woman that she should protect her health and not get exposed to the virus by going to work as an interpreter, to which she replies that she is under government orders to continue to work in spite of the risks: "just telling you that I love you. What can I do? It is my job."

The corpus contains several threads related to theme (7) "Language and communication: literacy and information gaps; seeking explanations from other Deaf," and it is here where the sensitive issue of limited literacy and general knowledge emerges. The striking feature of these examples is that the people involved, communicating within a safe "Deaf space," display no embarrassment or hesitation to ask for help. The more informed or more literate members step up immediately to perform their expected roles of providing support to those who have asked for explanations, as in the following example: One member has been told that he needs a cholesterol blood test for pain in his legs, to which he responds, "To be honest, for the first time I see the words of cholesterol well what is it," to which a female member responds succinctly: "Cholesterol can get sick, bile and fat. There are two kinds – good and bad."

Corpus excerpts illustrating theme (8) "Accessibility issues; misunderstandings with hearing people" were generally fewer in number and more placid and non-confrontational than I had anticipated, accustomed as I am to interacting with more "activist" Deaf in other countries who have much greater legal entitlement to access and are more outspoken in expecting accommodation to Deaf communication needs. In the corpus under study, there were relatively few expressions of frustration at dealing with the hearing world, possibly because everyone was under more or less stringent lockdown orders and therefore had fewer face-to-face contacts and communicative encounters with hearing people outside their personal network.

On theme (9) "Seeking or offering pandemic-related help," several threads were initiated in the corpus. In late June, when lockdown measures were relaxed, several of the members took trips to lakes within driving distance and posted pictures of themselves wading in the water. In Nur-Sultan at that time, it had become difficult to obtain certain medicines to treat symptoms of COVID-19 or "pneumonia" as it was being labelled. When one member heard that two other group members were staying for a few days in another town, she asked them to try to buy packages of paracetamol for her. That text thread, accompanied by images of the needed product, stretched over several days as the search continued. The efforts of the travelers were in vain, as pharmacies in the small town were also out of stock. However, several of the group members persevered on behalf of their friend, inquiring at various pharmacies. Eventually one person managed to obtain the medicine, although in limited quantity because there were restrictions on how much one customer could buy.

A unique deaf-centric pandemic-related thread that showed up in the corpus was images of special "masks for deaf." One such mask manufactured in Indonesia was featured on the German news channel DW (Deutsche Welle) and was apparently widely shared among Deaf people worldwide. One person in the WhatsApp group forwarded the news item, which featured a see-through transparent window around the mouth area to enable lip-reading. From Spain, an image of a another deaf-specific mask was uploaded to the group displaying the words "Soy Sordo" in Spanish (*I am deaf*) on one half of the mask and the international symbol of deafness on the other half, alerting hearing people that the deaf mask-wearer would not be able to communicate if the hearing person's mouth were covered with a mask.

Deaf people are said to live in a "Deaf world," but the WhatsApp group members clearly display their sense of belonging to a wider world as well. Illustrating theme (10) "Social responsibility and assistance to others (non-group members)," a female member states she does not want to engage with the group that day, saying "April 1 is a day of jokes [but] I understand clearly the pain for Italy and China and the world has taken a lot of people from life. I don't want to laugh on April 1st. At least the coronavirus would go away would be better. Laughter is not my day today."

Another thread related to social responsibility emerges when a male member mentions having talked for the first time with a homeless person. He says he feels sorry for the homeless and "I will help giving them 200 tg at least" ("tg" stands for tenge, the Kazakh currency). A female joins the thread, recounting how she too had given money to a homeless person:

> I waited for the bus in winter, it was cold here. I saw the homeless person he didn't have money. People didn't stop and then he asked everyone money for the bus. I had my last 500 tenge. I gave it to him and he was very grateful.

She goes on to say that someone who had seen her act of kindness then offered her 500 tg, which shocked her because, as she says, "it was my help" to give to the homeless person. The female member does not say so, but it seems that the other bus passenger, having noticed that a deaf person had given money to the homeless person, then "took pity" on her as a deaf person and gave her the equivalent amount, which shocked her because she does not consider herself needy and she is certainly not a beggar.

Under theme (11) "Miscellaneous topics of conversation," many topics were raised in the group over the 14 weeks. These topics reflect the embeddedness of the WhatsApp group members in the local Central Asian culture and their knowledge and engagement with the Kazakh cultural context. One posting clearly reflected the status of Kazakhstan as a former Soviet republic familiar with Soviet film productions when a member uploaded a brainteaser consisting of emoticons symbolizing old Soviet movies, asking other group members to figure out the references. Another example of the prevalence of the Soviet legacy in Kazakhstan occurred when the hearing woman posted to the group saying she had "goosebumps" while interpreting WWII films commemorating Victory Day (celebrated annually on May 9). When asked to explain, she briefly recounted the film contents as being "the story how Hitler attacked, how the CIA informed Stalin, how Kazakhstan people suffered" for the USSR's war effort. Another thread discussed some negative Kazakh perceptions of Uzbek cultural practices such as bride "kidnapping" and a preference for sons over daughters, cultural practices which one member reminded the group are actually still found in modern Kazakhstan. On other days, similar to the worldwide trend during the pandemic confinement period, group members showed videos of home food preparation and discussed their preferred regional or family specialties.

With respect to theme (12) "International network of online resources," most of the evidence of the WhatsApp group members' engagement with Deaf people in other countries can be found in the forwarded multimedia posts to the group to be viewed as images. Many of the forwarded images or recordings originated with Deaf signers using RSL, from either Russia or other RSL-using countries under the influence of the former Soviet Union. Posts from further afield included images of Indonesian Deaf women making masks with transparent windows enabling Deaf people to read lip movements or see facial expressions. Uploads from abroad also included blogs by Deaf people from India talking about problems of child labor and by Deaf people from the Arab world explaining their situation during the pandemic. Other posts consisted of humorous videos from international Deaf signers – possibly of the "fake news" variety – talking about such topics as killer insects, marital relations, or unusual – perhaps staged – street events in their countries.

Illustrative of online pandemic-era initiatives providing new opportunities for Deaf people to socialize within a signing, accessible platform was the show "Kitchen," live-streamed on May 30, 2020, featuring two Deaf performers. Andrey Dragunov, a Deaf Moscow-based Russian performer known as "Finger Dancer," and Igor Sapega, a London-based professional Deaf chef, teamed up to offer a transnational participatory cooking class. Andrey functioned as the emcee, chatting in IS with international Deaf viewers, while Igor's Ukrainian wife Laura coordinated communication from London with Andrey and the international participants in several sign languages.

During the pandemic's strict confinement period when people were unable to attend cultural events, locked-down hearing audiences worldwide were able to enjoy musicians and artists presenting impressive synchronized home-based, live-streamed opera performances or concerts. In the Deaf world, however, there had been no event equivalent to the live-streamed concerts available for hearing people until the cooking show debuted. International Deaf festivals previously scheduled to be held in the USA, Egypt, and Kyrgyzstan in 2020, the equivalent of cultural and sporting events in the hearing world, were cancelled for the remainder of the year.

This live cooking show, created in response to strict pandemic lockdown measures, was a significant event for the Deaf worldwide. The event attracted 2,253 viewers in real time and the recorded version had received over 18,000 views on Instagram as of August 2020. This Deaf-accessible visual space with entertaining content offered Deaf people, including Kazakh Deaf viewers, a unique opportunity to experience international connections online as a substitute for cancelled offline events.

A stellar example of the international communication network among Deaf people occurred on the final day of data collection, July 4, 2020. On that day, a compelling post was forwarded by one of the Kazakh WhatsApp group members, which provides a fitting conclusion to this study of how these nine members of the Kazakh Deaf community experienced the spring 2020 coronavirus pandemic. The post featured a young Deaf man lying on a bed in Bishkek, Kyrgyzstan, while being supplied with oxygen through a nose tube. The young man was obviously distressed and had a fearful look on his face as he labored to sign a warning message in RSL from his sick bed, indicating his emotional stress over his illness and repeatedly telling all Deaf people how important it is to wear a mask to protect themselves and to protect others from catching the virus. He concluded by saying he was fighting the virus and hoping for the best. Reactions from the Kazakh WhatsApp group upon seeing this video were to repost it again within the group and to make comments on it ranging from "horror" to "no words."

The video recorded by this COVID-infected Deaf man served to underscore the ultimate danger threatening the well-being of everyone during the pandemic period. Hearing people had regularly been seeing and hearing such testimonies of infected people on a daily basis through the media, but on this occasion the group members were exposed to a vivid personal account in sign language by a Deaf person. The posting brought home the reality of suffering experienced by someone who catches the virus.

Thus this signed video message originating in Kyrgyzstan, sent to a circle of that infected man's Deaf friends, who then forwarded it to their own circle of Deaf friends, ultimately including the unspecified Deaf friend who forwarded the message to a member of the "Antistress" group in Kazakhstan, who in turn posted it to his own friends in the Nur-Sultan Deaf community, dramatically underscores the sense of connectivity of Deaf people in ever-expanding circles of friendship and mutual support.

Conclusion

Although this WhatsApp group cannot be taken as representative of all Deaf people in Kazakhstan, the data suggest that Kazakhstani Deaf conform to many cross-national Deaf cultural norms, primary among which is proficiency in their national sign language rather than the majority spoken language as their primary and most efficient means of daily communication. However, they are clearly sufficiently literate in written Russian to rely on text messages for approximately 63% of their postings in this online medium, the remainder of which consisted of uploaded images or recorded video messages in Russian Sign Language.

Because this study was conducted in the context of the COVID-19 pandemic, there was an undercurrent of stress and uncertainty present in many of the postings. This context naturally gave rise to numerous instances in which Deaf in-group solidarity was in evidence. Deaf in-group solidarity extended to encompass forwarded postings to the WhatsApp group of information made available online by Deaf people in other countries regarding precautionary measures to take. Whether such outreach to foreign sources of information would be a normal reaction for members of this group when not under the stress generated by the pandemic is an open question. Within the group itself, the content and style of the postings reflects a significant degree of trust in and reliance on each other and Deaf-enculturated hearing friends to provide access to up-to-date information. This was particularly evident in pandemic-related questions such as following the ever-increasing rates of infection and mortality, staying informed about constantly evolving government lockdown measures in response to infection and hospitalization rates, and finding out how to obtain government subsistence payments or distribution of free food.

In addition, content of the group's 14,066 postings over the four-month period provided ample evidence of group members' willingness to support each other emotionally on days when anxiety, uncertainty, confinement fatigue, or concern over unwell family members suspected of being infected with the coronavirus caused high levels of psychological duress.

The interactions documented under both the pandemic-related themes and the Deaf culture themes are all indicative of what Buzolits et al. (2021) term "prosocial behaviors," i.e., positive responses at the interpersonal level in the service of "trauma stewardship." These interactions also provide examples of negative responses, which Buzolits et al. (2021) classify as "trauma exposure responses." The most salient of these in the corpus were feelings of helplessness and hopelessness, minimizing one's own situation compared to the suffering of others, hypervigilant activities such as frequently paying attention to media coverage of infection rates and death tolls, uploading of purportedly humorous but often grim or gruesome video scenes as a distraction from the tedium of daily life under lockdown measures, and expressions of grief and loss.

As this chapter goes to press in the latter half of 2020, the WhatsApp group, which was the primary focus of the study, continues to actively function. The number of infected cases is on the rise around the world. In Kazakhstan, the public health situation is still worrisome as of the time of writing as hospitals have reached bed capacity and testing capacity has been depleted. Nur-Sultan, Almaty, and other urban centers are under a new wave of restrictions in an effort to contain the spread of the virus. International border controls are still in place, as is intercity travel. While the sense of solidarity and mutual support among this group seems solid, how the members of the group will weather the pandemic collectively over an extended period remains to be seen. Based on the continuing flow of messages, it appears they are creating their own "pandemic bubble," i.e., a circle of trusted friends with whom they occasionally interact offline as the pandemic persists and confinement protocols remain in place.

To my knowledge, this is the first study of any aspect of the Kazakhstani Deaf community published in English. The field is thus wide open for future studies to constitute a baseline of information about the country's Deaf communities. Surveys of the Deaf population and their educational and employment status would be a starting point, but finer-grained ethnographic studies of the social, cultural, and personal networks would also reveal much about the lives of Deaf Kazakhstanis.

The most critical need appears to be for a committed constellation of engaged Kazakhstani Deaf community members to coalesce around the goal of collectively asserting their needs and aspirations within the appropriate political context of their country. If collaboration with academic researchers and a sense of ownership of the results of that research can serve to ignite such a spark among the Deaf of Kazakhstan, then scholars will have served not only the valid purpose of dissemination of knowledge but also the higher purpose of facilitating access to human rights.

Note

1 It is customary to refer to Deaf people with a capitalized "D" in English when referring to individuals who consider themselves members of a cultural group rather than as patients with a deficiency to be "cured" by medical professionals. The term "deaf," written with a lowercase "d," refers only to the medical diagnosis of hearing loss.

References

Bauman, H-Dirksen L., ed. 2008. *Open Your Eyes. Deaf Studies Talking*. Minneapolis: University of Minnesota Press.

Buzolits, Johanna, Ann Abbey, Kate Kittredge, and Ann E. C. Smith. 2021. "Managing Trauma Exposure and Developing Resilience in the Midst of COVID-19." In *COVID-19: Global Pandemic, Societal Responses, Ideological Solutions*, edited by J. Michael Ryan, 209–20. London: Routledge.

Crasborn, Onno, and Anja Hiddinga. 2015. "The Paradox of International Sign: The Importance of Deaf-Hearing Encounters for Deaf-Deaf Communication across Sign Language Borders." In *It's a Small World: International Deaf Spaces and Encounters*, edited by Michele Friedner and Annelies Kusters, 59–69. Washington, DC: Gallaudet University Press.

Friedner, Michele, and Annelies Kusters, eds. 2015. *It's a Small World: International Deaf Spaces and Encounters*. Washington, DC: Gallaudet University Press.

Green, E. Mara. 2014. "Building the Tower of Babel: International Sign, Linguistic Commensuration, and Moral Orientation." *Language in Society* 43: 445–65.

Hiddinga, Anja, and Onno Crasborn. 2011. "Signed Languages and Globalization." *Language in Society* 40 (4): 483–505.

Ladd, Paddy. 2003. *Understanding Deaf Culture: In Search of Deafhood*. Clevedon, UK: Multilingual Matters.

Lane, Harlan. 1984. *When the Mind Hears: A History of the* Deaf. New York: Random House.

Moody, William. 1987. "International Gestures." In *Gallaudet Encyclopedia of Deaf People and Deafness*, edited by John V. Van Cleve, Vol. 3, 81–82. New York: McGraw Hill.

———. 2002. "International Sign: A Practitioner's Perspective." [Registry of Interpreters for the Deaf-RID]. *Journal of Interpretation*, 1–47.

Nanda, Serena. 2021. "Inequalities and COVID-19." In *COVID-19: Global Pandemic, Societal Responses, Ideological Solutions*, edited by J. Michael Ryan, 109–23. London: Routledge.

Padden, Carol, and Thomas Humphries. 1988. *Deaf in America: Voices from a Culture*. Cambridge, MA: Harvard University Press.

Plumlee, Marilyn. 2009. "International Sign: Its Use as an International Conference Lingua Franca." *The Journal of Translation Studies* 10 (4): 301–41.

Pursglove, Michael, and Anna Komarova. 2003. "The Changing World of the Russian Deaf Community." In *Many Ways to Be Deaf*, edited by Leila Monaghan, Constanze Schmaling, Karen Nakamura, and Graham H. Turner, 249–59. Washington, DC: Gallaudet University Press.

Ryan, J. Michael. 2021. "COVID-19: Social Consequences and Cultural Adaptations." In *COVID-19: Social Consequences and Cultural Adaptations*, edited by J. Michael Ryan, 1–8. London: Routledge.

Saville-Troike, Muriel. 1989. *The Ethnography of Communication*. 2nd ed. New York: Basil Blackwell Publishers.

Senghas, Richard J., and Leila Monaghan. 2002. "Signs of Their Times: Deaf Communities and the Culture of Language." *Annual Review of Anthropology* 31: 69–97. DOI: 10.1146/annurev.anthro.31.020402.101302.

Supalla, Ted, and Rebecca Webb. 1995. "The Grammar of International Sign: A New Look at Pidgin Languages." In *Language, Gesture, and Space* (International Conference on Theoretical Issues in Sign Language Research), edited by Karen Emmorey and Judy S. Reilly, 333–52. Hillsdale, NJ: Erlbaum.

Wilcox, Sherman, ed. 1989. *American Deaf Culture: An Anthology*. Burtonsville, MD: Linstok Press.

15

PEOPLE'S EXPERIENCES AND ATTITUDES DURING THE COVID-19 PANDEMIC IN THE UNITED STATES AND POLAND[1]

Magdalena Szaflarski

Countries around the world have responded differently to the coronavirus (COVID-19) outbreak. Reasons for these variations are rooted in specific sociocultural contexts, healthcare systems, and geopolitical locations. As a result of unique societal conditions, COVID-19 experiences and public views of the crisis are also expected to vary. However, similarities in experiences and attitudes are also expected due to the nature of the virus (SARS-CoV-2) being constant and requiring similar responses. In addition, countries located within regional or geopolitical blocs and ones with similar ideologies may show comparable social experiences and attitudes. Much remains to be learned about the COVID-19 social milieu from cross-cultural perspectives.

This study compares people's COVID-19 experiences and attitudes in the United States and Poland. The United States has a history of relatively stable democratic and market systems and has been a global power. However, right-wing tendencies have been strengthening in the United States over the last two decades, leading up to and reinforced by the election of Donald Trump, a populist president (Conway et al. 2018; Conway, Repke, and Houck 2017). Poland has had a violent modern history, being a central site of World Wars I and II and Soviet-style communism (1945–1989). Since 1989, Poland has built a Western-style democratic state and market-based economy, one of the most successful within the former Soviet bloc (Petrova 2012). Poland is a member of the European Union (EU), but in recent years has moved toward populism and nationalism, aligning the state close with the Roman Catholic Church, de-liberalizing, and departing ideologically and practically from the EU (Fomina and Kucharczyk 2016; Przybylski 2018; Rupnik 2018). This is where the contemporary US and Polish societies overlap: Both currently have populist-type rule and are socially split along the right-wing and liberal/progressive lines. Attacks on the media and distrust in science have strengthened in both countries (American Association of University Professors

(AAUP) 2017; Iyengar and Massey 2019; Rotkiewicz 2018), impacting COVID-19 national responses, messaging, and public attitudes (*The Lancet* 2020; Breczko 2020).

The first US COVID-19 case was reported on January 20, 2020, and a US ban on arrivals of foreign nationals from China was implemented on January 30 (Centers for Disease Control and Prevention [CDC] 2020; Muccari, Chow, and Murphy 2020). The White House Coronavirus Task Force was announced on February 29. Poland's first case was reported on March 4. Within a week, Poland banned large gatherings and mandated all schools and educational institutions to close, including preschools and daycare centers (Pinkas et al. 2020). Around that time, many US states also announced school closures. On March 13, both countries declared a national state of emergency, but while the United States focused on international travel bans and formulating a national strategy, Poland moved quickly to a national stay-at-home order on March 24 and additional requirements (face masks, social distancing) and restricted mobility by March 31, following the EU recommendations. As the cases began to surge in New York City, Poland had already been almost completely shut down.

In late March, the US states begun issuing new stay-at-home orders and extending school closings. By early April, about 95% of those in the country were under lockdown. While US cases surged through April and May, Poland implemented a national face mask and social distancing order in mid-April and began loosening restrictions (onet.pl 2020). Public places and nonessential businesses reopened by mid-May under strict rules of social distancing, mask wearing, and quarantine of positive coronavirus cases. The US states started to reopen in May, too, but with delayed and poorly articulated and poorly followed national reopening guidelines. Social gatherings and travel around the Memorial Day holiday in late May resulted in increases in infections observed by mid-June. By the end of June, most US regions showed rising infections, with another wave of spikes following the July 4th holiday. By mid-July, all but six states reported increases in new cases, and almost 70,000 new cases were added in the country in one day (CDC 2020). Increases in hospitalizations were also noted in all age groups.

The coronavirus trends in the United States and Poland are shown in Figure 15.1. The differences between the two countries based on the data available are striking. The impact of coronavirus in Poland so far has been markedly lower than in the United States. Poland's relatively low COVID-19 impact is likely due to the early mandatory closings and stay-at-home orders and their strict continuation for about two months. Businesses deemed less safe, such as movie theaters and fitness clubs, remained closed for about three months. Strict rules for reopening have also likely kept infections down.

This study aims to provide further understanding of how country context, along with personal beliefs (political, religious) and sociodemographic factors (e.g., age, socioeconomic position), shape people's coronavirus-related experiences and attitudes. The issues are examined using online survey data collected in June and July of 2020 from individuals 18 years and older in the United States and Poland.

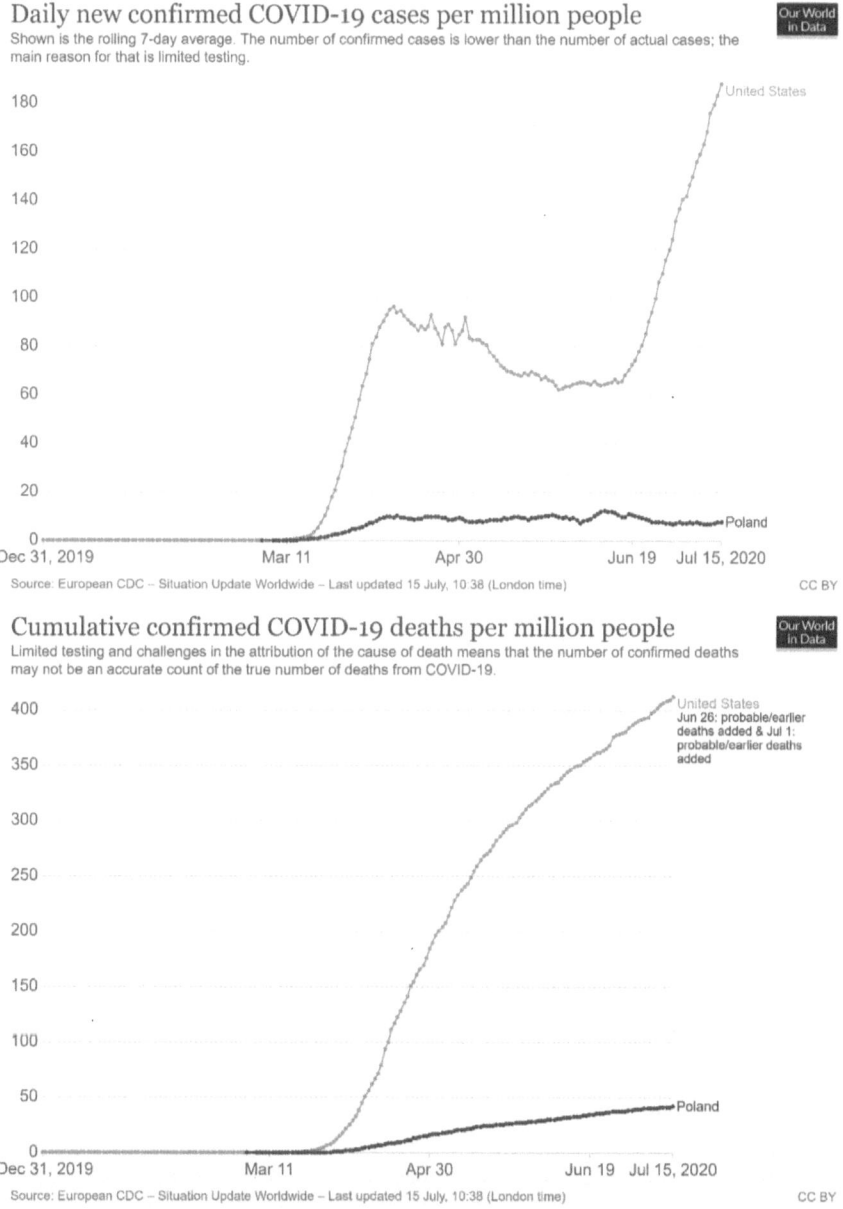

FIGURE 15.1a–15.1b   Comparison of COVID-19 Trends in the United States and Poland

Theoretical framework

A conceptual framework for this study is shown in Figure 15.2. Two types of factors are proposed to shape COVID-19 attitudes/experiences: ideological and sociodemographic. They are briefly reviewed in the next sections.

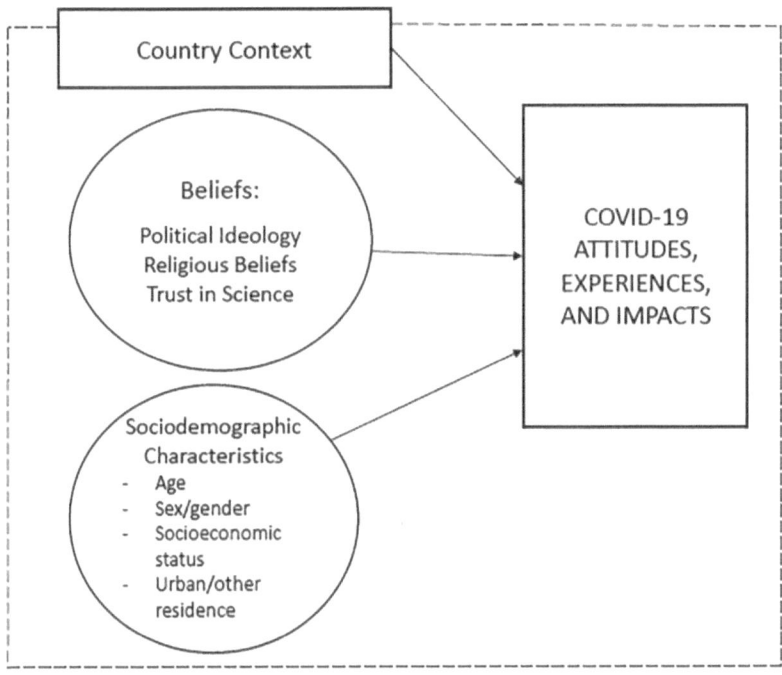

FIGURE 15.2   Conceptual Model of Factors Shaping COVID-19 Attitudes and Experiences

Political ideology and COVID-19

Conservatives in the United States and Poland seem to be less concerned than liberals are with COVID-19. Recent polls found that only 35% of US conservatives (versus 68% of liberals) are concerned about the virus (Malloy and Schwarts 2020) and that only 42% of Republicans feared that they or someone in their family might be exposed to coronavirus, compared to 73% of Democrats and 64% of Independents (McCarthy 2020). Emerging social science research (Conway et al. 2020) also shows that conservatives perceive COVID-19 as less of a threat than liberals do, and that they desire less governmental COVID-19 restrictions and are more frustrated with restrictions at any level of government, compared with their liberal counterparts. Conservatives also trust federal government information about the pandemic more than they do state and city governments, which may be explained by the former being currently more conservative and the latter more liberal. Furthermore, conservatives generally feel the impacts of the pandemic less than liberals do, and they are less likely to follow the news.

Social scientists note that "conservatives' relative apathy" towards the pandemic actually goes against prior research showing strong relationships between conservative ideology and threat (Conway et al. 2020), especially physical threat such as disease (Conway and Repke 2019; Crawford 2017). However, the COVID-19 perceptions observed in the United States may be consistent with common cultural perceptions of the current conservative-liberal divide among people in that country (Kristian 2020). In the midst of the pandemic, Republicans and Democrats in the United States have moved markedly apart in coronavirus concern, with the majority of Republicans and few Democrats saying "the worst is behind us" (Pew Research Center 2020b). Researchers have also explored how the COVID-19 threat promotes social conservatism and right-wing presidential candidates in the United States and Poland (Karwowski et al. 2020) and strengthens the triple threat of neoliberalism, nationalism, and neoconservatism in societies more broadly (Ryan 2021a).

Religious beliefs and COVID-19

In addition to political views, religious beliefs are likely to shape perceptions of the COVID-19 pandemic and social responses. First, religion has been a dominant sociocultural force throughout human history. It has influenced personal lives and shaped governments, often making a strong mark on a society's laws and policy (Cuevas and Dawson 2020). As others have noted, religions "provide a frame of reference for understanding and interpreting the world" (Hunsberger and Jackson 2005, 815, cited in Cuevas and Dawson 2020). Second, religion and religiosity are strongly associated with political ideology. The evidence is particularly strong for the relationship between conservatism and religious beliefs, which has also been shown to be stable across cultures and different religions (Cuevas and Dawson 2020; Hall, Matz, and Wood 2010). In the United States under Trump, conservative evangelical churches have been aligned with populist ideas against the lockdowns, creating "a political theodicy of rage" (Turner 2021). Third, religion and science have been increasingly at odds, with some religious conservatives refusing to have their children vaccinated or denying science on the health impacts of climate change or even hazards of smoking (McLintic 2019). Religiosity may then make some people less trusting of science-based information about COVID-19. Anti-quarantine protests in the United States reflect "a political climate that is increasingly hostile to rational, scientific, and medical expertise" (Meeker 2021, this volume). Even though Christians have strong support of the current national governments in both the United States and Poland, the situations of religious institutions in these countries during the COVID-19 pandemic have differed. The Polish Roman Catholic Church (the main religious institution in Poland) was not immediately included in the restrictions on large gatherings, but within a matter of two to three weeks, worship services were ordered to be limited, first to 50 and then to only five participants (Pinkas et al. 2020). Church leaders supported governmental efforts and encouraged individual churches to transition to virtual worship activities. A study of different denominations in Poland during the pandemic shows that churches have largely limited or totally suspended their in-person activities (Sulkowski and Ignatowski 2020). In contrast, most US states granted religious exemptions to COVID-19 social distancing rules during the lockdown (Pew Research Center 2020a). Only ten states prohibited in-person religious gatherings in any form. In some states, churches resisted state orders or sued states for the right to congregate. A number of COVID-19 outbreaks have since been linked to religious gatherings. The Trump administration has also been pushing for the reopening of churches, especially Christian churches, which has been viewed as politically motivated.

Sociodemographic factors and COVID-19

A third group of factors worth exploring in relation to COVID-19 attitudes/experiences are sociodemographic characteristics. For example, experiences vary with age. Older adults have the highest mortality from and severity of the disease linked to the virus, but younger people are currently more likely to be infected and contributing to the virus spread. In the United States, older adults tend to see the virus as a major threat to their personal health while younger adults worry about their job and finances (Schaeffer and Rainie 2020). Around the world, economic and income-based inequalities related to COVID-19 are a significant concern (Ryan 2021b; Nanda 2021; Parsons 2021). There are also race, age, sex/gender, and geographic differences in views on mask wearing (Pew Research Center 2020b). For example, women and urban residents in the United States are more likely to support mask wearing compared to men and residents of nonurban areas. Cross-national research has also identified groups experiencing the highest levels of stress during the pandemic: younger ages, women, single people, and those living with children (Kowal et al. 2020).

Hypotheses

Based on the past theory and literature, this study proposes that COVID-19 attitudes/experiences among adults in the United States and Poland will vary by country, political ideology, religiosity, trust in science, and several sociodemographic factors. Specifically, I hypothesized that (1) experiences and impacts will be less negative in Poland than in the United States and (2) conservatism, religiosity, and low trust in science will be associated with (a) positive views of conservative governments' responses to COVID-19, (b) more trust in such governments' messaging and less trust in science-based approaches, and (c) stronger opposition to rules that place restrictions on personal freedoms. Furthermore, vulnerable groups (e.g., elderly, women, and low-income individuals) were expected to feel more COVID-19 threat and impact.

Methods

Data

The study is based on cross-sectional data collected through an online survey conducted in June and July of 2020. The study used a snowball sample via online and social media platforms. Specifically, the researcher's professional and personal online and social media networks in the United States and Poland were engaged to recruit participants aged 18 years and older. The online questionnaire was constructed and administered in English and Polish and included 67 structured items. Measures of COVID-19 experiences, behaviors, and views have been adapted from other recent COVID-19 studies and public health toolboxes (National Institutes of Health [NIH], CDC). Demographic and other information about respondents (including ideology and religiosity) were also collected. All items required a response to eliminate missing data. A panel of five bilingual native-Polish and English speakers (three scientists and two laypersons) translated/reviewed the Polish version of the questionnaire. The average time of completion was less than 20 minutes. Completions were monitored for the demographic representation in the survey. Special efforts were made through repetitively targeting residents of Poland, men, and young and older adults. The final analytic US-Poland sample was 538 respondents. The study was approved by the Institutional Review Board at the University of Alabama at Birmingham.

Measurement

Dependent variables. The dependent variables included perceptions of COVID-19 threat (three items) and federal/national government response (11 items) as well as personal COVID-19 experiences (six items) and impacts (five items). Measures of these constructs were adapted from Conway and colleagues (Conway, Woodard, and Zubrod 2020), who validated and refined them in three different US-based samples. The recommended short versions of the measures (scales) were adapted with minor changes in the current study. Examples of 7-point Likert or Likert-type survey items include: "I am afraid of the coronavirus (COVID-19)" (threat), "I support government measures to restrict the movement of citizens to curb the spread of coronavirus (COVID-19)" (response), "I have had coronavirus (COVID-19)-like symptoms at some point in the last two months" (experiences), and "I have lost job-related income due to the coronavirus (COVID-19)" (impacts). Some of the scales or subscales were non-normally distributed and were transformed into categorical variables (see Tables 15.2 and 15.3).

Independent variables. Country of residence was a binary variable (USA/Poland), with USA as a reference category. Political ideology and religiosity were each assessed with one 7-point Likert-type item: "Do you think of yourself as liberal or conservative?" (1 "very liberal" to 7 "very conservative") and "How religious are you?" (1 "not at all" to 7 "very"). The final measures were categorical (low, moderate, high) due to non-normal distributions. Trust in scientific information about COVID-19 combined two 7-point Likert-type items asking, "Do you trust the following people (scientists, doctors) for information about the coronavirus (COVID-19)?"

Four age groups were constructed: 18–29 years, 30–49 years (reference category), 50–64 years, and 65 and older, to allow comparison with previously published data (Schaeffer and Rainie 2020). Respondents were asked about sex assigned at birth: male (reference) or female, and how they identify their gender, and all but two respondents identified as man/woman. Race (White, Black, other) and Hispanic/Latinx ethnicity are noted in the descriptive results, but the numbers were insufficient to include in the analysis.

Marital status was coded as married/domestic partner versus other (reference). Children at home was dummy-coded. Socioeconomic position was assessed with college versus less than college education (reference category) and financial status ("How do you assess your financial status relative to other people in your country?" on a scale from 1 "very low" to 7 "very high"). Residence location had three categories: urban, suburban, and small town/rural area. A dummy-coded urban vs. other variable was used in multivariable analyses.

Analysis

Percentage distributions were computed for categorical variables and means and standard deviations for continuous variables. Cross-tabulations and Pearson chi-square tests were used to compare variable distributions between the country subsamples. Independent-samples t-test (two-tailed) was conducted for continuous variables to compare differences in means between the two countries. Because of the numerous data points available in this study, the multivariable analysis for this chapter focused on examining explanatory factors in COVID-19 perceived threat and support of COVID-19 restrictions. These multivariable estimations used ordinary least squares (OLS) regression. Explanatory factors were added in a nested fashion, starting with the country variable, followed by blocks of ideology and sociodemographic factors. Significance level of .05 was applied.

Findings

The descriptive statistics for the full sample and the US and Poland subsamples are presented in Table 15.1. A slight majority of the respondents (54%) resided in the United States. Of all participants, 92% were White, 75% identified as female, and 80% were college educated. The majority fell into the middle groups, 30–49 and 50–64 years old, but the Poland subsample was somewhat younger. The Poles were also significantly less likely to be married/living with a domestic partner and have children less than 28 years of age living at home and more likely to reside in urban or rural areas (vs. suburbs) compared to the US-based respondents. Trust in scientific information on COVID-19 was generally high among all respondents: 84% expressed higher levels of trust. The majority of respondents (60%) assessed their religiosity as low and 25% as high. The US-based respondents were more likely to be conservative than the Polish respondents, but the Poles were more likely to be moderate ideologically.

The US-Poland comparison of the measures of COVID-19 perceived threat, government response, impacts, and experiences is presented in Tables 15.2 and 15.3. There were a few differences between the US and Polish respondents. The

TABLE 15.1 Percentage Distributions of Social Characteristics in the Full Sample and in the US and Poland Subsamples

	All	USA	Poland	Sig. diff.
	n = 538	n = 291	n = 247	
Country				
USA	54.1			
Poland	45.9			
Age group				
18–29	16.7	9.6	25.1	<.001
30–49	49.1	49.8	48.2	
50–64	27.0	33.0	19.8	0.001
65+	7.2	17.8	6.9	
Sex/gender				
Male	25.1	23.7	26.7	
Female	74.9	76.3	73.3	
Race				
White	92.0	86.9	98.0	<.001
Black	2.6	4.8	0.0	<.001
Other	5.4	8.2	2.0	0.002
Hispanic/Latino	2.6	3.8	1.2	
College educated	80.1	82.8	76.9	
Married/domestic partner	66.2	73.2	57.9	<.001
Children <18 at home	39.8	47.7	31.2	<.001
Residence location				
Urban	52.4	41.9	64.8	<.001
Suburban	25.8	39.9	9.3	<.001
Rural	21.7	9.9	25.9	<.001
Political ideology				
Liberal	39.8	40.9	38.5	
Moderate	49.1	45.0	53.8	0.047
Conservative	11.2	7.6	3.5	0.020
Religiosity				
Low	60.2	38.8	40.9	
Moderate	35.5	34.0	36.8	
High	24.9	27.1	22.3	
Trust in science/medicine				
Low	15.8	15.8	15.8	
High	84.2	84.2	84.2	

US respondents had significantly higher levels of perceived threat but lower tolerance for punishing people for violations of the COVID-19 social rules (Table 15.2). However, the Poles were much more likely to be upset about the government limiting personal freedoms due to COVID-19 (Table 15.3). The support for government-sponsored research toward COVID-19 treatment and vaccine was generally high among all respondents, but people in the United States were somewhat more supportive than the Poles (92% vs. 84%).

The COVID-19 impacts were somewhat lesser among people in Poland than in the United States. Some financial impacts were felt by both groups, with slightly

TABLE 15.2 Mean Scores on COVID-19 Perceived Threat, Government Response, and Experiences: Continuous Measures

	USA		Poland		Sig. diff★
	Mean	SD	Mean	SD	
COVID-19 perceived threat	4.3	1.7	3.7	1.6	<0.001
Support for actual or potential government actions against COVID-19					
Restrictions	5.5	1.8	5.2	1.6	
Punishment for violations	3.5	1.9	4.7	1.8	<0.001
Stimulus	5.4	1.6	5.2	1.3	
Government untruthful	4.8	1.7	4.9	1.8	
Experiences					
Following news about COVID-19	3.6	1.7	3.5	2.0	

★ t-test (two-tailed)

TABLE 15.3 Percentage Distributions of Categorical Measures of COVID-19 Government Response, Impacts, and Experiences

	USA	Poland	Sig. diff.★
Reaction to limiting freedoms			<.001
Not upset	59.8	25.5	
Somewhat upset	28.5	40.1	
Upset	11.7	34.4	
Government response			
Support research on cure/vaccine	92.2	83.8	0.003
Impacts			
Financial			
Low	60.8	53.0	
Moderate	21.3	28.3	
High	17.9	18.6	
Resource			<.001
Low	55.7	83.4	
Moderate	74.7	25.3	
High	21.0	7.3	
Psychological			0.004
Low	40.5	53.0	
Moderate	37.1	33.6	
High	22.3	13.4	
Experiences (none/little vs. some)			
Personal	15.5	15.0	
Within social circle	19.2	12.1	0.026

★ Pearson chi-square test

less than half of the respondents reporting moderate or high financial impact of COVID-19. However, the Poles reported significantly fewer problems with access to necessities and less psychological impact than the US respondents did. While a small group of all respondents (15%) had personal experiences with COVID-19, the US respondents were more likely than their Polish counterparts to know someone who had been infected or had COVID-like symptoms. The levels of following the news about COVID-19 was similar by country (Table 15.2).

Table 15.4 shows findings about the hypothesized associations between a group of explanatory factors and perceived COVID-19 threat. The nested models are presented as Models 1–4. First, living in Poland is associated with a significantly lower level of perceived threat than is living in the United States, before and after adjustments for all other factors. Second, conservative ideology is also associated with lower perceived threat compared to liberal ideology, before and after all adjustments. Moderate ideology is also associated with lower threat but no longer after adjustment for trust in science. With political ideology in the model, religiosity is not associated with perceptions of COVID-19 threat. Interestingly, there are few associations between demographic factors and perceptions of threat. In the final model only being female is detrimental to perceived threat: After adjusting for all other factors, women's level of perceived threat is higher than men's. The final model (Model 4) explained 14% variation in perceived COVID-19 threat.

Table 15.5 presents findings about associations between the hypothesized explanatory factors and support for COVID-19 restrictions. No consistent significant differences were found in the view on restrictions by country, which is consistent with the bivariate results. However, conservatism was associated with less support of restrictions, and moderate orientation also but not after adjusting for trust in science, similar to the findings for perceived threat. Low trust in science was associated with less support for restrictions. Among sociodemographic variables, college-educated respondents were more likely to support restrictions than were those with less than college education. Family effects were inconsistent, but, after adjusting for all covariates, people with children at home supported restrictions more than did those without children. This model explained 24% of variation in views on restrictions.

Discussion

In this sample of residents of the United States and Poland, we found some interesting similarities and differences in people's attitudes, impacts, and experiences related to the coronavirus pandemic. Perceptions of threat and personal impacts appear generally lower in Poland than in the United States. However, views of government responses to the pandemic are in many ways similar.

This study has several limitations that need to be taken into account when interpreting the findings. The main study limitation (due to lack of resources) is a convenience sample. The data collection was monitored for sociodemographic

TABLE 15.4 Factors Associated With COVID-19 Perceived Threat in the United States and Poland

	Model 1			Model 2			Model 3			Model 4		
	b	Std. Error	Sig.	b	Std. Error	Sig.	b	Std. Error	Sig.	b	Std. Error	Sig.
Country (ref: USA)	−0.589	0.143	**<.001**	−0.648	0.140	**<.001**	−0.599	0.149	**<.001**	−0.569	0.145	**<.001**
Moderate ideology				−0.386	0.160	**0.016**	−0.327	0.161	**0.043**	−0.216	0.158	0.173
Conservative ideology				−1.455	0.264	**<.001**	−1.375	0.267	**<.001**	−0.997	0.269	**<.001**
Moderate religiosity				0.014	0.170	0.933	−0.007	0.171	0.965	−0.020	0.166	0.906
High religiosity				0.010	0.202	0.962	−0.092	0.206	0.656	−0.096	0.201	0.632
Ages 18–29							−0.271	0.228	0.235	−0.392	0.223	0.079
Ages 50–64							0.117	0.175	0.505	0.126	0.170	0.461
Ages 65+							0.284	0.292	0.332	0.178	0.285	0.531
Female							0.419	0.165	**0.011**	0.452	0.161	**0.005**
College educated							0.120	0.184	0.515	0.029	0.180	0.871
Income							**0.032**	0.059	0.589	−0.010	0.058	0.863
Married/domestic partner							−0.097	0.177	0.584	−0.020	0.173	0.908
Children <18 at home							−0.206	0.163	0.206	−0.200	0.158	0.206
Urban							**−0.036**	0.147	0.806	−0.062	0.143	0.666
Low trust in science										−1.105	0.199	**<.001**
R-square	0.031			0.095			0.118			0.168		
Adj. R-square	0.029			0.087			0.095			0.144		
df	1			5			14			15		
Sig. F change	<.001			<.001			0.141			<.001		

TABLE 15.5 Factors Associated With Favoring COVID-19 Restrictions in the United States and Poland

	Model 1			Model 2			Model 3			Model 4		
	b	Std. error	Sig.	b	Std. error	Sig.	b	Std. error	Sig.	b	Std. error	Sig.
Country (ref: USA)	-0.253	0.150	0.093	-0.330	0.145	**0.023**	-0.287	0.152	0.060	-0.239	0.142	0.093
Moderate ideology				-0.471	0.165	**0.005**	-0.408	0.165	**0.014**	-0.229	0.155	0.140
Conservative ideology				-1.774	0.273	**<.001**	-1.628	0.274	**<.001**	-1.016	0.263	**<.001**
Moderate religiosity				0.041	0.175	0.813	-0.033	0.175	0.849	-0.053	0.163	0.745
High religiosity				-0.081	0.209	0.698	-0.203	0.212	0.338	-0.209	0.196	0.287
Ages 18–29							0.123	0.234	0.600	-0.073	0.218	0.739
Ages 50–64							-0.007	0.179	0.970	0.008	0.166	0.964
Ages 65+							0.462	0.299	0.124	0.292	0.279	0.296
Female							0.403	0.169	**0.018**	0.456	0.157	**0.004**
College educated							0.075	0.189	0.691	-0.072	0.176	0.682
Income							0.150	0.060	**0.013**	0.083	0.056	0.144
Married/domestic partner							-0.450	0.181	**0.014**	-0.325	0.169	0.055
Children <18 at home							0.307	0.167	0.066	0.316	0.155	**0.041**
Urban							-0.002	0.150	0.988	-0.043	0.140	0.756
Low trust in science										-1.787	0.194	**<.001**
R-square	0.005			0.101			0.138			0.258		
Adj. R-square	0.003			0.093			0.115			0.237		
df	1			5			14			15		
Sig. F change	<.001			<.001			0.010			<.001		

distributions, and outreach efforts were implemented to achieve a good representation by national/population standards. However, in the end, the sample is not representative of the US and Poland's populations. The majority of the respondents are female and college-educated, and very few represent racial/ethnic minorities. The latter is an important weakness of these data, as US racial and ethnic minorities have been especially vulnerable during the pandemic (Laster Pirtle 2020; Schaffer 2021; Ramsari 2021). On the other hand, racial and ethnic comparisons are not particularly relevant to the US-Poland comparison, as Poles are more racially and ethnically monolithic. However, I recognize that minority populations have grown lately in Poland (e.g., migrants/migrant workers from the former Soviet republics), and it would be important to know how they fare during the pandemic. In addition, the measures of COVID-19 attitudes/experience used in this study are based on limited prior research (Conway, Woodard, and Zubrod 2020). Some of them did not perform well, possibly due to the sample not being representative or incomplete measure validation to date. Further analyses of psychometric properties of these measures and validation in other samples and populations are warranted. This is also a cross-sectional study, and further longitudinal data are needed to understand how coronavirus attitudes/experiences change over time during this still evolving pandemic.

These limitations notwithstanding, this study provides a glimpse into how people in two countries, the United States and Poland, which represent different geopolitical regions, have fared during the pandemic and how they assess their conditions. It is not surprising to see lesser impacts of the pandemic in Poland considering the lower burden of COVID-19 there compared with the United States (Figure 15.1). However, it is interesting that reported financial impacts are similar between the two countries, as the United States has seen historic job losses and unemployment (Pew Research Center 2020c) while jobs are also vulnerable (Doerr and Gambacorta 2020) but more secure in Europe, possibly due to more progressive labor laws. In addition, the study participants reported problems with accessing basic resources, but more so in the United States than Poland. Poland's food and other essential supplies have been more plentiful than in the United States, even though there was a rush to hoard items in both countries early in the epidemic (Kirk and Rifkin 2020). The findings of psychological impacts also being higher in the United States than in Poland are likely linked to other social factors, especially job loss and other changes in employment, but also isolation (Kowal et al. 2020; Lieberoth et al. 2020).

However, residents of Poland and the United States seem to perceive their governments' actions during the pandemic similarly. Many support restrictions, and, especially in Poland, some support punishment for rule violations. In the United States, more than a half of the nation supports restrictions and safety guidelines, but more Democrats than Republicans (Pew Research Center 2020b). Polls in Poland show that the majority of people (62%) had positive views of government responses early in the pandemic (TVP Info 2020). However, a June poll (rp.pl 2020) shows lower support (42%), so support may be dropping. The presidential elections under way in Poland and the ideological split in the country may be affecting social attitudes. At the same time, Poles in this comparative study, more so than Americans, appear to feel oppression, and many are concerned that their personal freedoms are taken away. Poles may feel that way because of Poland's long struggle for democracy in the modern era and many fearing authoritarian tendencies (Rupnik 2018). The American society is also ideologically split, and freedom supporters are plentiful and pose a great threat to the fight against COVID-19 by resisting public health guidelines (Meeker 2021, this volume; Welna 2020).

There were few sociodemographic differences in attitudes, impacts, and experiences during the pandemic. Polls show different pandemic-related concerns by age. The older age groups are concerned about their health impacts, while younger age groups worry about jobs and incomes (Schaeffer and Rainie 2020). Other research has also explored how high-risk senior women may be vulnerable in terms of social isolation and loneliness during the pandemic (Porter 2021, this volume). In the current study, we found little impact of demographic factors on attitudes/experiences. However, as in previous research (Kowal et al. 2020), this study found women to be more vulnerable than men. Poles with lower incomes have been reported to be twice as likely as those with higher incomes to be critical of the government response (rp.pl 2020). However, women and people aged 25–34 years were less likely to be critical. These mixed findings call for additional research.

This study provides new information about people's COVID-19 experiences and attitudes from a comparative perspective, building on other emerging literature (DeWees and Miller 2021; Fikry et al. 2021), but further work is needed. There are multiple directions for future research, with the data from the current study and beyond. In addition to measurement studies noted previously, future studies could investigate mediation mechanisms between ideological factors and COVID-19 attitudes/experiences. In other research, COVID-19 experiences and impacts did not consistently mediate the relationship between political ideology and perceived COVID-19 threat as did COVID-specific political beliefs (Conway et al. 2020). The authors argue that these findings point to the following: (1) conservatives' lack of concern is motivated by desired political outcomes and (2) as experiences and impact of COVID grow, the ideological effect on COVID-19 threat diminishes. These potential explanations require further attention, as does the role of religious beliefs and trust in science. For example, in this study, moderates' perceived threat of coronavirus was not higher than that of liberals if their trust in science was high. Thus, trust in science possibly mitigated perceptions of threat and social responses. Most of all, long-term/longitudinal data are needed from different societal contexts to more fully understand how people fare and perceive the pandemic under social conditions and pandemic trajectories.

Note

1 I would like to thank all of the study participants for taking their time to complete the survey and my colleagues, friends, relatives, and others in the United States and Poland for assistance with survey distribution. I am especially grateful to Ludwika Jakubowska-Burek,

PhD, MEng, Jerzy P. Szaflarski, MD, PhD, Ludwika and Marek Nowak, and Basia A. and Ember Szaflarski for their help with survey construction, translation, pilot testing, and/or distribution.

References

American Association of University Professors (AAUP). 2017. "National Security, the Assault on Science, and Academic Freedom." www.aaup.org/report/national-security-assault-science-and-academic-freedom.

Breczko, Boleslaw. 2020. "Niepokojące Dane. Polacy Nie Wierzą, Że Koronavirus Powstał Naturalnie." *Wirtualna Polska (WP) Tech*, April 4. https://tech.wp.pl/niepokojace-dane-polacy-nie-wierza-ze-koronawirus-powstal-naturalnie-6505447842072193a.

Centers for Disease Control and Prevention (CDC). 2020. "Coronavirus Disease 2019 (COVID-19): Cases and Deaths in the U.S." July 15. www.cdc.gov/coronavirus/2019-ncov/cases-updates/us-cases-deaths.html.

Conway, Lucian Gideon, III, Shannon C. Houck, Laura Janelle Gornick, and Meredith A. Repke. 2018. "Finding the Loch Ness Monster: Left-Wing Authoritarianism in the United States." *Political Psychology* 39: 1049–67.

Conway, Lucian Gideon, III, and Meredith A. Repke. 2019. "The Psychological Contamination of Proenvironmental Consensus: Political Pressure for Environmental Belief Agreement Underlines Its Long-Term Power." *Journal of Environmental Psychology* 62: 12–21.

Conway, Lucian Gideon, III, Meredith A. Repke, and Shannon C. Houck. 2017. "Donald Trump as a Cultural Revolt Against Perceived Communication Restriction: Priming Political Correctness Norms Causes More Trump Support." *Journal of Social and Political Psychology* 5: 244–59.

Conway, Lucian Gideon, III, Shailee R. Woodard, and Alivia Zubrod. 2020. Social Psychological Measurements of COVID-19: Coronavirus Perceived Threat, Government Response, Impacts, and Experiences Questionnaires. *PsyArXiv*, April 7. https://doi.org/10.31234/osf.io/z2x9a.

Conway, Lucian Gideon, III, Shailee R. Woodard, Alivia Zubrod, and Linus Chan. 2020. "Why Are Conservatives Less Concerned About the Coronavirus (COVID-19) Than Liberals? Testing Experiential Versus Political Explanations." Pre-print at www.researchgate.net/publication/340627232_Why_are_Conservatives_Less_Concerned_about_the_Coronavirus_COVID-19_than_Liberals_Testing_Experiential_Versus_Political_Explanations/link/5ea33bb3299bf112560c1f8b/download.

Crawford, Jarret T. 2017. "Are Conservatives More Sensitive to Threat Than Liberals? It Depends on How We Define Threat and Conservatism." *Social Cognition* 35 (4): 354–57.

Cuevas, Joshua A., and Bryan L. Dawson. 2020. "An Integrated Review of Recent Research on the Relationships Between Religious Belief, Political Ideology, Authoritarianism, and Prejudice. *Psychological Reports* 1–38 (May 18). http://dx.doi.org/10.1177/0033294120925392.

DeWees, Mari, and Amy C. Miller. 2021. "The Costs of Care: A Content Analysis of Female Nurses' Media Visibility and Voices in the United States, China, and India During the COVID-19 Pandemic." In *COVID-19: Global Pandemic, Societal Responses, Ideological Solutions*, edited by J. Michael Ryan, 221–3. London: Routledge.

Doerr, Sebastian, and Leonardo Gambacorta. 2020. "COVID-19 and Regional Employment in Europe." *BIS Bulletin* (16). www.bis.org/publ/bisbull16.pdf.

Fikry, Noha, Nada M. Ahmed, Malin E. Almeland-Grohn, Laila ElKoussy, Mostafa A. ElSharkawy, Farah Seifeldin, and Ahmed Sharaf Younis. 2021. "COVID-19, the Pand(m)emic: Social Media Explorations from the Arab World." In *COVID-19: Global Pandemic, Societal Responses, Ideological Solutions*, edited by J. Michael Ryan, 234–47. London: Routledge.

Fomina, Joanna, and Jacek Kucharczyk. 2016. "Populism and Protest in Poland." *Journal of Democracy* 27 (4): 58–68.

Hall, Deborah L., David C. Matz, and Wendy Wood. 2010. "Why Don't We Practice What We Preach? A Meta-Analytic Review of Religious Racism." *Personality and Social Psychology Review* 14 (1): 126–39.

Hunsberger, Bruce, and Lynne M. Jackson. 2005. "Religion, Meaning, and Prejudice." *Journal of Social Issues* 61 (4): 807–26.

Iyengar, Shanto, and Douglas S. Massey. 2019. "Scientific Communication in a Post-Truth Society." *Proceedings of the National Academy of Sciences, USA* 116 (16): 7656–61. https://doi: 10.1073/pnas.1805868115.

Karwowski, Maciej, Marta Kowal, Agata Groyecka, Michal Białek, Izebela Lebuda, Agnieszka Sorokowska, and Piotr Sorokowski. 2020. "When in Danger, Turn Right: Does Covid-19 Threat Promote Social Conservatism and Right-Wing Presidential Candidates?" *Human Ethology* 35: 37–48. https://doi.org/10.22330/he/35/037-048.

Kirk, Colleen P., and Laura S. Rifkin. 2020. "I'll Trade You Diamonds for Toilet Paper: Consumer Reacting, Coping and Adapting Behaviors in the COVID-19 Pandemic." *Journal of Business Research* 117: 124–31.

Kowal, Marta, Tao Coll-Martin, Gozde Ikizer, Jesper Rasmussen, Kristina Eichel, Anna Studzinska, Karolina Koszlkowska, Maciej Karwowski, Arooj Najmussaqib, Daniel Pankowski, Andreas Lieberoth, and Oli Ahmed. 2020. Who Is The Most Stressed During COVID-19 Isolation? Data From 27 Countries." Preprint at https://psyarxiv.com/qv5t7/.

Kristian, Bonnie. 2020. "Coronavirus and the End of the Conservative Temperament." *The Week*, March 15. https://theweek.com/articles/902015/coronavirus-end-conservative-temperament.

The Lancet. 2020. "Reviving the US CDC." *Lancet* 395 (10236): 1521. https://doi: 10.1016/S0140-6736(20)31140-5.

Laster Pirtle, Whitney N. 2020. "Racial Capitalism: A Fundamental Cause of Novel Coronavirus (COVID-19) Pandemic Inequities in the United States." *Health Education and Behavior* 47 (4): 504–8.

Lieberoth, Andreas, Siang-Yi Lin, Sabrina Stockli, Hyemin Han, Marta Kowal, Stavroula Chrona, and Rebekah Gelpi. 2020. "Stress and Worry in the 2020 Coronavirus Pandemic: Relationships to Trust and Compliance with Preventive Measures Across 45★ Countries." *Royal Society Open Science* Stage One Registered Report. Revised Manuscript (RSOS-200589). https://osf.io/6t3mb/.

Malloy, Tim, and Doug Schwartz. 2020. "Biden Crushes Sanders in Democratic Race, Quinnipiac University National Poll Finds; More Disapprove of Trump's Response to Coronavirus." *Quinnipiac University Poll.* https://poll.qu.edu/images/polling/us/us03092020_untz23.pdf.

McCarthy, Justin. 2020. "U.S. Coronavirus Concerns Surge, Government Trust Slides." GALLUP Politics, March 16. www.news.gallup.com/poll/295505/coronavirus-worries-surge.aspx?utm_source=alert&utm_medium=email&utm_content=morelink&utm_campaign=syndicat.

McLintic, Alan. 2019. "The Motivations Behind Science Denial." *New Zealand Medical Journal* 132 (1504): 88–94.

Meeker, James K. 2021. "The Political Climate of the Plague: The Ironic Resistance of Anti-Quarantine Protesters." In *COVID-19: Social Consequences and Cultural Adaptations*, edited by J. Michael Ryan, 109–21. London: Routledge.

Muccari, Robin, Denise Chow, and Joe Murphy. 2020. "Coronavirus Timeline: Tracking the Critical Moments of COVID-19." July 17. www.nbcnews.com/health/health-news/coronavirus-timeline-tracking-critical-moments-covid-19-n1154341.

Nanda, Serena. 2021. "Inequalities and COVID-19." In *COVID-19: Global Pandemic, Societal Responses, Ideological Solutions*, edited by J. Michael Ryan, 109–23. London: Routledge.

onet.pl. 2020. "Koronawirus. Rozwój Pandemii Dzień po Dniu." July 20. https://wiadomosci.onet.pl/kraj/koronawirus-jak-rozwijala-sie-epidemia-w-polsce-i-na-swiecie-kalendarium/xgt8wcd.

Parsons, Ryan. 2021. "Business as Usual: Poverty, Education, and Economic Life Amidst the Pandemic." In *COVID-19: Global Pandemic, Societal Responses, Ideological Solutions*, edited by J. Michael Ryan, 139–50. London: Routledge.

Petrova, Tsveta. 2012. "How Poland Promotes Democracy." *Journal of Democracy* 23 (2): 133–47.

Pew Research Center. 2020a. "Most States Have Religious Exemptions to COVID-19 Social Distancing Rules." April 27. www.pewresearch.org/fact-tank/2020/04/27/most-states-have-religious-exemptions-to-covid-19-social-distancing-rules/.

———. 2020b. "Republicans, Democrats Move Even Further Apart in Coronavirus Concerns." June 25. www.people-press.org/2020/06/25/republicans-democrats-move-even-further-apart-in-coronavirus-concerns/?utm_source=Pew+Research+Center&utm_campaign=ee5b9608d5-EMAIL_CAMPAIGN_2020_06_26_02_16&utm_medium=email&utm_term=0_3e953b9b70-ee5b9608d5-400165853.

———. 2020c. "Unemployment Rose Higher in Three Months of COVID-19 Than It Did in Two Years of the Great Recession." June 11. www.pewresearch.org/fact-tank/2020/06/11/unemployment-rose-higher-in-three-months-of-covid-19-than-it-did-in-two-years-of-the-great-recession/.

Pinkas, Jaros Ław, Mateusz Jankowski, Łukasz Szumowski, Aleksandra Lusawa, Wojciech S. Zgliczyński, Filip Raciborski, Waldemar Wierzba, and Mariusz Gujski. 2020. "Public Health Interventions to Mitigate Early Spread of SARS-CoV-2 in Poland." *Medical Science Monitor* 26: e924730. https://doi: 10.12659/MSM.924730.

Porter, Lynnette. 2021. "High Risk or Low Worth? A Few Practical and Philosophical COVID-19 Issues Surrounding the Isolation of High-Risk Senior Women." In *COVID-19: Social Consequences and Cultural Adaptations*, edited by J. Michael Ryan, 256–69. London: Routledge.

Przybylski, Wojciech. 2018. "Can Poland's Backsliding Be Stopped?" *Journal of Democracy* 29 (3): 52–64.

Ramsari, Atefeh. 2021. "The Rise of the COVID-19 Pandemic and the Decline of Global Citizenship." In *COVID-19: Global Pandemic, Societal Responses, Ideological Solutions*, edited by J. Michael Ryan, 94–105. London: Routledge.

Rotkiewicz, Marcin. 2018. "Kto i Dlaczego Wierzy w Pseudonaukowe Bzdury." *Polityka*, December 4. www.polityka.pl/niezbednik/1773196,1,kto-i-dlaczego-wierzy-w-pseudonaukowe-bzdury.read.

rp.pl. 2020. "Sondaż: 41,5 Proc. Ocenia Negatywnie Walkę Rządu z Epidemią." *Rzeczpospolita*, June 13. www.rp.pl/Koronawirus-SARS-CoV-2/200619796-Sondaz-415-proc-ocenia-negatywnie-walke-rzadu-z-epidemia.html.

Rupnik, Jacques. 2018. "The Crisis of Liberalism." *Journal of Democracy* 29 (3): 24–38.

Ryan, J. Michael. 2021a. "The Blessings of COVID-19 for Neoliberalism, Nationalism, and Neoconservative Ideologies." In *COVID-19: Global Pandemic, Societal Responses, Ideological Solutions*, edited by J. Michael Ryan, 80–93. London: Routledge.

———. 2021b. "The SARS-CoV-2 Virus and the COVID-19 Pandemic." In *COVID-19: Global Pandemic, Societal Responses, Ideological Solutions*, edited by J. Michael Ryan, 9–19. London: Routledge.

Schaeffer, Katherine, and Lee Rainie. 2020. "Experiences with the COVID-19 Outbreak Can Vary for Americans of Different Ages." *Pew Research Center*, June 16. www.pewresearch.org/fact-tank/2020/06/16/experiences-with-the-covid-19-outbreak-can-vary-for-americans-of-different-ages/.

Schaffer, Scott. 2021. "Necroethics in the Time of COVID-19 and Blacks Lives Matter." In *COVID-19: Global Pandemic, Societal Responses, Ideological Solutions*, edited by J. Michael Ryan, 43–53. London: Routledge.

Sulkowski, Lukasz, and Grzegorz Ignatowski. 2020. "Impact of COVID-19 Pandemic on Organization of Religious Behavior in Different Christian Denominations in Poland." *Religions* 11 (254). https://doi:10.3390/rel11050254.

Turner, Bryan S. 2021. "Theodicies of the COVID-19 Catastrophe." In *COVID-19: Global Pandemic, Societal Responses, Ideological Solutions*, edited by J. Michael Ryan, 29–42. London: Routledge.

TVP Info. 2020. "62 Proc. Wyborców KO Dobrze Ocenia Działania Rządu w Walce z Koronawirusem." *TVP*, March 19. www.tvp.info/47188090/62-proc-wyborcow-ko-dobrze-ocenia-dzialania-rzadu-w-walce-z-koronawirusem.

Welna, David. 2020. "Self-Isolation Orders Pit Civil Liberties Against Public Good In Coronavirus Pandemic." *NPR*, March 17. www.npr.org/2020/03/17/817178765/self-isolation-orders-pit-civil-liberties-against-public-good-in-coronavirus-pan.

16

PERFORMING PRECARITY IN TIMES OF UNCERTAINTY

The implications of COVID-19 on artists in Malta

Valerie Visanich and Toni Attard

During the uncertain times of living in the current COVID-19 pandemic, the ground has shifted noticeably, in ways that could neither have been expected nor predicted. In the last couple of months, physical social distancing, closure of borders to international visitors, closure of schools and colleges, and lockdown communities became a global form of temporal certainty. The COVID-19 virus was first reported in the city of Wuhan in December 2019, and since has rapidly spread worldwide with mounting confirmed cases and deaths. This has resulted in unprecedented policy challenges on a global level. Governments, worldwide, are taking interventionist measures to control the spread of the virus and to provide a safety net for citizens and businesses directly hit by financial loss. The pandemic is, in effect, not only a health crisis but also a major economic shock, leading to the collapse in the prices of bonds and shares and threatening a deep global recession (Milne 2020). The scale of economic shock is resulting in a decline of household expenditure, followed by the secondary "multiplier" impacts of unemployment, loss of personal incomes, and corporate financial distress (ibid.). Yet, the magnitude of economic and health impacts is not the focus of this chapter. Instead, it will specifically address the impact on the cultural sector and the direct hit on artists.

Measures to restrict mass gatherings and efforts to normalize physical social distance, due to the virus, had direct implications of the whole cultural ecosystem. Economically, the pandemic triggered a collapse in revenues in various sectors, including the hotel and restaurant industries, tourism, recreation, and culture and in global and domestic supply chains (ibid.). Closures of theaters and cancellation of cultural events caused a sudden implosion of the cultural and creative sector, with a consequence of escalating levels of unemployment, especially for freelance artists. By early March 2020, it has been reported that at least 170,000 jobs were lost in the film industry in Hollywood and the UK due to the coronavirus pandemic (Pulver 2020).

This chapter explores the shared concerns of artists during these unprecedented times and the disruptions in their everyday life. Such analysis is framed on an understanding of the precarious working conditions of artists in general, often with working conditions that offer no form of protection and are underrepresented by unions or lobby groups. The intensification of the coronavirus curbs brought to the fore common themes on the livelihood of artists. This chapter focuses on two of them: first, the major shift in the everyday life and well-being of artists, and second, the financial loss experienced by artists. This chapter draws on an online survey held in mid-March 2020 with artists in Malta.[1] However, issues and recommendations are general ones and could be applied elsewhere.

Performing precarity within the "freebie" culture

Pierre Bourdieu (1998) stressed that precariousness at work is a new mode of domination in contemporary capitalism. More recently, there has been a burgeoning of the literature on the changes in the landscape of work, broadly defined in terms of liquid modernity (Bauman 2000, 2005), information society (Castells 2000), "new" capitalism (Sennett 1998, 2006; Boltanski and Chiapello 2005), or risk society (Beck 1992 [1986]; Beck, Joost, and Adam 2000). Most of these works historicize, map out geographically, and explain sociologically the new work experience, broadly characterized by decentralization and the self-disciplining subjects working on precarious short-term contracts within a neoliberal economic climate.

The term "precarity" is generally used in sociology and political economics, as well as in the media (Vosko 2006; Kalleberg 2009), to refer to insecure employment including through self-employed and short-term contracts. Precarious employment is considered as a multidimensional construct, differing across countries and relying on the explicit economic and social structure of the labor market (Benanch et al. 2016; Moscone, Tosetti, and Vittadini 2016).

The most common indicators of having precarious employment conditions are related to issues of limited workplace rights and social protection, powerlessness to exercise legally granted workplace rights, employment insecurity, low wages, individualized bargaining relations, and overall working environment (Benanch et al. 2016; Edralin 2014; Lewchak et al. 2003). Herein, we explore three indicators of precariousness applied in the everyday life of artists and their working conditions; namely, the nonstandard working conditions, the existence of a freebie culture, and the lack of representativeness of artists as a collective.

First, the precariousness of work within the creative economy is, in part, reflected in the infiltration model of nonstandard employment, defined by subcontracting, outsourcing, and other modes of flexploitation, which is a situation when people working with flexible working arrangements do not have a strong bargaining position (Gray 1998). As precarious workers, they have to live in a

> limbo of uncertainty, juggling their options, massaging their contacts, never knowing where their next project or source of income is coming from. The

resultant cycle of feast and famine is familiar to anyone whose livelihood folds into the creative economy.

(Ross 2008, 36)

Studying the lives of creative laborers, Rosalind Gill and Andy Pratt (2013) explored the precariousness, insecurity, and discontinuation in work due to

long hours and bulimic patterns of working, by the collapse or erasure of the boundaries between work and play, by poor pay, by high levels of mobility, by passionate attachment to the work and to the identity of creative labourer (e.g. web designer, artist, fashion designer), by an attitudinal mind-set that is a blend of bohemianism and entrepreneurialism, by informal work environments and distinctive forms of sociality, and by a profound experiences of insecurity and anxiety about finding work, earning enough money and "keeping up" in rapidly changing fields.

(ibid., 33)

Artists are habitually considered as an army of freelance and intermittent workers, engaging in casualized, temporary employment and subject to be underpaid or receive late payment. They are frequently subject to being the

least paid of the so-called professions and generally live under the poverty line. Artists dangle between self-employment, casual contract work, artists' grants, and the very remote possibility of success on the art market (a star system that promotes exceptionalism).

(Garrett and Jackson 2016, 6)

Second, the freebie culture in the arts accentuates artists' degree of precarity. In 2012, an "art strike" was self-declared by a number of Warsaw art institutions, as a systematic struggle against the freebie culture, to promote better working for artists (Sharp 2017). The strike kick started discussions on the right for a living wage for artists and resulted in the signing of an agreement in 2014 to guarantee a minimum wage for artists (Figiel 2014).

In Britain, the policy framework report published in 2011 by the Arts Council England had clarified the legal obligations of arts organizations in offering internship opportunities (Arts Council England 2011). It has also tackled the issue of unpaid labor within the cultural and creative industries.

More recently, in the beginning of 2020, the Arts Council in Ireland launched a new policy to facilitate the working and living conditions of artists and ensure that a career in the arts is viable (Falvay 2020). Such measure is aimed to combat the freebie culture of under-/nonpaid work of artists. The Irish Arts Council chair stated that this new policy aims to bring fair and equitable pay and bring to an end "the idea that it is acceptable to get artists to work as a 'freebie', or to offer work without proper payment because it might somehow enhance an artist's career." The campaign #PayTheArtist promotes fair payment to artists through new funding conditions.

Internships, including art-in-residency programs, exemplify practices of the freebie culture. For Ross Perlin (2011) in *Intern Nation*, internships are structurally designed to fit in with the normalization of precarious, networked workforce: "What structured training programs were to the bureaucratic firms of the mid-twentieth century, internships may well be to the new network capitalism of firms dealing in intangible goods" (Perlin 2011, 95).

Albeit being relevant platforms for mobility, intercultural exchange of ideas, and collaborative work, internships are also mechanisms of precarization (Leban 2017). The symbolic value of internships is through addressing the "skills gap" during or after graduation, often measured by the currency of experiences and exposure. Drawing from Gary Becker's (1964) human capital theory, Perlin (2011) highlights the contemporary purpose of internships, to accumulate contacts, social networks, and insider knowledge in the hope of future full-time employment.

Third, another indicator of precarity shared by artists is their lack of representation as a collective. One major setback in Poland to guarantee equitable wage for artists, following the art strike, was the fact that artists were unrecognized as a union (Figiel 2014). Artists are hardly represented as a group in their contestation of precariat conditions (Gill and Pratt 2013). The spirit of individualism, commonly shared by artists, makes it difficult to convince them to join together in a group. "Collective bargaining requires an obedient rank-and-file," says jazz critic and music historian Ted Gioia, "but is there a profession more resistant to this than art-making?" (Green 2019).

Situation in Malta

Similar to countries like Poland, the UK, and Ireland, the situation of inequitable remuneration for artists' work resonates with many artists across the world. In Malta, a small island state (122 square miles with a population around half a million) in the Mediterranean Sea, artists are also prone to experience under/late payment.

In another study by Toni Attard about artists' payments, a total of 83.7% of respondents claimed that late payment is the norm, whereas 54.5% stated that they currently have pending payments for artistic work invoiced more than 30 days ago (Attard 2020). A total of 40.7% were awaiting payment between €500 and €2,500 and 35.6% between €100 and €500. The top three debtors are public cultural organizations, private companies, and private individuals (ibid.).

The living conditions of artists were considerably aggravated as soon as emergency measures to combat the COVID-19 virus were put in place, particularly with the banning of all public gatherings and lockdown of cultural sites like theaters, museums, libraries, and exhibition halls. Additionally, all educational institutions, including those offering cultural education, were closed down. The archbishop of Malta also issued a directive to ban all external religious cultural celebrations, including those associated with the popular village *festa* (Micallef 2020). The *festa* is the annual village patron saint feast, celebrated in every village in Malta and Gozo.

The first case of the COVID-19 virus in Malta was reported on March 7, 2020. As of mid-October 2020, there were over 3,700 confirmed cases, with 41 mortalities. The public health authorities are seeking to extend as much as possible the duration of the pandemic to slow the spread so that the peak is lower and the Maltese health services will be able to better cope.

Numerous artists operate within a freelance "gig economy," often moving from one gig or project to another. Thus, such measures resulted in cancellations and postponements of events, which had a direct impact on artists' income. The Maltese government responded through interventionist measures to address the financial impact of COVID-19 on employees and businesses. In view of this, Arts Council Malta and other public cultural organizations responded to the needs of the sectors through a number of measures, such as online training, project funding, and online support.

Methodology

Prior to the inclusion of artists in measures to safeguard the self-employed during the pandemic, published on March 25, 2020 (ibid.), numerous artists shared their concerns on the implications of this virus on their work and income on social media. Such concerns were the impetus for us to conduct a survey between March 14 and 21, 2020.

This chapter sets out to explore the concerns of artists on the implications of the pandemic, surrounded by discourse on precarity in artists' employment conditions. An online survey was designed to measure in detail the impact of the virus on their work practices and livelihood. In the absence of sector-led associations, participants were chosen through an opt-in survey shared on social media platforms popular amongst artists in Malta. There are various reasons for opting for an online survey rather than conducting a full ethnography – what might have been considered as a more appropriate sociological tool to inform the recommendations made. First, an online survey is a reliable research method that allows automation and real-time access to instantaneous data, specifically needed during the fast-changing times during the pandemic. Second, other research methods, such as face-to-face inter-views, could not have been conducted because of governmental directives restrict-ing physical contact. It is noteworthy to point out that all ethical procedures have been followed and participants recruited were informed of their rights to remain anonymous.

The survey received 346 responses of which 167 respondents earn an income exclusively from the arts and 138 partially earn an income from the arts. A total of 41 respondents claim that they do not earn an income from the arts and therefore the total valid responses for the scope of the survey is 305. Respondents came from

In which artistic sectors do you mainly operate in?
305 responses

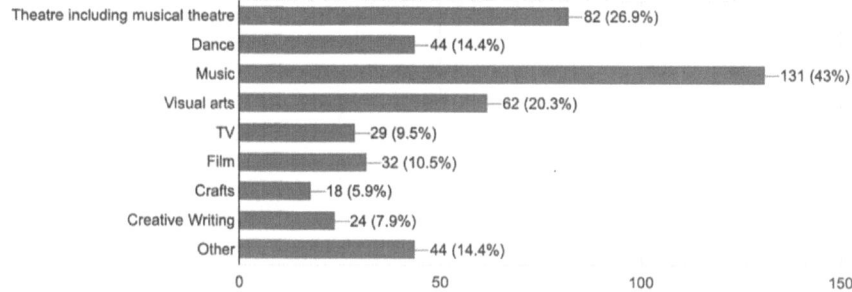

FIGURE 16.1   Artistic Sector of Sample

different artistic sectors, with a large number of respondents working within the music sector (43%) (Figure 16.1). All research participants were specifically chosen because they considered themselves artists.

Research outcome

Participants voiced their perceptions on various issues related to the inferences of the pandemic on their livelihood and income. The majority of participants (52.8%) maintained that the cultural activities providing them with a source of income were cancelled. In effect, public artistic events, such as performances, exhibitions, and concerts, are the main source for lost income. Herein we focus on two thematic areas extracted from the survey results: the shifts and disruptions in the everyday life and well-being of artists and the financial loss experienced.

Shifts in the everyday life

Zygumt Bauman's (2000) use of the liquidity metaphor is effective in the current context to describe the cultural, economic, and social uncertainties experienced on a global scale. The liquefaction is not only in the rapidity and mutability of a virus, but also in the uncertainty of the duration on the pandemic. As a result, there have been substantial shifts in the everyday life of individuals, on a cultural, social, and economic level.

In our survey, the majority of participants (95.7%) of respondents believe that the coronavirus is negatively affecting their work. When asked to select the artistic sectors that most represent their work, respondents were given the option to select multiple responses, since various artists operate across interdisciplinary practices. The majority of respondents work in music (43%), followed by theater (27%) and visual arts (20%). There were no significant differences in genre distribution between those whose income comes only from the arts and those earning partial income from the arts.

A total of 1,317 responses for seven different categories for activities were captured in the survey, with an average of 4.3 impacted activities per respondent. Respondents claim that more than half of the activities providing them with a source of income were cancelled. A number of events (38%) were postponed, other events were changed (3.9%), and some shifted online (5.2%) (Figure 16.2). The category of work related to artistic events also registers the highest percentage share of all postponed and cancelled events. Rehearsals, work in progress, and creative research register the highest percentage for activities that have changed, whereas arts education features as the predominant activity that shifted online. Despite the relevance of shifting to work-from-home mode during the pandemic, using various virtual meetings platforms, for artists it was not always possible to transfer work online. This was possible for activities related to arts education (43.5%). However, it was not possible to transfer private events (4.3%), such as gigs, online (Figure 16.3).

The casualization and short-contract working conditions, subject to postponement or termination during unfavorable times, have substantial influences on the artist's life satisfaction and well-being. One research participant reflected on the effect of such crisis on her/his well-being: "It is also important to safeguard the mental well-being of those who have been impacted severely by production cancellations and financial troubles." Fifty-three percent of artists were very concerned that this pandemic is having substantial impact on their personal well-being (Figure 16.4).

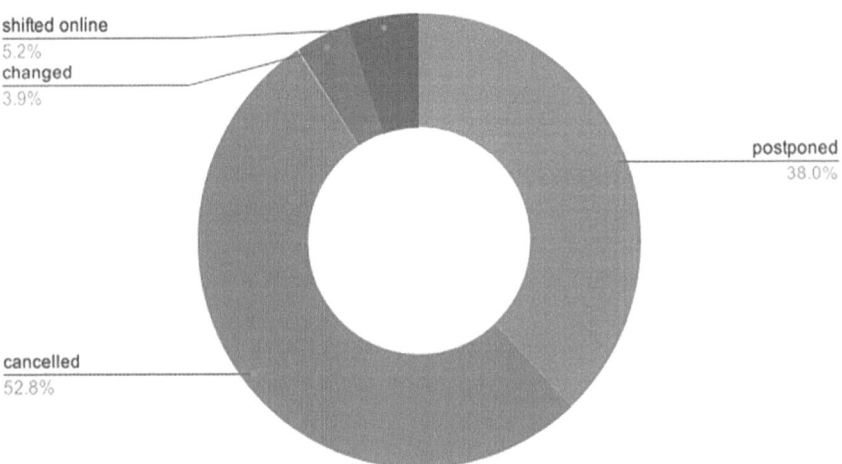

FIGURE 16.2 Impact on All Activities

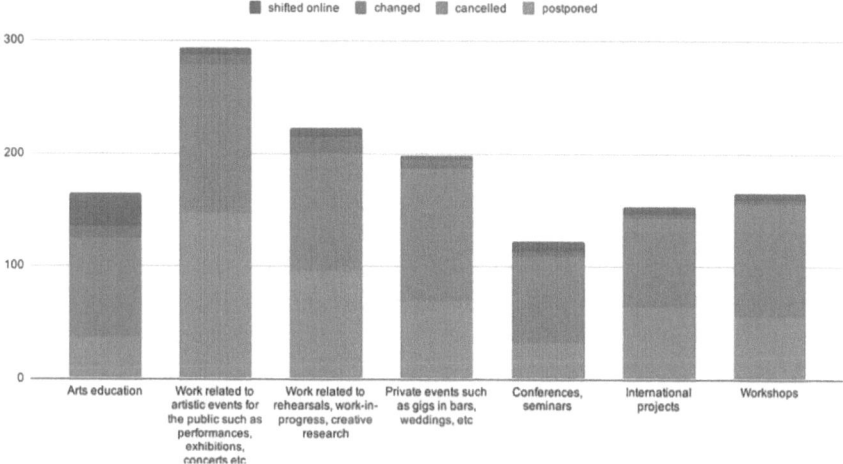

FIGURE 16.3 Activities Providing a Source of Income and Impact

Right now, how concerned are you about the impact of COVID-19 on your livelihood as an artist?

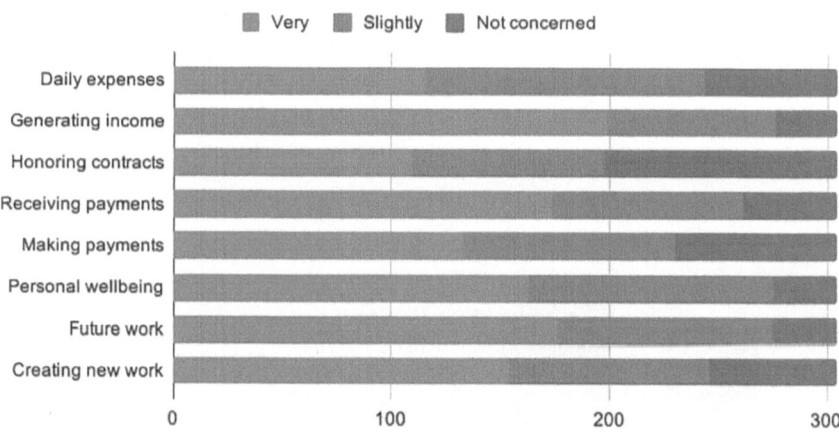

FIGURE 16.4 The Impact of the Pandemic on the Livelihood of the Artist

Financial loss

Perhaps the most jarring of all is that the pandemic continued to underpin the notion of inequalities in the rights for a living wage amongst workers. Moreover, economic inequality is contributing to chances of contracting and surviving from coronavirus (see Nanda 2021).

Reflecting the general nonstandard employment and precariat practices of artists, including working to the demands of the market and economic conditions, in times of crisis artists have to fully shoulder the financial burden when events are cancelled. A majority of participants (67.2%) maintained that they had already suffered financial losses, while 25.9% say it's too early to calculate these losses (Figure 16.5). A total of 32.5% of respondents state that most of their income for this period has been or will be lost, and 28.2% claim that all their income for this period has been or will be lost.

Concerning the total amount of income lost, 18.4% of respondents claim losses of more than €1,000 and 17% claim between €500 and €1,000 (Figure 16.6). Respondents claiming an income exclusively from the arts register higher losses that those claiming partial income. Those with partial income also claim to be the most unsure of the financial losses. Asked to forecast weekly financial losses should the current scenario be extended further, both categories of respondents claim mostly between €250 and €500 per week, followed by the €100 and €250 category for those earning an income exclusively from the arts. This continues to demonstrate how artists, working as freelancers, were harshly hit by the pandemic. Such a situation is likely to be exacerbated in the months ahead due to postponement of projects. One participant referred to this and stated,

> During the months of lockdown, I'm not generating money, even though I might continue with preparations. Also, if a current project/s is/are postponed to e.g. October, this means that in October I cannot accept new work. So I'm losing more money.
>
> *Anecdote by an artist participating in the survey*

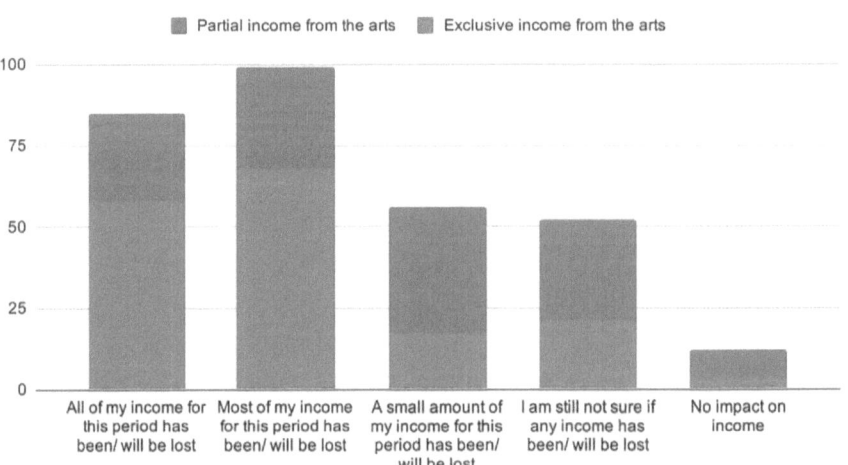

FIGURE 16.5   Impact on Income

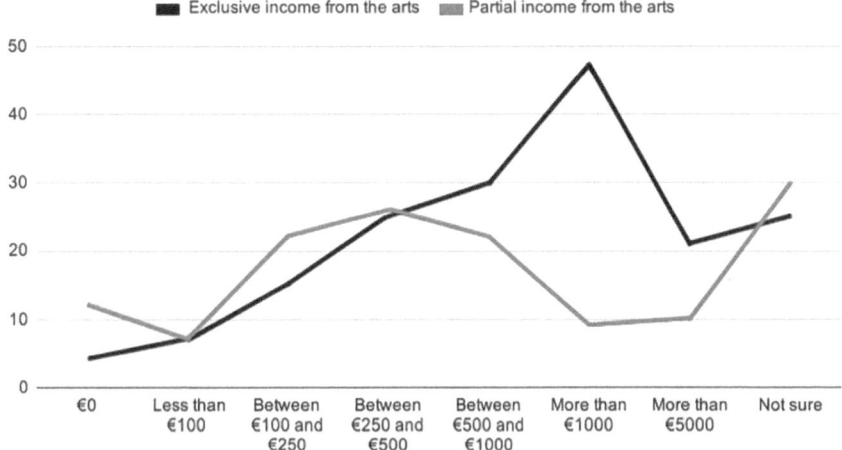

FIGURE 16.6 Financial Losses So Far

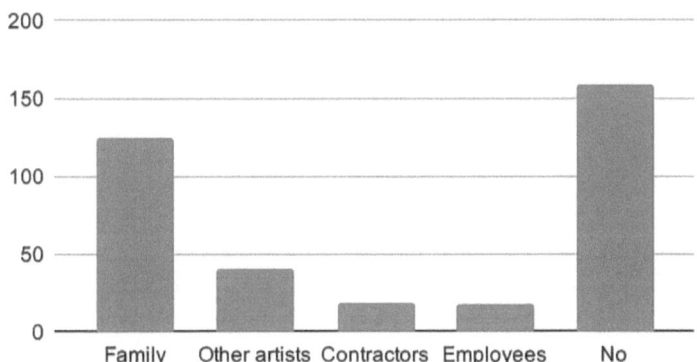

FIGURE 16.7 Dependents on Artist's Income

Whereas 52.1% of respondents stated that there are no dependents on their income, others claimed that their livelihood from the arts impacted their family (Figure 16.7). A high percentage (41%) of participants claimed that their family is dependent on their income from the arts.

Thus, such financial losses, when working on short-term contracts with no advance payment, reflect the nonstandard employment practices archetype of precarious work conditions. Respondents earning an income exclusively from the arts indicated that they had more financial dependents, including family members, other artists, contractors, and employees than for those earning only part of their income from the arts.

Generating income, future work, and receiving payments were the three main concerns of respondents at the time of responding to the survey. Honoring contracts featured as the least of concerns with 108 responses.

COVID wage supplement: governmental measures in Malta

Similar to other countries, with the introduction of wage subsidies to employers from all sectors whose business suffered financial losses due to the pandemic, Malta also implemented a similar scheme. Following consultation and open discussion with various sectors of workers who had their operations temporarily suspended, the "Covid Wage Supplement" was introduced. This measure, managed by the Malta Enterprise, Malta's economic development agency, provides a basic wage covering full-time employees and the self-employed (Malta Enterprise 2020).

The Covid Wage Supplement scheme established two lists classified by NACE codes, the Statistical Classification of Economic Activities in the European Community, identifying the sectors that can benefit. Through this scheme, people working in sectors identified in ANNEX A, whether full-time employees or self-employed/freelance, are entitled to a monthly supplement of €800. Part-time employees within these sectors are entitled to a monthly supplement of €500. Motion picture, video, and television program activities were originally excluded from this list; however, they were added to the revised list following feedback from the film and television industry. ANNEX A includes:

Motion picture video and television program activities
Motion picture video and television program post-production activities
Motion picture video and television program distribution activities
Motion picture projection activities
Sound recording and music publishing activities
Photographic activities
Cultural education
Performing arts
Support activities to performing arts
Artistic creation
Operation of arts facilities

Creative practitioners working in the sectors in ANNEX B, such as working in book publishing, publishing of newspapers and television, and radio broadcasting, who were considered to have been adversely but not drastically affected, are entitled to a monthly supplement of €160 in the case of full-time employees, and €100 in the case of part-time employees. Businesses in Gozo, Malta's sister island, listed in ANNEX B, can benefit from €320 per month in the case of full-time employees or self-employed, €420 for those self-employed who employ staff, and €200 per month for part-time employees.

Malta's creative sector is adopting its own measures to adapt to the situation. Arts Council Malta issued a call for feedback from its beneficiaries on March 20, 2020, to assess how they were impacted, and has relaxed obligations related to its funding agreements with artists, while fast-tracking payments in light of the situation (Arts Council Malta 2020). It has also assured its beneficiaries that project losses due to restrictions will be made up for. Public cultural organizations were directed by the Arts Council to support the sector by easing up on financial obligations and providing more flexibility in terms of logistics. Such measures are a step towards the safeguarding of artists during challenging times. It is also a worthy endeavor of initiating discussion for policy makers on having long-term measures to counteract exploitative and precariat conditions often faced by artist.

Discussion

In divergence to the neoliberal climate within the Anglo-American context in recent years, safety-net measures of wage supplements in various European countries are targeted at protecting citizens at risk of experiencing the hard-hit effects of the coronavirus pandemic. These measures continue to reinforce the state's obligation to protect citizens and offer social security during the churning labor market. This is needed especially when the pandemic brought about increased debt burdens that will continue to eat away at social spending – a kind of "blessing" to the neoliberal agenda to minimize state obligation (see Ryan 2021).

Recent discussions on having self-employed and freelance artists included in the wage supplement scheme is a step forward towards having creative practitioners fairly represented amongst other self-employed workers. Throughout recent years, one major barrier for the creative sector to improve its professional status has been the lack of collective sector-led voice of artists through unions and associations. Within this climate of uncertainties, industry-led associations opened up conversations with government to discuss financial measures, yet it became evident that there is an absence of an equivalent industry-led organization in Malta for the arts. Even though it is misguided to dismiss the autonomy of the self-employed artist and her/his attitude for self-direction and entrepreneurship, it is necessary for artists to be represented collectively by lobbying groups.

In spite of the resistance by some artists to engage in professional arts management, public policy measures are required to address a few of the challenges brought forth in this chapter. The public sector, as a major investor in the arts, needs to set an example by ensuring that fair and equitable conditions are offered to artists, providing contracts and payments on time. Public funding commitments, be they commissions or grants, should emphasize further the importance of appropriate remuneration for artists and their right to enjoy a living income from the artistic work they generate. Continuous advocacy within the private sector is also needed to ensure that the business community understands and values the contribution artists can make to the development of their enterprises.

In these exceptional circumstances, we propose a few immediate responses, inspired by the conversations held virtually with artists as well as from the observations that emerged from the results of the online survey. These recommendations include the need to mobilize, with immediate effect, an emergency fund for artists, prioritizing those earning an income exclusively from the arts, and to consider universal basic income as a funding model. Recommendations to public and private institutions receiving services from artists include fast tracking any pending payments to provide immediate liquidity to artists. Also, the commissioning of new work needs to provide advances to pay for research and development that may be performed at home. Equally relevant, funders and sponsors are recommended to shift any grants that will not be issued in the interim into solidarity grants that support the livelihood of artists. Building on the suggestions of Leban (2017), it is recommended that policy makers, at both the national and the EU level, acknowledge the precarious working conditions of the artists within the creative economy. This is necessary to safeguard the well-being of artists working through internship programs as well as artists doing nonpayment work within the freebie culture. It is worth noting the normalization in requests for free work within the arts. Every request for free work in the name of exposure and every underpaid offer undermines the value of the arts and the livelihood of the artist. It threatens the growth of artistic talent and reinforces a culture that free or underpaid work pays the bills.

While the collected data through online surveys informs the recommendations made in this chapter and provides a tentative engagement with artists in Malta, the authors are aware of the present time and physical presence limitations. It is suggested that a full ethnography with artists would be followed on to supplement this data and present a richer and more in-depth picture of the situation.

Conclusion

Sociologically, it is intriguing to see how the pandemic is impacting not only on socioeconomic structures, but also on everyday life in general. This chapter deals with the current concerns of artists during the coronavirus pandemic. In view of the multidimensional definition of precarious work, this chapter also acknowledges the precarious working and living conditions of artists within the creative economy. It specifically explores three indicators of precariousness applied in the everyday life of artists and their working conditions: their nonstandard practices, the freebie culture surrounding the arts, and the underrepresentation of artists as a collective.

The data presented in this chapter had initiated discussion on a national platform and prompted action through the "Covid Wage Supplement" in Malta, as a systematic allocation of governmental measure to artists and creative practitioners. Additional to the supplement, this chapter outlined the need for artists to secure contracts that protect their rights over a period of time and to be represented adequately by unions or lobby groups and/or sector-led associations. The introduction of these measures and policies are necessary for an equitable income to artists, particularly to support them during times when their livelihood is at stake.

Note

1 The data in this research was presented as part of a keynote delivery by one of the authors, Toni Attard, as the director of Culture Venture at the International Virtual conference COVID-19 crisis and emergency funding mechanism: what action plan for the cultural and creative sectors organized by Fondation Rambourg Tunisie and Culture Funding Watch.

References

Arts Council England. 2011. "Internship in the Arts." Accessed April 6, 2020. www.arts council.org.uk/sites/default/files/download-file/internships_in_the_arts_final.pdf.

Arts Council Malta (ACM). 2020. "COVID-19 Wage Supplement Notice." Accessed April 1, 2020. www.artscouncilmalta.org/news/covid-19-wage-supplement-notice.

Attard, Toni. 2020. "Paying the Artist." Accessed March 30, 2020. http://cultureventure. org/2020/03/03/paying-the-artist/.

Bauman, Zygmunt. 2000. *Liquid Modernity*. Cambridge: Polity Press.

Beck, Ulrich. 1992 [1986]. *Risk Society: Towards a New Modernity*. London: Sage.

Beck, Ulrich, Joost van Loon, and Barbara Adam. 2000. *The Risk Society and Beyond: Critical Issues for Social Theory*. London: Sage.

Becker, Gary. 1964. *Human Capital*. New York: Columbia University Press.

Benach, Joan, Alejandra Vives, Gemma Tarafa, Carlos Delclos, and Carles Muntaner. 2016. "What Should We Know About Precarious Employment and Health in 2025? Framing the Agenda for the Next Decade of Research." *International Journal of Epidemiology* 45 (1): 232–38.

Boltanski, L., and E. Chiapello. 2005. "The New Spirit of Capitalism." *International Journal of Politics, Culture, and Society* 18: 161–88.

Bourdieu, Pierre. 1998. *Acts of Resistance. Against the New Myths of Our Time*. Cambridge: Polity Press.

Castells, Manuel. 2000. *The Rise of the Network Society. The Information Age: Economy, Society and Culture*, Vol. I. Oxford: Blackwell.

Edralin, Divina. M. 2014. "Precarious Work Undermines Decent Work: The Unionized Hotels Workers Experiences." *DLSU Business and Economics Review* 24 (1): 13–26.

Falvay Deirdre. 2020. "Stop Exploiting Artists with 'Freebie' Culture, Arts Council Says." *The Irish Times*. Accessed April 6, 2020. www.irishtimes.com/culture/stop-exploiting-artists-with-freebie-culture-arts-council-says 1.4168716?mode=amp&fbclid=IwAR0Y PiAaIIkkoHDG8LvbVSl4vPFtcfZ8XaSnK7hHGe_17OB_CeWOp8SpSzc.

Figiel, Joanna. 2014. "On the Citizen Forum for Contemporary Arts." *Artleaks Gazette*. Accessed April 4, 2020. https://artsleaks.files.wordpress.com/2012/09/joanna_figiel_ artleaks_gazette_2.pdf.

Garrett, Rebecca, and Liza Jackson. 2016. "Art, Labour and Precarity in the Age of Veneer Politics." *Alternate Routes* 27. Accessed April 11, 2020. www.alternateroutes.ca/index. php/ar/article/view/22404, 283.

Gill, Rosalind, and Andy Pratt. 2013. "Precarity and Cultural Work in the Social Factory? Immaterial Labour, Precariousness and Cultural Work." *On Curating* (16). Accessed April 4, 2020. www.on-curating.org/issue-16.html#.WZmUeYpLeog, 26.

Gray, Anne. 1998. "New Labour – New Labour Discipline." *Capital & Class* 65: 1–8.

Green, Ken. 2019. "Artists Need Unions, Too: The Role of Organized Labor in Creative Industries." *Union Track*. Accessed April 5, 2020. www.uniontrack.com/blog/artists-unions.

Kalleberg, Arne. 2009. "Precarious Work. Insecure Workers: Employment Relations in Transition." *American Sociological Review* 74 (1): 1–22.

Leban, Sebastjan. 2017. "Art in Residency: Precarity or Opportunity? Seismopolite." Accessed April 7, 2020. www.seismopolite.com/art-in-residency-precarity-or-opportunity.

Lewchak, Wayne, Alice de Wolff, Andy King, and Michael Polanyi. 2003. "From Job Strain to Employment Strain: Health Effects of Precarious Employment." *Just Labour* 3: 23–35.

Malta Enterprise. 2020. "Covid Wage Supplement." Accessed April 4, 2020. https://covid19.maltaenterprise.com/employee-wage-support/?application-form-added.

Micallef, Keith. 2020. "Enthusiasts React to Church's Feasts Directive and 'Early Stage' Decision." *Times of Malta*, 26 March. Accessed March 30, 2020. https://timesofmalta.com/articles/view/enthusiasts-react-to-churchs-feasts-directive-and-early-stage-decision.780929.

Milne, Alistair K. L. 2020. "A Critical COVID-19 Economic Policy Tool: Retrospective Insurance." March 21. SSRN: https://ssrn.com/abstract=3558667 or http://dx.doi.org/10.2139/ssrn.3558667.

Moscone, Franscesco, Elisa Tosetti, and Georgio Vittadini. 2016. "The Impact of Precarious Employment on Mental Health: The Case of Italy." *Social Science & Medicine* 158: 86–95.

Nanda, Serena. 2021. "Inequalities and COVID-19." In *COVID-19: Global Pandemic, Societal Responses, Ideological Solutions*, edited by J. Michael Ryan, 109–23. London: Routledge.

Perlin, Ross. 2011. *Intern Nation: How to Earn Nothing and Learn Little in the Brave New Economy*. London and New York: Verso.

Pulver, Andrew. 2020. "At Least 170,000 Lose Jobs as Film Industry Grinds to a Halt Due to Coronavirus." *The Guardian*, March 19. Accessed April 10, 2020. www.theguardian.com/film/2020/mar/19/loss-of-jobs-income-film-industry-hollywood-coronavirus-pandemic-covid-19.

Ross A., 2008. "The New Geography of Work: Power to the Precari-ous?" *Theory, Culture and Society* 25: 31–49

Ryan, Michael, J. 2021. "The Blessings of COVID-19 for Neoliberalism, Nationalism, and Neoconservative Ideologies." In *COVID-19: Global Pandemic, Societal Responses, Ideological Solutions*, edited by Michael Ryan, 80–93. London: Routledge.

Sennett, Richard. 1998. *Corrosion of Character – The Personal Consequences of Work in the New Capitalism*. New York: WW. Norton and Company.

———. 2006. *The Culture of the New Capitalism*. London: Yale University Press.

Sharp, Rob. 2017. "What We Can Learn from Artistic Unions in Poland." *Art Market*, April 13. Accessed April 7, 2020. www.artsy.net/article/artsy-editorial-artists-unionize.

Vosko, Leah. 2006. "Precarious Employment: Towards an Improved Understanding of Labour Market Insecurity." In *Precarious Employment: Understanding Labour Market Insecurity in Canada*, edited by Leah Vosko, 3–39. Montreal: McGill-Queens University Press.

PART III

Unveiling social inequalities

17

ANTI-ASIAN RACISM, RESPONSES, AND THE IMPACT ON ASIAN AMERICANS' LIVES

A social-ecological perspective

Pamela P. Chiang

Since the mass outbreak of COVID-19 in late December in Wuhan, China, racist attacks and discriminatory behaviors towards Chinese and Asians in general have drastically grown in many parts of the world (Coates 2020; White 2020). In the UK hate crimes against Chinese people tripled between January and March of 2020, compared to the same period in 2018 and 2019 (Chadwick 2020; Devakumar et al. 2020). In the virtual world, a 900% increase of hate speech toward China and Chinese people on Twitter was observed; online posts against Asians have also increased by 200% on hate sites (Business Standard 2020; Schild et al. 2020). Although the outbreak of the coronavirus in the United States took place after its spread in Asia and Europe, racist attacks and hate crimes against Asians and Asian Americans in the US had already occurred in Asian communities before the first case was confirmed in the country on January 20, 2020, in Washington State (Holshue et al. 2020). From March 19 to May 20, 2020, more than 1,700 incidents of verbal and physical assaults were reported to AAPI STOP HATE, a website set up by the Asian Pacific Policy Planning Council (A3PCON) (2020). According to the New York City Commission on Human Rights, out of 248 complaints received from February to April 2020, more than 99 cases (40%) were about anti-Asian discrimination compared to only five reports during the same time frame in 2019 (Holcombe and Moghe 2020).

Drawing on the social-ecological perspective (Ungar 2002), this chapter examines the experience of anti-Asian racism among people of Asian descent in the United States during the pandemic, their responses to racism and attacks, and the extent to which their lives have been affected at various levels of the environment (micro: individual; mezzo: families and communities; and macro: societal/cultural/political systems). This framework, based on Bronfenbrenner's (1977) ecological perspective, is used to understand how people and their environment interact, and how human beings are shaped by and adapted to their environments and by the larger contexts in which settings are embedded. In addition, this chapter also examines current literature (e.g., newspapers, websites, articles, newsletters, etc.) to enhance the understanding of how community organizations and government agencies have responded to this spike in anti-racism against Asians due to COVID-19.

The forms of racist attacks against people of Asian descent in the United States are not limited to verbal assault, such as racial hashtags "Kung-Flu" and "Go back to your country," but also include physical assault, school bullying, harassment, and discrimination. Reports included being followed, having cars coughed on, being spat on, being barred from public transportation and services, job loss, and vandalism and property damage to Asian-owned businesses (Tessler, Choi, and Kao 2020; Thorbecke and Zaru 2020). Even Asian American health professionals, who were fighting coronavirus on the front lines, faced racist rejection or confrontation from their patients in the workplace and in the community (Jan 2020).

Studies have documented various reasons for the increased hate crimes against Asians and Asian Americans amid the pandemic. First, xenophobia has long existed in the history of the United States, in that when illness came from other countries, society tended to fear foreign-born people (Campbell and Ellerbeck 2020; Cheng 2020; Litam 2020; White 2020). Anti-Asian racism in the context of COVID-19 is arguably an extension of xenophobia in the 21st century in that it scapegoats people of Asian descent of the virus spread even when scientific evidence pointed out that COVID-19 in New York City originated from Europe, not from Asia (Mount Sinai 2020).

Another factor contributing to this wave of hate crimes is the continued misinformation disseminated by the media coverage that reinforced racial misrepresentation of Asian Americans in the pandemic (Litam 2020; Noel 2020). In early February 2020 when the first coronavirus case in New York City was discovered in Manhattan, *The New York Times* covered the news using images of Asians wearing face masks in a predominantly Asian community, Flushing, New York, instead of an image of Manhattan (Campbell and Ellerbeck 2020; Goldstein 2020).

The third force came from government officials' use of racist language that escalated the existing climate of hostility. On March 16, 2020, President Trump openly referred to coronavirus as the "China Virus," which was later found to be the point at which blame and Sinophobia increased tremendously on social media platforms (Jan 2020; Schild et al. 2020). During the same time, a national mental health crisis hotline reported a 39% increase in text messages for help from Asian Americans after President Trump's derogatory language (Filbin 2020). The president continued to use the term "Kung-Flu" in June, and so did other officials in the White House briefing (McEnany 2020).

While many anti-Asian racist incidents have been extensively covered in the news, hardly any literature has examined how individuals of Asian descent have responded to such attacks and how these have affected their lives during the pandemic when facing two wars at once – coronavirus and racism (Misra et al. 2020). In addition, even less literature has tracked what the federal and state governments as well as NGOs in the United States have done to respond to this heightened report of hate crimes since December of 2019. This chapter begins to fill that gap.

Survey study

Method

For five consecutive days from June 18 to June 22, 2020, the author launched an online survey in English in about ten social groups on Facebook in which primary members are Taiwanese, Chinese, and people of other Asian ethnicities living in the United States. The survey link was also distributed via emails and text messages throughout the author's personal networks to individuals who fit the survey criteria. Survey respondents were required to meet the following three criteria in order to participate in the online survey: (1) be at least 18 years of age or above; (2) be of Asian descent (Asian, Asian American, or with roots in East Asia, South Asia, or Southeast Asia); (3) had stayed or lived in the United States during the pandemic (from December 2019 to the time the survey was conducted in June 2020).

The survey included ten questions, separated into two categories: (1) five demographic questions addressed sex, age, ethnicity, state residency, and the length of residence in the US and (2) five main questions measured respondents' personal experience of racist attacks, harassment, or/and discrimination (or their family's or friend's experience), their awareness of racist attacks from the media and social media, their responses to such attacks, and the impacts that these have had on their lives. There is also an open-ended question in the end of the survey allowing respondents to elaborate. This study has been approved by the Institutional Review Board at the university with which the author was affiliated. All the survey respondents were provided with an electronic consent form to indicate their consent prior to participating.

Survey results

The final valid sample size was 249. The mean age was 39.2 (SD = 9.7). Most respondents were female (69%), and about one-third were male (31%). The majority were Taiwanese (77.9%); Chinese made up 15.3%, the rest were Korean (1.6%), Filipino (1.2%), Japanese (0.4), Indian Chinese, and Malaysian Chinese. In terms of the length of residency in the United States, more than half (58.7%) of respondents had lived in the US for at least a decade: nearly 30% had lived in the US for 10 to less than 20 years, 29% had lived in the US for 20 years and more, and 5.7% were born in the United States. As a result, most of the participants were not newly arrived immigrants, who may have had language barriers or adjustment

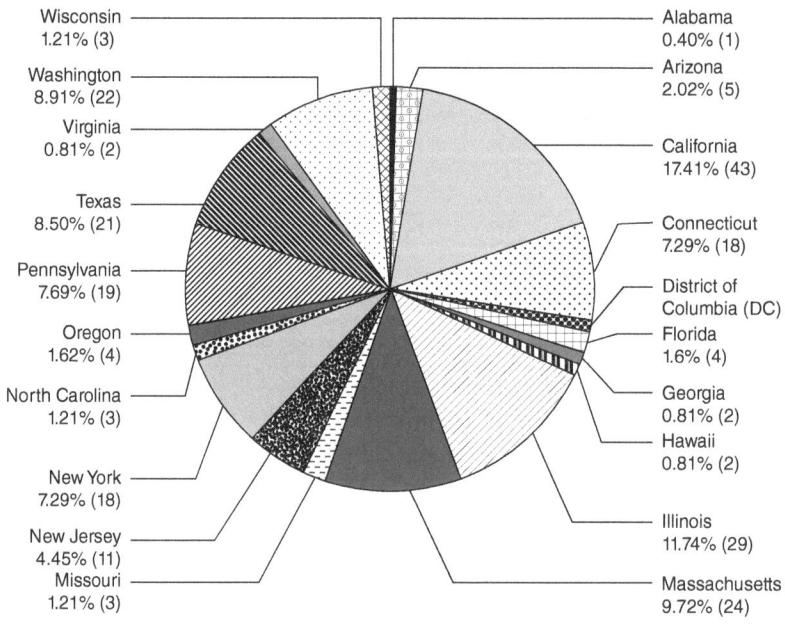

FIGURE 17.1 Distribution of State Residency

issues in the United States. As indicated by Figure 17.1, the majority of respondents were from the following states: Washington (8.9%), New York (7.3%), New Jersey (4.5%), California (17.4%), Connecticut (7.3%), Illinois (11.7%), and Massachusetts (9.7%). This distribution fits the outbreak in the United States that occurred in early March, when the majority of confirmed cases were on the East and West coasts and Illinois.

Experience of racist attacks and harassment

When asked to "check any of the following acts(s) that happened to you or to your family/friends/colleagues in relation to your (or their) Asian descent since December 2019 in the United States," as shown in Figure 17.2, more than half of respondents (51.8%) reported that neither their family or friends nor themselves personally experienced any racist attack. In other words, 48.2% of the respondents had personal experience or their family or friends did. The top reported racist act was "verbal harassment/assault" (38.2%), followed by "online message abuse on social media (Facebook, Twitter, etc.) (10.8%); the third most commonly reported attack was "physical harassment/assault" (6.4%).

In the narratives, venues in which respondents reported experiencing verbal microaggression and physical attacks included in parking lots, metro stations, and even schools and universities normally assumed to be safe environments. Instances

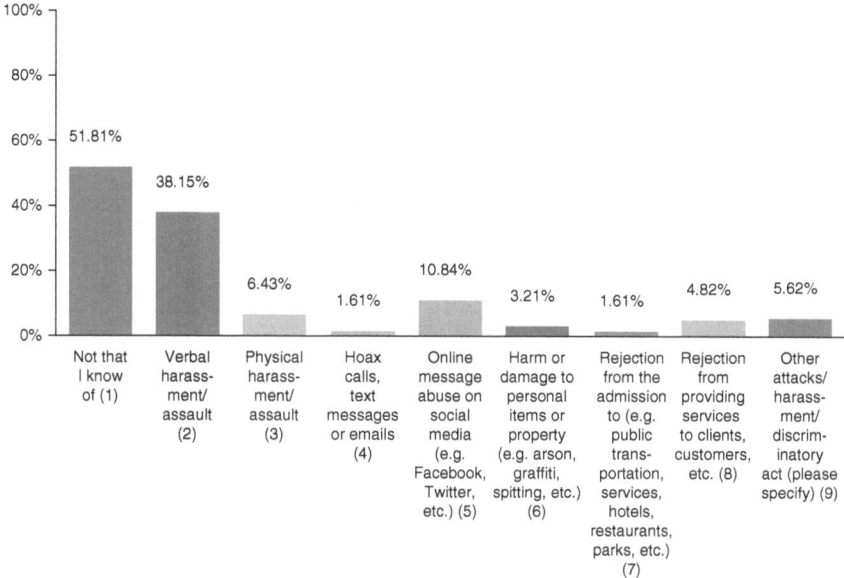

FIGURE 17.2 Racist Act(s) That Happened to Respondents or to Their Family/Friends/Colleagues in the United States During the Pandemic

include, "My kids 8 and 9 years old got attacks at school," "My professor teased me, 'did you bring virus back during the winter break?'" "My friend at the University received many anonymous mails saying to kill Asians," and "I was verbal attacked and threatened because of wearing a mask on NYC metro." Others received disparate treatment and unfriendly attitudes in restaurants or stores (e.g., scoffing, being treated in an unfriendly way compared to White customers, etc.). For example, "The deli worker won't talk to me and disinfected utensil station right after I stopped by"; "I got (an) assault note on my car."

Awareness of racist attacks learned from the media and social media

Compared to a lower rate of racist attacks on the individual or their family or friends (48.2%), respondents reported a much higher percentage of awareness of racist acts in the media and social media (84.7%), which had equal potential to instill fear in them and to affect how they fared and responded in their daily lives.

The top three types of racist attack they experienced via all forms of media are similar to their personal experience: "verbal harassment/assault" (77.5%)"; "physical harassment/assault" (62.3%); and "harm or damage to personal items or property (arson, graffiti, spitting, etc.)" (41.4%).

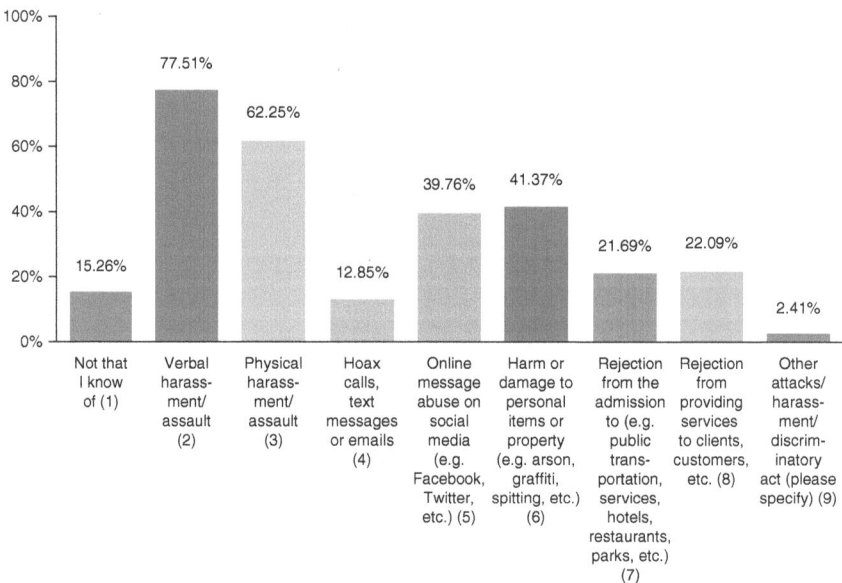

FIGURE 17.3 Racist Act(s) Learned in the Media and Social Media in the United States

Ways to respond

For those who personally experienced anti-Asian racism attack/harassment (an esti-mated 97 people), when asked how they responded to such acts/incidents, 80.4% of them reported they just walked away; 54.6% said they told their friends, family, colleagues, or posted it on social media. Only 16.5% reported it to authorities (e.g., police, guards, or other reporting system, etc.) and even fewer (3.1%) spoke with mental health professionals about their experience. Some reported (13.4%) that they called out or fought back on the spot or on social media, demonstrated by quotes such as "I called them out for their racism and had verbal arguments, then proceeded to walk away," "I confronted and talked to the person who initiated the act," and "I responded directly on social media to the person who attacked."

Life impact of racist attacks

In this question respondents were asked, "to what extent do you find the following statements to be true in your life?" (Answer choices included "a lot," "a moderate amount," "a little," and "not at all.") Respondents were given 11 statements and were asked to rate each statement that addressed the following: mental health con-dition, feeling about job security, how they did their grocery shopping, whether they ever tried to cover their Asian traits (by wearing a mask or sunglasses), reduc-tion of going out, reduction of going out alone, whether they had ever thought about leaving America, and involvement in social advocacy in the context of racism during the pandemic.

On the micro level, as shown in Figure 17.4, among responses that reporting these statements to be true (those who answered "a lot," "a moderate amount," and "a little"), the top three impacts were "I have become anxious, stressed or worried because of the concern for racist climate/acts" (79.9%); "I have become vigilant when going out because of the concern for racist climate/acts" (78.3%); and "I worried about the safety of my family members because of their Asian traits" (75.1%). The results show that the direct impact of racist attacks heavily weigh on people's mental health.

On the mezzo level, in terms of how people engaged in their community, in their workplace, or in the larger US society, pandemic-related racism also affected people's feelings, behavior, and intent to continue living in the US. For example, 51.8% reported that they reduced their engagement in the community or neighborhood "by going out less" and "by not going out alone but with company" (41.8%). As further, 43.7% of respondents affirmed, "I worried about my job opportunity/ security/performance evaluation because of my Asian descent," which supports in the early outbreak a disproportionately large number of applications for unemployment benefits by people of Asian descent (Thorbecke and Zaru 2020). An even more profound impact is that one-third (33.7%) of respondents even thought about moving (relocating) to their country of origin or to another country because of the concern for racist climate/acts. This is of great concern, as we know that the majority of the survey respondents had lived in the US for more than a decade, including those who were born in the United States.

Going beyond the individual and family life, a small percentage of people indicated that experience of racism first hand or in the media resulted in their

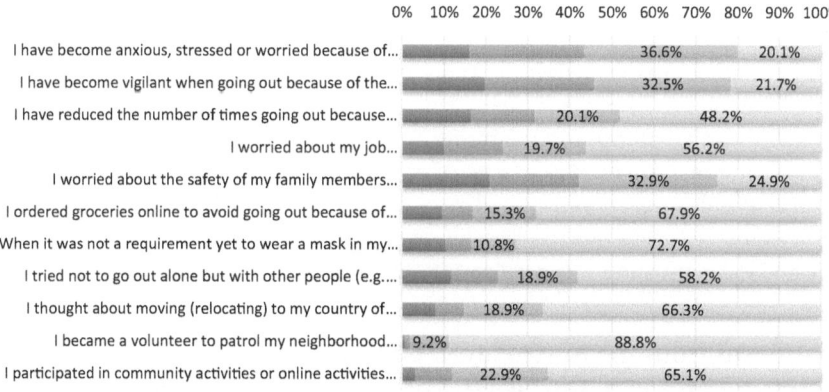

FIGURE 17.4 Life Impact of Racist Attacks

involvement in activism, advocacy, and mutual support in the community. For instance, about one-third (34.9%) indicated that they "participated in community activities or online activities to address anti-Asian racism." Another 11.24% of respondents agreed, "I became a volunteer to patrol my neighborhood because of the concern for racist climate/acts."

Interestingly, even though 27.3% of respondents indicated in the affirmative as to whether "they ever tried to cover their face by wearing a mask or sunglasses so that people cannot easily recognize their Asian traits when wearing a mask was not a requirement yet in their state," some respondents talked about their fear of wearing a facial mask (of their own will) and that they were racially attacked when the state's policy was not yet requiring people to wear a facial mask, which put those of Asian descent at a higher risk of being racially profiled (Leung 2020). For example, a respondent wrote, "before the official shelter in place order, people looked at me very strangely while I wear a mask at work"; another said, "reason for not wearing face masks, because we get stared at"; and "early on when government suggested not to wear a mask really put Asian American at risk."

Study limitations

There is scarcity of studies on people's responses to racism and the impact of racism on Asian Americans' lives since the outbreak of pandemic in late January 2020 in the United States. The study has strengths in that it not only addressed the aforementioned questions but also conducted primary research in the Asian community after most states' lockdown policies had nearly ended and states were partially reopened (Haffajee and Mello 2020). Despite the small sample size, the responses represent residents' voices from 19 states and the District of Columbia.

The study does, however, have limitations given the short time frame of data collection. For instance, respondents were offered an English version of the online survey. Only people with English literacy and access to certain social media platforms could participate in the survey. Further studies should consider offering the survey in other Asian languages in order to reach out to more Asian Americans whose English proficiency is limited. The study also received more responses from states with large outbreaks in the spring, and where large cities, such as Chicago, Seattle, Boston, San Francisco, Los Angeles, and New York, for example, are located. People's experience of and responses to racism and discrimination may greatly vary if they live in states with fewer people of Asian descent, less diversity of race and ethnicity, and more rural areas as opposed to metropolitan areas.

Responses from the macro level: efforts by the government and NGOs

On the macro level, what have state and federal governments, as well as Congress, and community-based organizations done in response to the rise of anti-Asian racism in the country despite President Trump's administration repeatedly using derogatory rhetoric to downgrade Asian Americans and their cultural heritage in the usage of the terms, "China Virus" and "Kung-Flu" since March 2020?

First of all, Congress and its members took steps to raise awareness and denounce the racism. On February 26, 2020, the Congressional Asian Pacific American Caucus (CAPAC) urged Congress members to share evidence-based information with their constituents in order to stop the xenophobia and misinformation related to COVID-19 (CAPAC 2020). On March 11, 2020, the National Council of Asian Pacific Americans (NCAPA) along with 260 NGOs wrote to the Speaker of the House and the Senate to "call for unity, and publicly denounce the increase in racist attacks and discrimination against the Asian American community" (NACPA 2020). In April, a dozen senators requested the U.S. Commission on Human Rights (USCCR) to take stronger actions to prevent and address anti-Asian racism in a letter (Yam 2020).

As for the federal government, rather than proactively take actions to prevent and to promote a uniform response, actions have been limited to reactively issuing guidelines and offering statements and warnings compared to the series of initiatives taken after the 9/11 terrorist attack in 2001 (Campbell and Ellerbeck 2020) and those during the SARS outbreak in 2003 (Person et al. 2004). For instance, the Centers for Disease Control and Prevention (CDC) released a statement for "Reducing Stigma" related to the spread of coronavirus (CDC 2020). In early March, the US Department of Education (2020) issued a coronavirus statement to educators to inform them of the increasing number of bullying against students of Asian descent and to ensure that CDC guidelines were followed after several bullying occurrences had already taken place in the nation (Capatides 2020). In spite of the FBI warning in late March about the surge of racist attacks against Asian Americans (Margolin 2020), it was not until May that the US Commission on Civil Rights (2020) issued recommendations to all civil rights commissions in the country that "it is also necessary for the federal government to communicate and act in a manner that demonstrates to communities that it will protect all Americans regardless of race, national origin, or other protected characteristics."

At the state level, a few states have shown more efforts than other states have in investigating anti-Asian racism and hate crimes. On March 23, 2020, the state of New York's Office of the Attorney General launched a hotline to report hate crimes and bias-based incidents "in the wake of rising reports of harassment and assaults, as well as rhetoric against Asian Americans" (New York Attorney General 2020). The New York City Commission on Human Rights (NYCCHR) organized a COVID-19 Response Team and launched a series of efforts to combat racist attacks and discrimination by putting ads in local media, on online texting platforms, and in shops in the community to encourage reporting of discrimination (Cheng 2020; Thorbecke 2020). The Asian American Commission of Massachusetts (2020) held numerous webinars and panels raising awareness during the Asian American and Pacific Islander Heritage month in May 2020 and launched an online reporting system for racial hostility. On April 30, 2020, the California Department of Justice (2020) issued a bulletin to law enforcement officials across the state to ensure the awareness of hate crime activity and the preparedness to respond to such crimes. The Seattle Police Department (2020) set up a reporting system for hate crimes and the Bias Crimes Unit within the Violent Crimes section to investigate these bias-based cases and to track and report trends on a monthly basis. Unfortunately, the federal government's approach to facing the nationwide issue of anti-Asian racism has been the same as its response to the nationwide surge of COVID-19: leaving localities and states alone to take mitigation measures in their own states and towns (Haffajee and Mello 2020).

In contrast, nongovernmental organizations have been a lot more proactive in making substantial efforts to tackle hate acts, to empower Asian Americans to cope with violence, as well as to promote neighborhood surveillance in Asian communities. For instance, the Asian Pacific Policy Planning Council (A3PCON 2020) in Los Angeles soon initiated a website to track hate crime reports against AAPI (STOP AAPI HATE) in March 2020. The Guardian Angels, a New York–based organization that mobilizes volunteers to patrol in many communities in the US and around the world, for the first time in 41 years recruited in Asian communities to protect residents in various Chinatowns (Chang 2020). Asian Americans Advancing Justice (AAJC 2020), a national organization that aims to improve the civil and human rights of Asian Americans, launched a series of online bystander intervention programs to train people to address xenophobic harassment, de-escalate conflict, and maintain self-care. The Lawyers' Committee for Civil Rights under Law (2020) in the District of Columbia offered a Stop Hate Project that provides hate crime victims with resources such as "pro bono attorneys, community organization, mental health services and access to counsel."

Community collaboration, however, will not be enough without the monitoring and intervening action of the virtual world on social media platforms by tech companies, especially when a lot of hate speech and human interaction turned into online activities during the lockdown in March 2020 (Croucher, Nguyen, and Rahmani 2020). Therefore, the gatekeeping of social media has become extremely important and time sensitive during the pandemic. In mid–March 2020 major companies such as Facebook, Reddit, Google, LinkedIn, Twitter, Microsoft, and YouTube issued a joint statement to fight against misinformation surrounding the coronavirus pandemic (Romm 2020; Shu and Shieber 2020). As false information has quickly spread online during the pandemic, which the World Health Organization (WHO) has termed an "infodemic" (Rithtel 2020), actions to limit misinformation while promoting accurate information should also apply to the spread of racist slurs, rumors, and verbal abuse spread online about people of Asian descent.

Conclusion

As the United States has been the country most severely hit by COVID-19, scapegoating one single race for the loss and grief caused by the spread of disease will not heal the nation but instead divides it further and undermines the harmony and collaboration it takes for the US society to recover. The stereotypes that continue to deem and treat Asian Americans as foreigners despite their immigration history in the United States since the 19th century and being the most rapidly growing immigrant group in the 21st century (US Census Bureau 2017) will only continue to obscure their contribution to a stronger and more diverse society.

The study results resonate with others in that the foremost impact of racism during the pandemic is the deterioration of individuals' mental health (Litam 2020). The results also suggest that people's feeling of safety in the community and in their workplace as well as their intentions of remaining in the United States have also been jeopardized. Even though pandemic-related racism has motivated people of Asian descent to become more involved in community organizations and volunteering (Tessler, Choi, and Kao 2020), particularly through NGOs in establishing mutual aid networks and self-defense as found in this study, combating anti-Asian racism during the pandemic has not ignited nationwide reckoning on the xenophobia that Asian Americans have long suffered in the United States for centuries. Continued efforts to raise more awareness and to advocate for the safety and well-being of Asians and Asian Americans in the United States are vital in the future.

The pandemic has already taken a toll on many people's physical and mental health; however, Asians and Asian Americans psychologically bear even more burdens due to the violence, assault, and discrimination in everyday life, in news, and on social media. As the findings revealed, only a very small percentage (3%) of people chose to seek out help from mental health professionals after encountering racist attacks or harassment. While it has been well-documented that Asian Americans in general have a low rate of mental health care utilization (Yee, Ceballos, and Lawless 2020), it is imperative to dismantle structural racism so that people of Asian descent feel comfortable and safe seeking mental health care in this critical time. For mental health care providers, it is important that they are aware of the contextual stress and strain on this racial group amid the pandemic and thus adopt culturally sensitive and trauma-based interventions in working with this population (Litam 2020). In the meantime, it may be more effective to offer community outreach meetings, services, and programs directly in Asian communities when the stigma and stereotype against Asian Americans persist in the larger context (Misra et al. 2020).

COVID-19 is not only a health pandemic but also a pandemic of anti-Asian racism and violence. Just as we need the federal government to respond to the COVID-19 spread in a swift and strong policy action (Haffajee and Mello 2020), we also need the national leadership in early and concerted efforts to address the various forms of racial discrimination against people of Asian descent in order to stop the spread and negative impact of this racism pandemic. No individuals, communities, or even a single state alone can mitigate xenophobia, hostility, and discrimination during the crisis and following the pandemic era while simultaneously trying to lessen the ramifications of coronavirus in the US society (Human Rights Watch 2020).

References

Asian Americans Advancing Justice. 2020. "As Trump Doubles Down on Racist Rhetoric at Tulsa Rally, Advancing Justice | AAJC and Hollabak! Train More than 10,000 to Address Anti-Asian and Anti-Asian American Harassment." Accessed June 1, 2020. www.advancingjustice-aajc.org/press-release/trump-doubles-down-racist-rhetoric-tulsa-rally-advancing-justice-aajc-and-hollaback.

Asian Pacific Policy and Planning Council (A3PCON). 2020. "Stop AAPI Hate Reporting Center." Accessed June 15, 2020. www.asianpacificpolicyandplanningcouncil.org/wpcontent/uploads/Press_Release_5_13_20.pdf.

Bronfenbrenner, Urie. 1977. "Toward an Experimental Ecology of Human Development." *American Psychologist* 32 (7): 513–31.

Business Standard. 2020. "Twitter Sees 900% Increase in Hate Speech Towards China Due to Coronavirus." Accessed June 1, 2020. www.business-standard.com/article/international/twitter-sees-900-increase-in-hate-speech-towards-china-due-to-coronavirus-120032800240_1.html.

California Department of Justice. 2020. "California Laws That Prohibit Hate Crimes and/or Provide Enhanced Penalties for Specified Hate-Related Acts." Accessed June 1, 2020. https://oag.ca.gov/system/files/attachments/press-docs/2020%20-%20Hate%20Crime%20Bulletin.pdf.

Campbell, Alexia Fernandez, and Alex Ellerbeck. 2020. "Federal Agencies Are Doing Little About the Rise in Anti-Asian Hate." *NBC News*, April 16. www.nbcnews.com/news/asian-america/federal-agencies-are-doing-little-about-rise-anti-asian-hate-n1184766.

Capatides, Christina. 2020. "Bullies Attack Asian American Teen at School, Accusing Him of Having Coronavirus." *CBS News*, February 14. www.cbsnews.com/news/coronavirus-bullies-attack-asian-teen-los-angeles-accusing-him-of-having-coronavirus/.

Centers for Disease Control and Prevention (CDC). 2020. "Reducing Stigma". Accessed June 11, 2020. www.cdc.gov/coronavirus/2019-ncov/daily-life-coping/reducing-stigma.html.

Chadwick, Johnathan. 2020. "'Playgrounds for Racism': Trust in Social Media Is Fulling Prejudice Against Chinese People During the Coronavirus Pandemic, Study Shows." *Daily Mail*, June 12. www.dailymail.co.uk/sciencetech/article-8414537/Social-media-fuelling-prejudice-against-Chinese-people-pandemic-study-claims.html?ITO=applenews.

Chang, Richard. 2020. "U.S. Asians, Harassed Over Coronavirus, Push Back on Streets, Social Media." *US News & World Report*, May 29. www.usnews.com/news/world/articles/2020-05-29/us-asians-harassed-over-coronavirus-push-back-on-streets-social-media.

Cheng, Shuliang Oliver. 2020. "Xenophobia Due to the Coronavirus Outbreak – A Letter to the Editor in Response to the Socio-Economic Implications of the Coronavirus Pandemic COVID-19): A Review." *International Journal of Surgery* 79 (July): 13–14. https://doi.org/10.1016/j.ijsu.2020.05.017.

Coates, Melanie. 2020. "Covid-19 and the Rise of Racism." *BMJ* 369 (April): 1384. https://doi.org/10.1136/bmj.m1384.

Congressional Asian Pacific American Caucus (CAPAC). 2020. "As Coronavirus Fears Incite Violence, CAPAC Members Urge Colleagues to Not Stoke Xenophobia." Accessed June 15, 2020. https://chu.house.gov/media-center/press-releases/coronavirus-fears-incite-violence-capac-members-urge-colleagues-not.

Croucher, Stephan M., Thao Nguyen, and Diyako Rahmani. 2020. "Prejudice Toward Asian Americans in the Covid-19 Pandemic: The Effects of Social Media Use in the United States." *Frontier in Communication* 5 (June): 39. https://doi.org/10.3389/fcomm.2020.00039.

Devakumar, Delan, Geordan Shannon, Sunil S. Bhopal, and Ibrahim Abubakar. 2020. "Racism and Discrimination in COVID-19 Responses." *The Lancet* 395 (April): 1194. http://dx.doi.org/10.1016/S0140-6736(20)30792-3.

Filbin, Bob. 2020. "Bob's Notes on COVID-19: Mental Health Data on the Pandemic." *Crisis Text Line.* Accessed June 1, 2020. www.crisistextline.org/data/bobs-notes-on-covid-19-mental-health-data-on-the-pandemic/.

Goldstein, Joseph. 2020. "New York City Eyes First Suspected Case of Coronavirus." *The New York Times*, February 3. www.nytimes.com/2020/02/01/nyregion/coronavirus-new-york-city.html?searchResultPosition=8.

Haffajee, Rebecca L., and Michelle M. Mello. 2020. "Think Globally, Acting Locally—the U.S. Response to Covid-19." *New England Journal of Medicine* 382: e75. http://doi.org/10.1056/NEJMp2006740.

Holcombe, Madeline, and Sonia Moghe. 2020. "NYC Launches Team to Combat Coronavirus Discrimination." *CNN*, April 22. www.cnn.com/2020/04/22/us/new-york-coronavirus-discrimination-harassment-response-team/index.html.

Holshue, Michelle L., Chas Debolt, Scott Lindquist, Kathy H. Lofty, John Wiesman, Hollianne Bruce, Christopher Spitters, et al. 2020. "First Case of 2019 Novel Coronavirus in the United States." *New England Journal of Medicine* 382: 929–36. https://doi.org/10.1056/NEJMoa2001191.

Human Rights Watch. 2020. "Covid-19 Fueling Anti-Asian Racism and Xenophobia Worldwide." Accessed May 12, 2020. www.hrw.org/news/2020/05/12/covid-19-fueling-anti-asian-racism-and-xenophobia-worldwide.

Jan, Tracy. 2020. "Asian American Doctors and Nurses Are Fighting Racism and the Coronavirus." *The Washington Post*, May 19. www.washingtonpost.com/business/2020/05/19/asian-american-discrimination/.

Lawyers' Committee for Civil Rights Under Law. 2020. "Stop Hate." Accessed June 20, 2020. https://lawyerscommittee.org/project/stop-hate-project/.

Leung, Hillary. 2020. "Why Wearing a Face Mask Is Encouraged in Asia, but Shunned in the U.S." *Time*, March 12. https://time.com/5799964/coronavirus-face-mask-asia-us/.

Litam, Stacey Diane Arañez. 2020. "Take Your Kung-Flu Back to Wuhan: Counseling Asians, Asian Americans, and Pacific Islanders with Race-Based Trauma Related to COVID-19." *The Professional Counselor* 10 (2): 144–56. https://doi.org/10.15241/sdal.10.2.144.

Margolin, Josh. 2020. "FBI Warns of Potential Surge in Hate Crimes Against Asian Americans amid Coronavirus." *ABC News*, March 27. https://abcnews.go.com/US/fbi-warns-potential-surge-hate-crimes-asian-americans/story?id=69831920.

McEnany, Kayleigh (@PressSec). 2020. "Under President, the Federal Government Has Been an Indispensable Partner to States as We Work to Defeat the China Virus." *Twitter*, July 21, 3:32 p.m. https://twitter.com/presssec/status/1285659032162897921?s=21.

Misra, Supriya, Phuong Thao D. Le, Emily Goldmann, and Lawrence H. Yang. 2020. "Psychological Impact of Anti-Asian Stigma Due to the COVID-19 Pandemic: A Call for Research, Practice, and Policy Responses." *Psychological Trauma: Theory, Research, Practice, and Policy.* http://dx.doi.org/10.1037/tra0000821.

Mount Sinai. 2020. "Mount Sinai Study Finds First Cases of COVID-19 in New York City Are Primarily from European and US Sources." *News Release.* June 2. www.mountsinai.org/about/newsroom/2020/mount-sinai-study-finds-first-cases-of-covid-19-in-new-york-city-are-primarily-from-european-and-us-sources-pr.

National Council of Asian Pacific Americans (NCAPA). 2020. "A Letter to House Leader-ship." Accessed June 16, 2020. https://d3n8a8pro7vhmx.cloudfront.net/ncapa/pages/89/attachments/original/1583935643/NCAPA_Letter_to_House_Leadership.pdf?1583935643.

New York Attorney General. 2020. "AG James Launched Hotline to Combat Coronavi-rus Hate Crimes and Xenophobic Rhetoric." Accessed March 23. https://ag.ny.gov/press-release/2020/ag-james-launches-hotline-combat-coronavirus-hate-crimes-and-xenophobic-rhetoric.

Noel, Tiffany Karalis. 2020. "Conflating Cutlure with COVID-19: Xenophobi Repercus-sions of a Global Pandemic." *Social Sciences & Humanities Open* 2 (1): 100044. https://doi.org/10.1016/j.ssaho.2020.100044.

Person, Bobbie, Francisco Sy, Kelly Holton, Barbara Govert, Arthur Liang, Brenda Garza, Deborah Gould, et al. 2004. "Fear and Stigma: The Epidemic within the SARS Outbreak." *Emerging Infectious Diseases* 10 (2): 358–63. https://doi.org/10.3201/eid1002.030750.

Rithtel, Matt. 2020. "W.H.O. Fights a Pandemic Besides Coronavirus: An 'Infodemic'." *New York Times*, February 6. www.nytimes.com/2020/02/06/health/coronavirus-mis information-social-media.html.

Romm, Tony. 2020. "White House Asks Silicon Valley for Help to Combat Coronavirus, Track Its Spread and Stop Misinformation." *Washington Post*, March 11. www.washing tonpost.com/technology/2020/03/11/white-house-tech-meeting-coronavirus.

Schild, Leonard, Chen Ling, Jeremy Blackburn, Gianluca Strnghini, Yang Zhang, and Savvas Zannettou. 2020. "Go Eat a Bat, Chang an Early Look on the Emergence of Sinophobic Behavior on Web Communities in the Face of COVID-19." *Computers and Society*, April 1–16. http://arxiv.org/pdf/2004.04046.pdf.

Seattle Police Department. 2020. "Hate Crime Unit." Accessed June 1. www.seattle.gov/police/information-and-data/bias-crime-unit.

Shu, Catherine, and Jonathan Shieber. 2020. "Facebook, Reddit, Google, LinkedIn, Microsoft, Twitter and YouTube Issue Joint Statement on Misinformation." Accessed June 1. https://techcrunch.com/2020/03/16/facebook-reddit-google-linkedin-micro soft-twitter-and-youtube-issue-joint-statement-on-misinformation/2020/03/16/face book-reddit-google-linkedin-microsoft-twitter-and-youtube-issue-joint-statement-on-misinformation/.

Tessler, Hannah, Meera Choi, and Grace Kao. 2020. "The Anxiety of Being Asian Ameri-can: Hate Crimes and Negative Biases During the COVID-19 Pandemic." *American Journal of Criminal Justice* (June): 1–1. https://doi.org/10.1007/s12103-020-09541-5.

Thorbecke, Catherine. 2020. "NYC Launches $100,000 Effort to Combat Anti-Asian Discrimination in COVID-19 Era." *ABC News*, May 26. https://abcnews.go.com/US/nyc-launches-100000-effort-combat-anti-asian-discrimination/story?id=70830974.

Thorbecke, Catherine, and Deena Zaru. 2020. "Why Asian American Unemployment Spiked 5,000% in NY During the Pandemic." *ABC News*, May 13. https://abcnews.go.com/Busi ness/asian-americans-face-coronavirus-double-whammy-skyrocketing-unemployment/story?id=70654426.

Ungar, Michael. 2002. "A Deeper, More Social Ecological Social Work Practice." *Social Service Review* 76 (3) (September): 480–97. https://doi.org/0.1086/341185.

U.S. Census Bureau. 2017. "Selected Characteristics of the Foreign-Born Population by Period of Entry into the United States: 2017 American Community Survey 1-Year Esti-mates." Accessed July 1, 2020. https://data.census.gov/cedsci/table?tid=ACSST5Y2017.S0501&q=S0501.

U.S. Commission on Civil Rights. 2020. "U.S. Commission on Civil Rights Unanimously Issues Recommendation to Secure Nondiscrimination in the COVID-19 Pandemic

Context, and Specifically to Address Anti-Asian Racism and Xenophobia." Accessed June 1, 2020. www.usccr.gov/press/2020/05-08-Anti-Asian-Discrimination.pdf.

U.S. Department of Education. 2020. "OCR Coronavirus Statement." Accessed June 1, 2020. https://content.govdelivery.com/accounts/USED/bulletins/27f5130.

White, Alexandre I. R. 2020. "The Art of Medicine: Historical Linkages: Epidemic Threat, Economic Risk, and Xenophobia." *The Lancet* 395 (April): 1250–251. http://dx.doi.org/10.1016/S0140-6736(20)30737-6.

Yam, Kimmy. 2020. "Senate Democrats Call for Federal Action on Anti-Asian Coronavirus Racism." *NBC News*, April 10. www.nbcnews.com/news/asian-america/warren-duckworth-hirono-call-federal-agencies-address-asian-america-coronavirus-n1181086.

Yee, Terence, Peggy Ceballos, and Alexis Lawless. 2020. "Help-Seeking Attitudes of Chinese Americans and Chinese Immigrants in the United States: The Mediating Role of Self-Stigma." *Journal of Multicultural Counseling and Development* 48 (1): 30–43. https://doi.org/10.1002/jmcd.12162.

18

THE IMPACT OF COVID-19 ON THE LIVES OF SEXUAL AND GENDER MINORITY PEOPLE

Matthew D. Skinta, Angela H. Sun, and Daniel M. Ryu

As of July 2020, over 14 million people have tested positive for COVID-19 world-wide and more than half a million have perished. During this pandemic, sexual and gender minority (SGM; i.e., lesbian, gay, bisexual, pansexual, transgender, nonbinary, etc.) people have experienced both blame and scapegoating related to historic animus, as well as an exacerbation of preexisting disparities within health-care systems. This chapter is grounded in minority stress theory, which proposes that the pervasive expression of societal anti–SGM animus may manifest through the internalization of negative social attitudes, behavioral patterns of concealment and interpersonal guardedness to protect the self against discrimination, and the direct harm of violence and prejudicial treatment (Meyer 2003; Hendricks and Testa 2012). This cumulative stress has been found to lead to a wide range of physical and psychological health disparities (e.g., Bränström, Hatzenbuehler, and Pachankis 2016; Burton et al. 2013). The first section explores the primary expres-sions of social bias that have been well-documented since the start of the pandemic: blame for COVID-19 due to moral/religious reasons or a broader association with disease; eruptions of violence toward SGM people under the guise of preventing the spread of COVID-19; expressions of bias that endanger SGM people in context of the broader pandemic; and the weakening of legal and administrative protections against discrimination while the public is focused on COVID-19.

The second half of the chapter will emphasize the direct effects of COVID-19 on the health and well-being of individuals in SGM communities. SGM people are overrepresented in contexts that present obstacles to complying with shelter-in-place orders or increase risk of virus exposure, including refugee and asylum seekers, homeless populations, and individuals who may not be out to family or those with whom they cohabit. SGM-specific disparities in healthcare access exist internationally and may be further exacerbated by the strain and restrictions of

COVID-19 upon healthcare services. COVID-related restrictions have also disrupted access to gender-affirming care for transgender patients and HIV-related care such as medication and pre-exposure prophylaxis (PrEP). The relatively quick progression of COVID-19 infection also poses challenges to ensuring that one is treated in accordance with their correct pronouns and name. Further, nondiscrimination policies in health care vary across borders, some of which are currently being undermined in the US and elsewhere in the world. This may lead to the rejection of care for SGM, particularly transgender and gender diverse patients, or a failure to acknowledge sexual minority relationship partners as medical decision makers. While it is too early to total the costs of the pandemic, it is likely that SGM communities will experience far-reaching disparate health outcomes not only as a direct result of the coronavirus, but also indirectly due to restricted access to HIV and non-COVID critical care, as well as broader sociopolitical consequences in response to or under cover of the pandemic.

Preexisting conditions: bias and health disparities

Minority stress theory is currently the most popular theory in psychological and public health research accounting for the impact of bias on the health and well-being of SGM people. Though minority stress theory had been first described in 1981 (Brooks 1981), it was not popularized until the work of Ilan Meyer over a decade later (Meyer 1995; Meyer 2003). Minority stress theory posits that when examining the impact of societal animus toward SGM people, there is no single source or response type that might be measured or articulated. That is, though bias, discrimination, and violence serve as stressors, only considering these overlooks internalized stigma (e.g., the acceptance of societal beliefs that pathologize SGM identities); expectation of rejection (e.g., the interpersonal guardedness that arises from an awareness others, including loved ones and family, may hold biased beliefs and be rejecting), and the stress of effortful concealment in a dangerous environment. More recent elaborations emphasize the role of resilience factors, such as community connectedness (Meyer 2015). The model has also been separately adapted for gender minority individuals to include gender-specific stressors, such as being misgendered by others as well as gender-specific resilience factors, such as pride in one's transgender or nonbinary experience (Hendricks and Testa 2012).

Minority stress theory is a helpful frame as it identifies factors that might be considered for intervention to mitigate bias as well as stressors to be considered when a new context suggests changes in the experience of stigma. In reminding researchers and interventionists that minority stress is a result of the environment and not individuals (Meyer 2019), we considered factors that illustrate actions taken by government and religious institutions that promote bias and increase health disparities, as well as widely disseminated speech that increases the likelihood of popular expressions of anti-SGM bias. Further, we have considered and described existing inequalities in healthcare systems that may be exacerbated or more pronounced during the current context of the pandemic. It is also important to consider the historical and societal projections toward SGM people that pervade most societies – sexual orientation and gender-diverse identities have been associated with wealth, vice, globalism, colonialism, or psychopathology (e.g., Kole 2007). The global impact and association between SGM identities and HIV, particularly in North America, Australia, and Europe, may also affect ideas about illness, contagion, and susceptibility that influence bias toward SGM people (e.g., Filip-Crawford and Neuberg 2016).

Health disparities

Prior to COVID-19, SGM people have reported difficulty accessing needed health services due to inequality in the workplace and health insurance sectors, the provision of substandard care or outright denial of care, as well as discrimination, stigma, violence, and rejection in their interactions with the healthcare system based on their sexual orientation or gender identity. Compared to the general population, SGM individuals in the United States are more likely to live in poverty and lack access to adequate medical care and paid medical leave. In the US, for example, 17% of SGM adults lack health insurance coverage compared to 12% of non-SGM adults (Whittington, Hadfield, and Calderón 2020). These problems are compounded for transgender adults and those of color: 22% of transgender adults, 23% of SGM adults of color, and 32% of transgender adults of color have no form of health coverage. Many SGM individuals work in industries that do not offer employer-sponsored health care, and even for those lucky enough to receive health benefits, same-sex spouses are offered significantly less coverage as compared to other-sex spouses (Dawson 2018). For transgender individuals, many insurance plans exclude or limit transition-related care as cosmetic, experimental, or unnecessary, despite the fact that such procedures are considered medically necessary. As a result, gender-affirming surgeries and hormone replacement therapy are prohibitively expensive for some of the most impoverished and stigmatized communities within the SGM population. Finally, minority stress is associated with a number of health behaviors that may lead to worsened healthcare outcomes, such as higher rates of smoking (Hoffman et al. 2018) and alcohol consumption (Livingston et al. 2017).

Further, many SGM individuals are reluctant to seek medical care due to negative experiences when seeking care (Kcomt et al. 2020). There is a lack of providers who are not only culturally competent, but also willing to work with SGM populations at all. Many SGM individuals receive substandard care or outright denial of care based on sexual orientation, gender identity, and gender expression. For transgender individuals, even seeking routine care has the potential for humiliation, discrimination, violations of privacy, and even violence. Nearly one-quarter (23%) of transgender individuals surveyed in the 2015 U.S. Transgender Survey avoided seeking needed health care due to fear of discrimination (James et al. 2016).

Each of these factors – access to health care, insurance in the United States, the possibility of mistreatment by medical providers, or humiliation in medical settings – may lead to deferred treatment and worsened outcome when an SGM individual notices symptoms that may indicate infection with COVID-19. Similarly, elevated rates of smoking, alcohol use, and underlying medical disorders may lead to a heightened risk of mortality that will not be clear until after the pandemic subsides and a greater examination of outcome data is possible.

Anti-SGM animus in response to COVID-19

Hate speech and targeted attacks from conservative religious and political leaders against the SGM community and persons living with HIV have increased alongside the spread of COVID-19. These attacks on the SGM community are particularly dangerous in the context of the pandemic, as support by political and religious institutions may result in exacerbations of preexisting bias when shelter-in-place orders and border controls already limit access to seeking safety or fleeing abusive and dangerous environments. Worldwide, religious and political figures have linked COVID-19 with divine sanction of abortion and gay marriage (OutRight Action International 2020). In Turkey, such claims were publicly supported by several political leaders, including President Erdogan (ILGA Europe 2020a). SGM people are not only scapegoated, but also stigmatized as vectors of disease during the COVID-19 pandemic (OutRight Action International 2020). In France, a gay couple found a threatening note telling them to vacate their home that linked the transmission of COVID-19 with being gay (Assunção 2020). These accusations incite discrimination and violence against SGM people, leading many to voice fears that they will be profiled and deprioritized for health care as the pandemic spreads (OutRight Action International 2020).

Anti-SGM violence exacerbated by or attributed to prevention of COVID-19

Violence against SGM people has also been reported under the guise of COVID-related public health prevention measures. In the Philippines, three SGM individuals among a group of curfew-violators were singled out by police for harassment and public humiliation in a live video streamed to Facebook (Juguilon 2020). In Belize, a young gay man living with HIV, Ulysease Roca Terry, was detained for breaking curfew. He described bullying and physical violence while in police custody, and he died days later from injuries believed to have been inflicted by the police (Channel5Belize 2020). In Panama, Peru, and Bogota, Columbia, quarantine schedules based on binary gender presentation (e.g., male days and female days) resulted in the denial of services, physical violence, arrest, and incarceration (Human Rights Watch 2020a). While these policies were rescinded in Peru after a week and in Bogota after a month, they remained in effect in Panama as of mid-July.

Lockdown measures isolate SGM individuals from community support systems, socialization, and work outside of the home and at times expose them to inescapable emotional and physical abuse from homophobic or transphobic family members (Cohen 2021; OutRight Action International 2020). This particularly impacts youth and young adults who may have been "out" at school or with peers while concealing their identity at home. Relatedly, job loss and school closures have also forced SGM people who previously lived independently to move back in with family – which for some would mean hiding their identities and facing discrimination, misgendering, threats, or acts of violence such as corrective rape or conversion therapy.

In Morocco, where homosexuality is illegal and the law does not prohibit discrimination on the basis of gender identity or sexual orientation, a campaign of "outings" have exposed the sexual identities of many gay men (Human Rights Watch 2020b). The outings began when a social media influencer instructed her female followers to create fake profiles on gay dating apps to identify gay men in their vicinity. As a result, numerous men received threatening messages and their photos were circulated on social media with homophobic captions and threats, which put them in danger of humiliation, blackmail, and violence. In several cases, men have been ejected from their homes amid a coronavirus lockdown, and in at least one verified report at the time of writing, has led to a young man's suicide (Parsons 2020).

Lockdowns have also removed the ability to escape or de-escalate abuse for those living with abusive partners (Toesland 2020). The prevalence of intimate partner violence is comparable or higher among SGM couples in comparison to heterosexual couples, though SGM people face unique barriers to seeking help (Rollè et al. 2018). Outing is both a method of abuse as well as a barrier to seeking help. Prior experiences of violence, discrimination, and rejection also make SGM victims less likely to seek help from medical or law enforcement communities when they are abused. The common misconceptions that intimate partner violence is a purely male-perpetrated, heterosexual experience can make it difficult for sexual minority men, women, and transgender individuals to access culturally competent services. In fact, SGM shelter services are rare or nonexistent in many regions, as most shelters do not admit men or transgender individuals and may not provide adequate protection against disclosing shelter locations to abusive women seeking partners who have fled. Confinement at home, together with the financial stress caused by the pandemic, greatly increases the risk of violence against survivors.

Even SGM-friendly homeless shelters are not exempt from violence. Under the guise of carrying out presidential initiatives to reduce public gatherings, police in Uganda raided a shelter for SGM youth. Twenty-three people were arrested with COVID-19-related charges, and though two were released for medical reasons, the rest were jailed for over 50 days and denied visitations, access to legal services (deemed not to be "essential"), and medication, despite the fact that some of the individuals were HIV positive (Reuters 2020).

Weakening legal protections in light of a distracted public

Many governments around the world took advantage of the immediate panic or distracted media to enact or repeal laws unrelated to the pandemic that would curtail the rights and liberties of SGM people and people living with HIV. In France, the parliament delayed voting on a long-promised bill that would have legalized reproductive assistance for same-sex couples and single women. While the government cited the strain of reduced legislative manpower due to COVID-19, others have called it a pretext to avoid the vote (Thorin 2020). The Constitutional Court of North Macedonia repealed an anti-discrimination law that protected SGM people, and the postponement of the country's parliamentary elections due to COVID-19 leaves the fate of this law particularly uncertain and urgent for its SGM citizens (ILGA Europe 2020b). At the time of writing, ministers in Boris Johnson's administration plan to throw out reforms to United Kingdom's gender identity laws that would have simplified the process for transgender people to change their birth certificate without the need for a medical diagnosis (Hunte 2020). In the US, the state legislatures of Idaho and Alabama passed laws denying transgender children gender-affirming medical care, school support, and involvement in school sports, as well as the ability to change their sex on their birth certificates (Charles 2020). At the federal level, the United States Department of Health and Human Services under Trump's administration completed a planned revision of Obama-era policies that prohibited healthcare discrimination based on sex and gender identity, by reinterpreting Section 1557 of the Affordable Care Act to prohibit nondiscrimination on the basis of biological sex (Simmons-Duffin 2020). In doing so, the administration has also affirmed a healthcare worker's right to deny care based on religious or moral objections. Such efforts have continued despite a Supreme Court ruling upholding the historic framing of discrimination according to sexual orientation and gender diversity constituting a prohibited form of sex discrimination under the law. During a public health crisis that disproportionately impacts the health and economic welfare of SGM people, the combination of attempted legal reversals and uncertainty pose new challenges for SGM people attempting to access health care from federally funded hospitals.

In several nations, governments have enacted laws that breach international human rights obligations to the legal recognition of gender identity and to remove HIV-specific criminal laws. The Hungarian parliament passed a bill that makes legal gender recognition impossible for transgender and intersex people, increasing their risk of harassment, discrimination, and exposure to violence whenever they use their identity documents (UNAIDS 2020). In Kazakhstan, the parliament proposed Amendment No. 539 to its health code, limiting transgender young people's access to essential trans-specific health care by increasing the age limit from 18 to 21 (ILGA-Europe, TGEU, and IGLYO 2020). In Poland, the legislature fast-tracked an amendment to the criminal law that significantly increased the penalties for HIV exposure, nondisclosure, and transmission (UNAIDS 2020). The criminalization of HIV not only violates the rights of persons living with HIV, it also undermines international efforts to curb the spread of HIV and ensure access to treatment (The Lancet HIV 2018). As the SGM community is disproportionately affected by HIV (the risk of acquiring HIV is 12 times higher for transgender people and 22 times higher among men who have sex with men), such laws should also be considered attacks against SGM people (UNAIDS 2019).

Direct effects of COVID-19 on individual health and well-being

In many parts of the world, SGM people face persecution, discrimination, violence, and even the risk of death penalties for their sexual orientation or gender identity (Itaborahy and Zhu 2012). The COVID-19 pandemic has occurred at the culmination of decades of increasing numbers of refugees and asylum seekers globally, particularly by SGM people attempting to flee violence or seek the security to live freely and openly (UNHCR 2018). With the closure of borders, individuals already fearing violence or persecution are trapped in place, with little recourse. Though the aforementioned degree of outings occurring in Morocco is not a global phenomenon, the fear of discovery and violence and the inability to escape across closed borders suggests a hidden human rights crisis that will not be fully understood while the pandemic continues. This is only one form of harm affecting vulnerable individuals, however, with changes in the implementation of healthcare access and provisions of treatment taking a toll on SGM people in every nation. In no domain is this more immediately clear than in the restrictions and challenges to receiving care by gender minority people and those living with HIV.

Barriers to gender-affirming care and HIV care due to COVID restrictions

Pandemic-related changes in hospital care have resulted in the interruption of both gender-affirming therapies as well as antiviral medication for HIV, including hour restrictions and availability of non–COVID-19-related services. The classification of medical treatment as "elective" or "essential" has postponed the initiation of gender-affirming therapies and cancelled gender-affirming surgeries postponed indefinitely (Mohan 2020). Hormone treatments and gender-affirming surgeries have been shown to alleviate distress around dysphoria and improve both mental health and quality of life for transgender individuals (Costa and Colizzi 2016; WPATH 2016; Wernick et al. 2019). For some, surgery cancellation may mean reapplying for procedures with their insurance, the cost of which may be prohibitive for a community that tends to have inconsistent access to insurance (Mohan 2020). For transgender individuals, the delay of gender-affirming medical care can be a matter of life or death, and indefinite postponement may give rise to hopelessness.

Hormone treatments have also been more difficult to access, as patients either cannot pick up their medications due to drug shortages or lockdown restrictions or are denied by pharmacies and health insurance as nonessential (OutRight Action International 2020). Transgender individuals who do not have their next supply of hormones have reported fears of detransitioning, which can heighten dysphoria, as well as concerns over social integration, personal safety, and health consequences (Mohan 2020). When researchers in the United States began to test the use of hormones in treating COVID symptoms, many transgender individuals in that country reported feeling that it underscored the deprioritization of transgender health care (Gulino 2020). Some even feared that should hormones be proven to be an effective treatment for COVID, the competing needs to support the COVID-19 response would further reduce access for transgender people. The sidelining of transgender medical care in the global health crisis underscores beliefs that the health and humanity of transgender patients are less valued than those of cisgender patients (Urquhart 2020).

People living with HIV around the world have also reported difficulties with accessing essential HIV-related care due to disruptions to the supply chain and to services due to the competing needs of COVID-19 care, as well as to distance, lack of transportation, fear of disclosure, and the distrust of the health system to maintain confidentiality (OutRight Action International 2020; World Health Organization 2020). In China, for example, it was estimated that 32.6% of individuals living with HIV were at risk of antiretroviral therapy (ART) discontinuation and about 48.6% did not know where to get ART drugs in the near future (Jiang, Zhou, and Tang 2020). Community-based organizations, such as the Wuhan LGBT center, have helped to maintain HIV services by organizing and delivering HIV medication from hospitals to those quarantined in their communities (often with family members unaware of their HIV status). However, in resource-poor settings such as sub-Saharan Africa, where two-thirds of the 37.9 million persons living with HIV reside (UNAIDS 2019), the COVID pandemic is expected to exacerbate the HIV pandemic in regions of the world that are medically and structurally vulnerable (Pinto and Park 2020). Social distancing, travel bans, state curfews, and the suspension of public transportation have together increased the costs of accessing critical medications, with some needing to travel on foot or pay their own way (OutRight Action International 2020). Although the WHO recommends multi-month prescriptions to reduce pharmacy and doctors' visits, concerns over medication shortages has meant that clinics are unwilling or unable to dispense more than a month's supply at a time (OutRight Action International 2020; Pillinger 2020). In addition, many persons living with HIV report being afraid of going to healthcare facilities where HIV services are located, as they do not want to be associated with those tested positive for COVID-19 or to be associated with those who live and work in proximity to COVID patients (OutRight Action International 2020). Disruptions, even short-term, might negatively impact the health of people living with HIV and their potential to transmit, as well as lead to death. Researchers who modeled three-month and six-month disruptions of HIV medication projected up to a two-fold increase in mother-to-child transmission and over half a million adult HIV-related deaths over the next year (Jewell et al. 2020).

Discrimination by medical providers in the context of COVID-19

Pre-COVID-19, studies have shown the prevalence of SGM individuals delaying or avoiding necessary health care due to anticipation of discrimination, mistreatment, or choosing not to disclose their SGM identities to providers, even when that information may be medically relevant (Göçmen and Yılmaz 2017). Healthcare inaccessibility may have far-reaching sequelae, as transgender individuals who delay health care due to fear of discrimination have poorer overall health and mental health outcomes (Seelman et al. 2017). These trends are particularly dangerous in the context of a global pandemic in which testing, early prevention, and appropriate medical care are necessary for individual and community well-being.

Healthcare providers, situated within local and international sociopolitical contexts, demonstrate anti-SGM sentiment in their work – even when governmental protections exist. Müller (2017) found that despite a constitutional right to non-discrimination in healthcare and policy-related efforts to improve SGM health care in South Africa, individuals continue to experience homophobia and transphobia from healthcare workers. Examples of experiences of SGM communities within healthcare systems include refusal of care, expressions of anti-SGM sentiment (e.g., moral judgement, ridicule, insults, blaming SGM identities for the individual's disease/healthcare needs), violations of confidentiality, forced religious practices, and poor-quality care (Müller 2017; Rispel et al. 2011; Stevens 2012).

Particularly when healthcare systems are overstressed and inaccessible in the context of COVID-19 and as frontline healthcare providers experience burnout, preexisting stigma and discrimination towards SGM communities may surface in deeply harmful ways. This process is particularly relevant to SGM populations who have both current and historical community trauma related to illness and disease. Lessons learned from the conceptualization of HIV highlight both explicit and implicit perpetuations of oppression in the way we communicate about COVID-19:

> Illnesses have been constructed as both evil predators and personal responsibilities, contributing to social rejection . . . Military metaphors – including such terms as targets and fighting – frame illnesses as society's invasive, wicked infiltrators that spur paranoia and command social order, and in turn can exacerbate pre-existing social inequities.
>
> *(Logie and Turan 2020, 1)*

SGM populations carry a context of being the pathologized and stigmatized "other" within healthcare systems and at times socially experienced (including by providers) as the cause of illnesses like HIV and COVID-19, while also experiencing stigma in the form of conceptualizing SGM identities themselves as disease. Further, due to sequelae of systematic oppression, SGM populations as a whole may be more likely to rely on income sources that subject them to a higher risk of infection (e.g., service industry, contract work, day labor, sex work, community work) – which may result in more stigma and blame towards individuals who present to hospital systems having contracted COVID-19.

Finally, the well-documented lack of training around SGM-specific care and interpersonal bias towards SGM communities more broadly might disincentivize providers from providing care to individuals who are deemed "difficult" or "complicated," as healthcare providers are forced to make quick and difficult choices around who receives healthcare resources. This may include names, pronouns, and identities that may or may not match forms of identification used in healthcare settings (and related barriers with insurance) or partner/family structures for visitation or shared medical decision-making that may differ from cisheteronormative standards.

Conclusion

The COVID-19 pandemic and subsequent closed borders, shelter-in-place orders, prohibitions on gathering, and carefully managed, finite medical resources all impact SGM people in specific, deleterious ways. This chapter has only reviewed some of the impacts that have been documented to different degrees during the beginning of the pandemic; time will yet reveal the full cost to the SGM community if a second wave strikes those nations that have managed to suppress the spread, and many large nations such as the United States, Russia, and Brazil, as of the time of writing, have not yet managed to control even the initial wave of the pandemic.

Some sites of resistance and protest have shown promise in responding to the enactments of the previously detailed bias. For example, in wealthier regions such as North America and Europe, the judiciary has served as a powerful buffer against discriminatory legal changes. In June 2020, the United States Supreme Court ruled that sexual orientation and gender identity are protected under federal legislation prohibiting sex discrimination (Barnes 2020), which may serve to slow government efforts to enshrine discrimination into federal healthcare rules. The following month, the European Court of Human Rights ruled against the Hungarian ban on gender marker changes in the case of a foreign citizen who had been granted asylum, though the logic of the ruling suggests the law may be completely overturned in a future case (Reid-Smith 2020). Judicial relief typically requires a legal framework and social context that recognizes SGM personhood and autonomy, which does not apply to all cases described in this chapter.

Many of the broader threats described are ones that pre-date COVID-19 and that suggest the importance of ongoing activism in the domains of both policy and social change. Greater access to health care and training and educational standards for doctors and nurses to enhance ethical, nondiscriminatory practice are key targets. Additionally, while some nations have greater legal obstacles or are dangerous for SGM citizens, both the United States and European Union have a poor history of consistently accepting SGM asylum seekers. Following the well-publicized arrests and murders of gay and lesbian people in Chechnya begun in 2017, for example, the United States has not accepted a single asylum seeker from the region. Across North America, Europe, and Australia, SGM asylum seekers are routinely challenged over their alignment with the evaluator's gender stereotypes. It can ultimately be hoped that the magnification of bias during the pandemic, as well as supportive court rulings and the gradual re-engagement of legislative bodies, serve as helpful reminders that advocacy for policy change can continue prior to the end of the pandemic.

References

Assunção, Muri. 2020. "Same-Sex Couple Told to Vacate Their Home in France: 'Homosexuals Are the First to Be Contaminated by COVID-19'." *Nydailynews.Com*, April 1. www.nydailynews.com/coronavirus/ny-coronavirus-same-sex-couple-asked-vacate-house-20200401-cv737gkd4rf6nl5jiuvxykubnq-story.html.

Barnes, Robert. 2020. "Supreme Court Says Gay, Transgender Workers Protected by Federal Law Forbidding Discrimination." *Washington Post*, June 15. www.washingtonpost.com/politics/courts_law/supreme-court-says-gay-transgender-workers-are-protected-by-federal-law-forbidding-discrimination-on-the-basis-of-sex/2020/06/15/2211d5a4-655b-11ea-acca-80c22bbee96f_story.html?arc404=true&tid=a_inl_manual.

Bränström, Richard, Mark L. Hatzenbuehler, and John E. Pachankis. 2016. "Sexual Orientation Disparities in Physical Health: Age and Gender Effects in a Population-Based Study." *Social Psychiatry and Psychiatric Epidemiology* 51 (2): 289–301.

Brooks, Virginia R. 1981. *Minority Stress and Lesbian Women*. Lexington, MA: Lexington Books.

Burton, Chad M., Michael P. Marshal, Deena J. Chisolm, Gina S. Sucato, and Mark S. Friedman. 2013. "Sexual Minority-Related Victimization as a Mediator of Mental Health Disparities in Sexual Minority Youth: A Longitudinal Analysis." *Journal of Youth and Adolescence* 42 (3): 394–402.

Channel5Belize. 2020. "An Investigation Is Launched into the Death of Fashion Designer Ulysease Roca." *Channel5Belize.com*, April 20. https://edition.channel5belize.com/archives/201612.

Charles, Carl. 2020. "It's Never Okay to Attack Trans Youth, but Especially Not During a Global Health Crisis." *Lambda Legal*, March 31. www.lambdalegal.org/blog/20200331_laws-attacking-trans-youth-coronavirus.

Cohen, Li. 2020. "Coronavirus Closed Down Colleges – Now Some SGM Students Fear an Abusive 'War Zone' at Home." April 16. www.cbsnews.com/news/coronavirus-SGM-college-students-homelessness-abuse-campuses-closed/.

Costa, Rosalia, and Marco Colizzi. 2016. "The Effect of Cross-Sex Hormonal Treatment on Gender Dysphoria Individuals' Mental Health: A Systematic Review." *Neuropsychiatric Disease and Treatment* 12: 1953–66. https://doi.org/10.2147/NDT.S95310.

Dawson, Lindsey. 2018. "Access to Employer-Sponsored Health Coverage for Same-Sex Spouses: 2018 Update." *KFF* (blog). October 29. www.kff.org/disparities-policy/issue-brief/access-to-employer-sponsored-health-coverage-for-same-sex-spouses-2018-update/.

Filip-Crawford, Gabrielle, and Steven L. Neuberg. 2016. "Homosexuality and Pro-Gay Ideology as Pathogens? Implications of a Disease-Spread Lay Model for Understanding Anti-Gay Behaviors." *Personality and Social Psychology Review* 20 (4): 332–64.

Göçmen, İpek, and Volkan Yılmaz. 2017. "Exploring Perceived Discrimination Among SGM Individuals in Turkey in Education, Employment, and Health Care: Results of an Online Survey." *Journal of Homosexuality* 64 (8): 1052–68.

Gulino, Elizabeth. 2020. "Why This New Coronavirus Study Is Creating A Lot Of Controversy." April 29. www.refinery29.com/en-us/2020/04/9751077/trans-coronavirus-estrogen-sex-hormone-therapy.

Hendricks, Michael L., and Rylan J. Testa. 2012. "A Conceptual Framework for Clinical Work with Transgender and Gender Nonconforming Clients: An Adaptation of the Minority Stress Model." *Professional Psychology: Research and Practice* 43 (5): 460–67.

Hoffman, Leah, Janine Delahanty, Sarah E. Johnson, and Xiaoquan Zhao. 2018. "Sexual and Gender Minority Cigarette Smoking Disparities: An Analysis of 2016 Behavioral Risk Factor Surveillance System data." *Preventive medicine* 113: 109–15.

Human Rights Watch. 2020a. "Panama: Set Transgender-Sensitive Quarantine Guidelines." *Human Rights Watch*, April 23, 2020. www.hrw.org/news/2020/04/23/panama-set-transgender-sensitive-quarantine-guidelines.

———. 2020b. "Morocco: Online Attacks Over Same-Sex Relations." *Human Rights Watch*. April 27. www.hrw.org/news/2020/04/27/morocco-online-attacks-over-same-sex-relations.

Hunte, Ben. 2020. "Gender Recognition Act: SGM Political Group Anger at Trans Law 'Changes'." *BBC News*, June 20, sec. UK. www.bbc.com/news/uk-53101071.

ILGA Europe. 2020a. "Joint Statement: End Hate Speech and Targeted Attacks Against LGBTI People in Turkey." May 9. https://ilga-europe.org/resources/news/latest-news/joint-statement-end-hate-speech-and-targeted-attacks-against-lgbti-people#_ftn1.

———. 2020b. "ILGA-Europe and ERA Joint Statement on the Decision of the Constitutional Court of North Macedonia to Repeal the Law on Prevention of and Protection against Discrimination." May 29, 2020. https://ilga-europe.org/resources/news/latest-news/decision-constitutional-court-north-macedonia-lppd.

ILGA-Europe, TGEU, and IGLYO. 2020. "Joint Statement Calling on the Parliament of Kazakhstan to Protect Trans People's Rights to Health and Legal Gender Recognition | ILGA-Europe." June 10. https://ilga-europe.org/resources/news/latest-news/joint-statement-calling-parliament-kazakhstan-protect-trans-peoples.

Itaborahy, Lucas Paoli, and Jingshu Zhu. 2012. *State-Sponsored Homophobia: A World Survey of Laws: Criminalisation, Protection and Recognition of Same-Sex Love*. Geneva, Switzerland: International Lesbian Gay Bisexual Trans and Intersex Association.

James, Sandra E., Jody L. Herman, Susan Rankin, Mara Keisling, Lisa Mottet, and Ma'ayan Anafi. 2016. *The Report of the 2015 U.S. Transgender Survey*. Washington, DC: National Center for Transgender Equality. https://transequality.org/sites/default/files/docs/usts/USTS-Full-Report-Dec17.pdf.

Jewell, Britta L., Edinah Mudimu, John Stover, Sherrie L. Kelly, and Andrew Phillips. 2020. "Potential Effects of Disruption to HIV Programmes in Sub-Saharan Africa Caused by

COVID-19: Results from Multiple Mathematical Models." https://doi.org/10.6084/m9.figshare.12279914.v1.

Jiang, Hongbo, Yi Zhou, and Weiming Tang. 2020. "Maintaining HIV Care During the COVID-19 Pandemic." *The Lancet HIV* 7 (5): e308–9. https://doi.org/10.1016/S2352-3018(20)30105-3.

Juguilon, Allena Therese. 2020. "Barangay Captain Makes SGM+ Quarantine Violators Do Lewd Acts as Punishment." *Rappler*, April 7. www.rappler.com/nation/257292-barangay-captain-SGM-quarantine-violators-lewd-acts-punishment.

Kcomt, Luisa, Kevin M. Gorey, Betty Jo Barrett, and Sean Esteban McCabe. 2020. "Healthcare Avoidance Due to Anticipated Discrimination Among Transgender People: A Call to Create Trans-Affirmative Environments." *SSM-Population Health*: 100608.

Kole, Subir K. 2007 "Globalizing Queer? AIDS, Homophobia and the Politics of Sexual Identity in India." *Globalization and health* 3 (1): 1–16.

The Lancet HIV, The Lancet. 2018. "HIV Criminalisation Is Bad Policy Based on Bad Science." *The Lancet HIV* 5 (9): e473. https://doi.org/10.1016/S2352-3018(18)30219-4.

Livingston, Nicholas A., Annesa Flentje, Nicholas C. Heck, Allen Szalda-Petree, and Bryan N. Cochran. 2017. "Ecological Momentary Assessment of Daily Discrimination Experiences and Nicotine, Alcohol, and Drug Use Among Sexual and Gender Minority Individuals." *Journal of Consulting and Clinical Psychology* 85 (12): 1131.

Logie, Carmen H., and Janet M. Turan. 2020. "How Do We Balance Tensions Between COVID-19 Public Health Responses and Stigma Mitigation? Learning from HIV Research." *AIDS and Behavior*: 1–4.

Meyer, Ilan H. 1995. "Minority Stress and Mental Health in Gay Men." *Journal of Health and Social Behavior* 36 (1): 38–56.

Meyer, Ilan H. 2003. "Prejudice, Social Stress, and Mental Health in Lesbian, Gay, and Bisexual Populations: Conceptual Issues and Research Evidence." *Psychological Bulletin* 129 (5): 674–97.

Meyer, Ilan H. 2015. "Resilience in the Study of Minority Stress and Health of Sexual and Gender Minorities." *Psychology of Sexual Orientation and Gender Diversity* 2 (3): 209–13.

Meyer, Ilan H. 2019. "Rejection Sensitivity and Minority Stress: A Challenge for Clinicians and Interventionists." *Archives of Sexual Behavior*. Advance online publication. DOI: 10.1007/s10508-019-01597-7.

Mohan, Megha. 2020. "Coronavirus: Transgender People 'Extremely Vulnerable' During Lockdown." *BBC News*, April 29, sec. World. www.bbc.com/news/world-52457681.

Müller, Alex. 2017. "Scrambling for Access: Availability, Accessibility, Acceptability and Quality of Healthcare for Lesbian, Gay, Bisexual and Transgender People in South Africa." *BMC International Health and Human Rights* 17 (1): 16.

OutRight Action International. 2020. "Vulnerability Amplified: The Impact of the COVID-19 Pandemic on SGMQ People." *OutRight Action International*, May 6. https://outrightinternational.org/content/vulnerability-amplified-impact-covid-19-pandemic-SGMq-people.

Parsons, Vic. 2020. "A Gay Man Has Tragically Died by Suicide After Being Hunted Down and Outed Thanks to a Trans Influencer." *PinkNews – Gay News, Reviews and Comment from the World's Most Read Lesbian, Gay, Bisexual, and Trans News Service* (blog). April 27. www.pinknews.co.uk/2020/04/27/gay-morocco-man-death-suicide-outed-trans-influencer-sofia-talouni-grindr-facebook/.

Pillinger, Mara. 2020. "Lessons from the HIV Policy Lab: Tracking National HIV Policies and ART Access Amidst COVID-19 | O'Neill Institute." May 8. https://oneill.law.georgetown.edu/lessons-from-the-hiv-policy-lab-tracking-national-hiv-policies-and-art-access-amidst-covid-19/.

Pinto, Rogério M., and Sunggeun Park. 2020. "COVID-19 Pandemic Disrupts HIV Continuum of Care and Prevention: Implications for Research and Practice Concerning Community-Based Organizations and Frontline Providers." *AIDS and Behavior*, April. https://doi.org/10.1007/s10461-020-02893-3.

Reid-Smith, Tris. 2020. "Top European Court Deals Major Blow to Hungary's Anti-Trans Law." *Gaystarnews*, July 17. www.gaystarnews.com/article/top-european-court-deals-major-blow-to-hungarys-anti-trans-law/.

Reuters. 2020. "Court Orders Release of Jailed SGM+ Ugandans After Coronavirus Charges Dropped." May 18. www.reuters.com/article/us-health-coronavirus-uganda-SGM-idUSKBN22U2DO.

Rispel, Laetitia C., Carol A. Metcalf, Allanise Cloete, Julia Moorman, and Vasu Reddy. 2011. "You Become Afraid to Tell Them That You Are Gay: Health Service Utilization by Men Who Have Sex with Men in South African Cities." *Journal of Public Health Policy* 32 (1): S137–S151.

Rollè, Luca, Giulia Giardina, Angela M. Caldarera, Eva Gerino, and Piera Brustia. 2018. "When Intimate Partner Violence Meets Same Sex Couples: A Review of Same Sex Intimate Partner Violence." *Frontiers in Psychology* 9 (August). https://doi.org/10.3389/fpsyg.2018.01506.

Seelman, Kristie L., Matthew J. P. Colón-Diaz, Rebecca H. LeCroix, Marik Xavier-Brier, and Leonardo Kattari. 2017. "Transgender Noninclusive Healthcare and Delaying Care Because of Fear: Connections to General Health and Mental Health Among Transgender Adults." *Transgender Health* 2 (1): 17–28.

Simmons-Duffin, Selena. 2020. "Transgender Health Protections Reversed By Trump Administration." *NPR*, June 12. www.npr.org/sections/health-shots/2020/06/12/868073068/transgender-health-protections-reversed-by-trump-administration.

Stevens, Marion. 2012. *Transgender Access to Sexual Health Services in South Africa*. Cape Town: Gender Dynamix.

Thorin, Marion. 2020. "Le projet de loi 'PMA pour toutes' pourrait attendre." *Ouest-France.fr.* May 22. www.ouest-france.fr/societe/famille/pma/le-projet-de-loi-pma-pour-toutes-pourrait-attendre-6843337.

Toesland, Finbarr. 2020. "Coronavirus Restrictions Highlight SGM Domestic Abuse Crisis." *NBC News*, April 17. www.nbcnews.com/feature/nbc-out/coronavirus-restrictions-highlight-SGM-domestic-abuse-crisis-n1186376.

UNAIDS. 2019. "Global HIV & AIDS Statistics – 2019 Fact Sheet." www.unaids.org/en/resources/fact-sheet.

———. 2020. "UNAIDS Condemns Misuse and Abuse of Emergency Powers to Target Marginalized and Vulnerable Populations." April 9. www.unaids.org/en/resources/presscentre/pressreleaseandstatementarchive/2020/april/20200409_laws-covid19.

UNHCR: The UN Refugee Agency. 2018. "Global Trends: Forced Displacement in 2017." www.unhcr.org/en-us/statistics/unhcrstats/5b27be547/unhcr-global-trends-2017.html.

Urquhart, Evan. 2020. "If I Get Sick With COVID-19, Don't Tell My Doctor I'm Transgender." *Slate Magazine*, April 24. https://slate.com/human-interest/2020/04/transgender-health-care-covid-coronavirus-privacy.html.

Wernick, Jeremy A., Samantha Busa, Kareen Matouk, Joey Nicholson, and Aron Janssen. 2019. "A Systematic Review of the Psychological Benefits of Gender-Affirming Surgery." *The Urologic Clinics of North America* 46 (4): 475–86. https://doi.org/10.1016/j.ucl.2019.07.002.

Whittington, Charlie, Katalina Hadfield, and Carina Calderón. 2020. "The Lives and Livelihoods of Many in the LGBTQ Community Are At Risk Amidst COVID-19 Crisis." *Human Rights Campaign*, March 20. http://hrc.im/COVID19brief.

World Health Organization. 2020. "The Cost of Inaction: COVID-19-Related Service Disruptions Could Cause Hundreds of Thousands of Extra Deaths from HIV." *World Health Organization*, May 11. www.who.int/news-room/detail/11-05-2020-the-cost-of-inaction-covid-19-related-service-disruptions-could-cause-hundreds-of-thousands-of-extra-deaths-from-hiv.

WPATH. 2016. "WPATH Policy Statements: Position Statement on Medical Necessity of Treatment, Sex Reassignment, and Insurance Coverage in the U.S.A." *WPATH*. December 21. www.wpath.org/newsroom/medical-necessity-statement.

19

VIOLENCE, VIRUS, AND VITRIOL

The tale of COVID-19

Monita H. Mungo

The world watched as officials in Wuhan City, Hubei Province of China, closed off the heavily populated city as a containment strategy for the transmission of 2019-nCoV (novel coronavirus) which caused the city to be deemed the epicenter in late January 2020. It was during that same time, January 20, 2020, that the first case of the novel coronavirus was discovered in the United States in Washington state (World Health Organization, January 2020). The politicization of the coronavirus began almost immediately. President Trump, who was in the middle of a highly polarized impeachment trial, as well as conservative news outlets, minimized the potential risks and spread of the novel coronavirus as being a ploy to divert attention from an impeachment process that was not successful for the Democrats. Further minimization efforts compared the new virus to the flu, although Dr. Anthony Fauci, director of the National Institute of Allergy and Infectious Diseases, described it as being ten times more lethal than the seasonal flu, which has a vaccine (Peters and Grynbaum 2020). The spread of the novel coronavirus, and the United States' governmental response, illustrates structural violence and its grave consequences. As the novel pathogen continues to baffle top scientists and medical professionals regarding exposure, acquisition, and mortality, the social impact and implications of the disease have laid bare the United States' infrastructure, unmasking stark inequalities and misguided ideologies for the world to see.

Structural violence

Structural violence provides an important framework for analyzing the social implications of the coronavirus pandemic. In the United States, structural violence is a direct result of the maintenance of the social and economic structure of society that preserves the dividing line that separates the weak from the powerful, the poor from the rich, and the inferior from the superior, while wreaking havoc and harm on those who cannot afford to pay or lack the ability to earn their way up the social mobility ladder. Structural violence, as described by Johan Galtung (1969), is characterized by both a passive phenomenon that occurs as a result of larger social processes that collude to harm people and a deliberate action by actors in power who wield it to maintain social stratification (Lee 2016). Violence is used to describe the preventable harm that occurs; it is structural because it is embedded in the way society is organized. Unlike physical violence, which can be observed and often has an apparent perpetrator and victim, structural violence is difficult to see, and assigning blame to one individual is challenging. It is camouflaged in social practices, policies, safety guidelines, and prevention recommendations that distribute power, access, and opportunity unequally, harming many victims simultaneously. To some degree, structural violence is experienced by all citizens, but more noticeable effects are seen in groups labeled as poor and minority, especially in times of crisis. In addition, structural violence goes unnoticed because its effects are seen as "ordinary difficulties" that people encounter (Lee 2016, 110), such as catching a virus.

Virus: the politicization of a pandemic

The severity of the novel coronavirus has arguably been lost on many citizens of the United States as a result of the divisive political nature in that country. In the beginning, when the scientific and medical communities proliferated messages of information, concern, and prevention, the novel coronavirus was considered a Democratic hoax by President Trump; a "fraud" and "another attempt to impeach the president" by a popular conservative cable news channel; and nothing more than another type of flu virus by social media and radio news icons (Peters and Grynbaum 2020). The amount of misinformation and wanton disregard for science rendered the United States exposed. Lived experience was ignored while reports continued to broadcast daily about China and Italy, where exponential growth in confirmed cases and deaths occurred. Because the divisive nature of the current political climate has been normalized, US citizens must fend for themselves for viable information to keep themselves and loved ones safe. While there are less polarizing and more scientifically based media outlets, the challenge is determining what sources can be trusted, since the way information is disseminated in the United States is also politicized. In this context, instead of being blissful, ignorance is dangerous, with the potential to be deadly. The spread of misinformation is a deliberate action of power wielded by several actors who are to blame for many citizens not complying with recommended precautions to safeguard themselves and others. The resulting harm is unwitting, contagious citizens going about their daily lives infecting others (Ryan 2021). The perpetrator of harm is difficult to accuse since misinformation and fact distortion are normalized and widespread, involving many actors such as news media shows and government officials. The violence perpetrated on American citizens as a result of a politically divisive country has caused harm in ways that are only beginning to be quantified. As a start, we can count the total number of confirmed cases of COVID-19 infections and deaths.

From the beginning, the federal response from the United States government has been one of chaos, confusion, contradiction, and distortion that resulted in deadly consequences. Over 70 days passed from the date when the Centers for Disease Control and Prevention (CDC) learned about cases of COVID-19 occurring in Wuhan in late December 2019 to the first announcement made by President Trump outlining the public health and safety guidelines for the country in mid-March. During that time frame, the United States had more than 4,600 cases of confirmed infections and more than 100 deaths (World Health Organization 2020). Until a vaccine is created, tested, and approved, slowing the spread of the virus in the United States has become the goal; evidence from China shows that lockdowns substantially slowed the spread of the virus in Wuhan (Kraemer et al. 2020). However, prevention efforts in the US have been hindered because of politics. A study by Painter and Qui (2020) showed that political beliefs affected compliance with social distancing orders. Specifically, Republicans and "misaligned Democrats" were less likely to comply. Since social distancing has been found to be a significant factor in slowing the spread of the novel coronavirus (Baldwin and Weder di Mauro 2020), compliance with this preventative measure is important. Adherence to other recommended preventive measures to reduce the probability of exposure such as hand washing, mask wearing, and avoiding public gatherings has also been shown to depend on political party affiliation. Fowler and Utych (2020) found that Democrats are more likely to comply with recommendations even when it disrupts their lives than are Republicans. As a result of the declared national emergency, Allyn and Sprunt (2020) found that 38% of Democrats compared to 26% of Republicans changed their travel plans; 59% of Democrats compared to 40% of Republicans cancelled plans to avoid large gatherings; and 60% of Democrats compared to 37% of Republicans decided to eat at home more often.

Racism and structural violence work together to wreak havoc during crises. Not only is the current pandemic highlighting the consequences for public health as a result of political polarization, it is also illuminating numerous problems in the social infrastructure such as disseminating information and strategies that are racially sensitive. As a preventative measure, public health officials have recommended wearing face coverings while in public spaces. To facilitate compliance, the CDC has posted instructions on making face coverings from materials such as old t-shirts or bandanas (Centers for Disease Control and Prevention 2020). It is important to note that the purpose for disseminating instructions on how to make a homemade face covering was to discourage the general public from purchasing medical grade masks needed in hospitals. While the recommendation seems ordinary, it does not consider the history of racism and how it operates in society. Without face coverings, Black men have a higher rate of being harassed by business owners, employees, and police (Smiley and Fakunle 2016), as well as being feared by everyone else. Add a homemade bandana, and it has the makings of a deadly outcome, especially in communities where police utilize aggressive tactical policies (Dewey 2021, this volume). The recommendation by the CDC is a passive phenomenon intended to provide safety measures to protect the general public. However, coupled with racism, safety measures and public protection collude to add harm to an already dangerous situation. Camouflaged as a public health recommendation, face coverings are potentially harmful for Black citizens generally, and Black men specifically, as a result of racial biases that evoke fear, suspicion, and feelings of imminent danger from seeing a Black man with a face covering. Viral videos and news stories can attest to the racial politics of adherence to the public health recommendation (de la Garza 2020; Taylor 2020). Wearing a mask while Black increases the potential of racial profiling regardless of public health guidelines and the threat of a deadly virus. Further, conflating race and crime endangers Black men and increases scrutiny and suspicion when wearing a face mask, forcing them to choose between protecting themselves against a deadly virus and avoiding the potential physical and psychological damage of being confronted by police (Dewey 2021, this volume; Natividad 2020). Thus, for some, the threat of a Black man wearing a face covering is more frightening than the threat of a deadly virus. Moreover, President Trump invokes the relationship between racism and structural violence by referring to the coronavirus as the "Chinese flu" and the "Chinese virus" (Shafer 2020), resulting in racist attacks, both verbally and physically, against Asian Americans (Chiang 2021, this volume). Not only does the label stigmatize Chinese Americans as being the cause and carriers of the novel coronavirus, it also invokes a historical stereotype about immigrants as disease carriers, which exposes them to hate, anger, and harassment by other citizens who are fearful and prejudiced.

In addition to prevention strategies that added additional risk to racialized citizens, other issues exposed the country's infrastructure as being woefully unprepared. The medical community did not have the required protective gear to minimize their exposure while treating patients with COVID-19. As a world superpower, the United States has access to more resources, expertise, and experience to have had better outcomes from a global pandemic than many of the countries that fared better. However, the public health system is fragmented from the medical system, which hampered the procurement of much needed resources such as basic medical equipment and testing supplies. Instead of a coordinated federal response to support the medical community, states battled for personal protection equipment as many hospitals and clinics were experiencing shortages while the number of confirmed COVID-19 cases and deaths increased. Moreover, according to a letter from the American Nurses Association to Congress, there was confusion about the recommendations received by the CDC regarding medical equipment use. The letter states, "We are concerned that C.D.C. recommendations are based solely on supply chain and manufacturing challenges. It's also concerning that these recommendations do not offer strategies to address the limited manufacturing and supply chain of necessary personal protective equipment" (Jacobs, Richtel, and Baker 2020). In addition, the American College of Emergency Physicians urged the White House "to ramp up production of medical gear through the Defense Production Act powers, and . . . increase distributions from the Strategic National Stockpile, a repository of critical medical supplies for public health emergencies" (Jacobs, Richtel, and Baker 2020). Medical supplies from the stockpile were distributed at rates less than what was needed, and the concerns about the confusing recommendations were not addressed. When the federal government abandoned the medical community, healthcare workers, schools, chain stores, and volunteer citizens around the country answered the call with donations of supplies, including masks made at home with personal sewing machines. At a time when the number of confirmed cases and deaths were steadily rising, healthcare workers risked exposure as a result of a dysfunctional federal response to the global pandemic. As a product of human decision, structural violence is preventable as well as correctable through human agency and ingenuity. Through a competent and coordinated response, the federal government has access, resources, and opportunity to resolve the inadequate supply of medical equipment. Inaction and slow reaction during a time of global uncertainty is a choice with harmful consequences. When harm such as death occurs, citizens blame weak individual bodies and not the social structure that created unequal conditions, such as unavailable testing and inadequate amounts of medical supplies. The established social arrangement compels citizens to blame each other and not the social structure that contributes to their harm.

Another harmful factor in the social structure is an economic system that allows for inequality. During times of crisis, inequality will undoubtedly intensify. The preventive measures taken to restrict the spread of the novel coronavirus have disparate effects on lower socioeconomic groups, including the loss of income and health insurance (assuming they had either to begin with) and housing and food security (Nanda 2021). The stay-at-home orders mandated by many states were enacted to help slow the spread of the novel coronavirus. However, this preventative measure does not consider the vast number of citizens who simply cannot comply, such as the "essential" low-skilled workers, or those who live in multiple-generation homes and thus find quarantining a challenging endeavor. According to the U.S. Bureau of Labor Statistics (2019), individuals who more likely to have the ability to work from home are male, White, and college educated. White Americans are twice as likely as African Americans or Latino Americans to have the option to work remotely. The latter two groups comprise a large number of restaurant, retail, and grocery employees who do not have the option to work at home.

Structural violence operates through systemic disparities (Lee 2016, 112) exposing its effects on marginalized groups. Crises increase these effects. Before the global pandemic, low-income workers were already feeling the pinch of an unequal society as a result of low wages, lack of health insurance, and rising cost of living. As a result of the pandemic, the economic disparity has worsened. With the closing of many industries such as restaurants and retail stores, the workers are at a higher risk of experiencing housing instability as well as job and food insecurity at a time when the resources at food pantries and other nonprofit agencies that assist with food and other social services are being stretched. While helpful in the short-term, state officials' attempts to halt housing evictions and utility shut-offs along with the one-time federal stimulus money are band-aids attempting to cover the massive bullet wound of the disparate economic impact of the novel coronavirus. With no other moderation on capitalism's inequality to help low-income workers' ability to comply with preventive strategies such as the stay-at-home order, citizens experienced increased angst to get to work because of concerns for lost wages and the consequences that follow. Protests erupted across the United States challenging the stay-at-home orders. Some protested because they felt their local government was infringing on their rights (Meeker 2021, this volume; Blum, Smith, and Sanford 2021, this volume) and others demonstrated because they feared the future since "staying home without work or income is hard" (Bosman, Tavernise, and Baker 2020).

Notwithstanding the economic inequality that the pandemic is bringing to the forefront, it is also exposing some deeply rooted beliefs that society has propagated for far too long. For example, the fallacy of meritocracy has been revealed as a result of the new labels "essential worker" and "hero" and their lists of low-skilled jobs that are sustaining society, as has the belief that if individuals work hard then they will be rewarded with the things that society values most: a good job, money, opportunities, and power. As a social ideal, meritocracy focuses on the notion of an independent spirit fortified with self-determination, while ignoring the myriad ways that an unequal social structure interferes with a good work ethic. Meritocracy makes the individual responsible for the social problems that shrink opportunities to be successful, while relieving governmental policies and politicians of their accountability. Society assigns value to job categories such as unskilled, low skilled and skilled, setting up different opportunities and choices that are available for each category. Assigned as low value, unskilled and low-skilled workers must contend with low wages, unaffordable health care, low probability of advancement, and food and transportation insecurity. When accounting for race, gender, and ability in that same group, the available opportunities and choices lessen. The essential services deemed necessary to help society survive during the global pandemic include the unskilled and low-skilled employees of grocery stores, delivery and transit companies, as well as factories and distribution centers. While these services are deemed essential, the highly used phrases of "essential worker" and "hero" ignores that these are the same employees that were overworked, underpaid, and lacked health care (Rho, Brown, and Fremstad 2020) before the pandemic. During the pandemic, the phrases, as inspirational and motivational as they may seem, reflect a paradox in the economic system: How can one be essential, heroic, low-skilled, and underpaid?

Vitriol: a crisis of leadership

During times of change and crisis, strong, effective, and empathetic leadership is extremely important. Even when a nation is in chaos and fearful, an effective leader can unite citizens under a common cause. After September 11, 2001, the uniting cause was a national pride that extended across many divisions of politics, race, class, and ideologies. Then president George W. Bush attempted to calm fears and strengthen vulnerabilities by displaying important leadership characteristics such as integrity, confidence, empathy, emotional intelligence, and the ability to communicate. The success of his attempt can be debated. However, those leadership skills are now arguably missing from the United States' management of the global pandemic. As a result, harm through either illness, death, loss of job, loss of income, or any other unnamed but avoidable injury is inflicted on citizens by a new pathogen, coupled with the lack of a coherent and cohesive federal response. The negligence of leadership is contributing to structural violence in the United States.

At the height of the first wave of the spread of the novel coronavirus, President Trump used language that compared the global pandemic to war. Consistent with this narrative were statements made at various news briefings and other events that spoke to his being a wartime president, with the novel coronavirus as the "enemy" we are fighting. In mid-March, after declaring a national emergency, when there were over 6,400 confirmed cases of infection and over 100 deaths (COVID-19 Dashboard), Mr. Trump announced, "One day, we'll be standing possibly up here and say we won" (Brady 2020a). Seven days later, when there were more than 53,500 confirmed cases of infection and over 1,000 deaths (COVID-19 Dashboard), Mr. Trump referred to the global pandemic as "a historic battle of an invisible enemy" (Brady 2020b). In early May, when confirmed cases reached over 1.2 million and deaths were over 73,000 (COVID-19 Dashboard), Mr. Trump conceded that this is the

> worst attack we've ever had. This is worse than Pearl Harbor. This is worse than the World Trade Center. There's never been an attack like this. And it should have never happened. It could have been stopped at the source. It could have been stopped in China.
>
> *(Oval Office 2020)*

In addition, he used wartime measures to combat the "invisible enemy" such as closing borders, restricting travel, and utilizing the Defense Production Act to compel factories to mass produce emergency supplies (Abutaleb et al. 2020). As a "wartime" president leading the charge against an "invisible enemy," he failed to do the most important job of the commander in chief: provide soldiers on the front line with the necessary ammunition to be victorious. Instead, he incited chaos and confusion amongst the ranks, rendering essential workers, medical staff, and citizens at large vulnerable to a pathogen wreaking havoc on the world.

President Trump and other government officials consistently contradicted their narrative of a well-planned war by their actions and words. For example, in early March, Mr. Trump toured the CDC and announced to reporters, "Anybody who wants a test will get a test" (White House Briefing Statement 2020). This statement was not true when it was uttered and did not become true for at least a few months, depending on the state. In late April, Vice President Mike Pence, who also leads the White House's coronavirus task force, toured the Mayo Clinic without wearing a mask, although they are required to enter the facility (Carlisle 2020). During that time, the United States had surpassed the one million mark for confirmed infections and had over 58,000 deaths (COVID-19 Dashboard). Effective leaders communicate messages consistently with their words and actions. Inconsistent and contradictory messages create confusion. In a politically polarized environment, the intention of the message is sidelined and the message itself becomes a smaller battle in the larger war. Polls showed that Republicans more than Democrats were influenced by the president's reactions and dismissiveness, so much so that they refused to take the coronavirus seriously, change travel plans, and follow social distancing guidelines (Abutaleb et al. 2020). In the context of a global pandemic, inconsistent messaging harms citizens, and a politically polarized environment exploits them to participate in their own mass contamination and murder.

Conclusion

The novel coronavirus crisis provides a sociological perspective of the many facets of a global pandemic. Beyond the medical implications of a new pathogen, it is highlighting the social illnesses already inflicting violence on citizens. A slow and uncoordinated federal response heightened the violence, while messages of confusion and contradiction deepened its impact. This combination solidified the United States as the country with the most confirmed cases of infection and deaths (COVID-19 Dashboard). The United States actively projects and works to protect its reputation across the globe as having a good infrastructure. An incompetent and incoherent federal response to a global crisis challenged and weakened that reputation. Mired in political polarization, ineffective or inadequate efforts to slow the spread of the novel coronavirus have harmed many citizens. The harm has been simultaneous, unequally distributed, and caused by negligence.

In its simplest explanation, structural violence is inflicted by policies, practices, and ordinary daily rituals mandated by a social structure or social institution. Structural violence prevents citizens from meeting their basic needs. It is less visible than physical violence, but it can be just as deadly. The harm from structural violence is subtle and is often overlooked. When it results in death, the cause is linked to the physical reason, such as being infected by the novel coronavirus, rather than assigning blame to the social structure for the lack of testing and medical supplies, fueling racial stereotypes, misinformation from government agencies, and deficient financial support for low-income citizens. Because deficiency in the social structure is common and expected, citizens blame each other and not the social structure that contributes to their harm. As a novel pathogen continues to elude top experts in the scientific and medical communities, its social impact has displayed stark inequalities and misguided ideologies. The structural violence inflicted on citizens as a result of the politicization of a global pandemic continues to threaten lives, especially the most vulnerable in society.

References

Abutaleb, Yasmeen, Josh Dawsey, Ellen Nakashima, and Greg Miller. 2020. "The U.S. Was Beset by Denial and Dysfunction as the Coronavirus Raged." *The Washington Post.* www.washingtonpost.com/national-security/2020/04/04/coronavirus-government-dysfunction/?arc404=true&itid=lk_inline_manual_11.

Allyn, Bobby, and Barbara Sprunt. 2020. "Poll: As Coronavirus Spreads, Fewer Americans See Pandemic As A Real Threat." *NPR, Special Series: The Coronavirus Crisis.* www.npr.org/2020/03/17/816501871/poll-as-coronavirus-spreads-fewer-americans-see-pandemic-as-a-real-threat/.

Baldwin, Richard, and Beatrice Weder di Mauro. 2020. "Economics in the Time of COVID-19." *VOX, CEPR Policy Portal.* https://voxeu.org/content/economics-time-covid-19.

Blum, Dinur, Stacy L. Smith, and Adam G. Sanford. 2021. "Toxic Wild West Syndrome: Individual Rights vs. Community Needs." In *COVID – 19: Social Consequences and Cultural Adaptations*, edited by J. Michael Ryan, 122–33. London: Routledge.

Bosman, Julie, Sabrina Tavernise, and Mike Baker. 2020. "Why These Protesters Aren't Staying Home for Coronavirus Orders." *The New York Times.* www.nytimes.com/2020/04/23/us/coronavirus-protesters.html.

Brady, James. 2020a. "Remarks by President Trump, Vice President Pence, and Members of the Coronavirus Task Force in Press Briefing." *The White House.* The United States Government, March 17. www.whitehouse.gov/briefings-statements/remarks-president-trump-vice-president-pence-members-coronavirus-task-force-press-briefing-4/.

———. 2020b. "Remarks by President Trump, Vice President Pence, and Members of the Coronavirus Task Force in Press Briefing." *The White House.* The United States Government, March 24. www.whitehouse.gov/briefings-statements/remarks-president-trump-vice-president-pence-members-coronavirus-task-force-press-briefing-10/.

Carlisle, Madeleine. 2020. "Ignoring Policy, Mike Pence Tours Mayo Clinic Without Mask." *Time.* https://time.com/5828743/mayo-clinic-pence-mask/.

Centers for Disease Control and Prevention. 2020. "How to Make Cloth Face Coverings to Help Slow Spread." www.cdc.gov/coronavirus/2019-ncov/prevent-getting-sick/how-to-make-cloth-face-covering.html.

Chiang, Pamela P. 2021. "Anti-Asian Racism, Responses, and the Impact on Asian Americans' Lives: A Social-Ecological Perspective." In *COVID-19: Social Consequences and Cultural Adaptations*, edited by J. Michael Ryan, 215–29. London: Routledge.

"COVID-19 Dashboard." Johns Hopkins University and Medicine Coronavirus Resource Center. https://coronavirus.jhu.edu/map.html.

Dewey, Jodie. 2021. "The Solution Is the Problem: What a Pandemic Can Reveal About Policing." In *COVID-19: Social Consequences and Cultural Adaptations*, edited by J. Michael Ryan, 61–71. London: Routledge.

Fowler, Luke, and Steve Utych. 2020. "Who Is Most Likely to Voluntarily Comply with COVID-19 Public Health Recommendations?" *The Blue Review*. www.boisestate.edu/bluereview/who-is-most-likely-to-voluntarily-comply-with-covid-19-public-health-recommendations/.

Galtung, Johan. 1969. "Violence, Peace, and Peace Research." *Journal of Peace Research* 6 (3): 167–91.

Garza, Alejandro de la. 2020. "For Black Men, Homemade Masks May Be a Risk All Their Own." *Time*. https://time.com/5821250/homemask-masks-racial-stereotypes/.

Jacobs, Andrew, Matt Richtel, and Mike Baker. 2020. "'At War with No Ammo': Doctors Say Shortage of Protective Gear Is Dire." *The New York Times*. www.nytimes.com/2020/03/19/health/coronavirus-masks-shortage.html.

Kraemer, Moritz U. G., Chia-Hung Yang, Bernardo Gutierrez, Chieh-Hsi Wu, Brennan Klein, David M. Pigott, Louis du Plessis, et al. (2020). "The Effect of Human Mobility and Control Measures on the COVID-19 Epidemic in China." *Science* 368 (6490): 493–97.

Lee, Bandy. 2016. "Causes and Cures VII: Structural Violence." *Aggression and Violent Behavior* 28: 109–14.

Meeker, James K. 2021. "The Political Nightmare of the Plague: The Ironic Resistance of Anti-Quarantine Protesters." In *COVID-19: Social Consequences and Cultural Adaptations*, edited by J. Michael Ryan, 109–21. London: Routledge.

Nanda, Serena. 2021. "Inequalities and COVID-19." In *COVID-19: Global Pandemic, Societal Responses, Ideological Solutions*, edited by J. Michael Ryan, 109–23. London: Routledge.

Natividad, Ivan. 2020. "Among the Reasons COVID-19 Is Worse for Black Communities: Police Violence." *Berkeley News*, April 23. https://news.berkeley.edu/2020/04/23/one-reason-covid-19-is-worse-for-black-communities-police-violence/.

Oval Office. 2020. "Remarks by President Trump at Signing of a Proclamation in Honor of National Nurses Day." *The White House*. The United States Government. May 6. www.whitehouse.gov/briefings-statements/remarks-president-trump-signing-proclamation-honor-national-nurses-day/.

Painter, Marcus, and Tian Qui. 2020. "Political Beliefs and Compliance with Social Distancing Orders." *VOX, CEPR Policy Portal*. https://voxeu.org/article/political-beliefs-and-compliance-social-distancing-orders.

Peters, Jeremy W., and Michael Grynbaum. 2020. "How Right-Wing Pundits Are Covering Coronavirus." *The New York Times*. www.nytimes.com/2020/03/11/us/politics/coronavirus-conservative-media.html.

"Remarks by President Trump After Tour of the Centers for Disease Control and Prevention." 2020. *The White House*. The United States Government, March 7. www.whitehouse.gov/briefings-statements/remarks-president-trump-tour-centers-disease-control-prevention-atlanta-ga/.

Rho, Hye, Hayley Brown, and Shawn Fremstad. 2020. "A Basic Demographic Profile of Workers in Frontline Industries." *Center for Economic and Policy Research*. https://cepr.net/a-basic-demographic-profile-of-workers-in-frontline-industries/.

Ryan, J. Michael. 2021. "The SARS-CoV-2 Virus and the COVID-19 Pandemic." In *COVID-19: Social Consequences and Cultural Adaptations*, edited by J. Michael Ryan, 9–19. London: Routledge.

Shafer, Ronald G. 2020. "Spain Hated Being Linked to the Deadly 1918 Flu Pandemic. Trump's 'Chinese Virus' Label Echoes That." *The Washington Post*. www.washingtonpost.com/history/2020/03/23/spanish-flu-chinese-virus-trump/.

Smiley, C., and D. Fakunle. 2016. "From 'Brute' to 'Thug:' The Demonization and Criminalization of Unarmed Black Male Victims in America." *Journal of Human Behavior in The Social Environment* 26 (3–4): 350–66.

Taylor, Derrick Bryson. 2020. "For Black Men, Fear That Masks Will Invite Racial Profiling." *The New York Times.* www.nytimes.com/2020/04/14/us/coronavirus-masks-racism-african-americans.html.

U.S. Bureau of Labor Statistics. 2019. "Table 1. Workers Who Could Work at Home, Did Work at Home, and Were Paid for Work at Home, by Selected Characteristics, Averages for the Period 2017–2018." www.bls.gov/news.release/flex2.t01.htm.

"World Health Organization Novel Coronavirus (2019-nCoV) Situation Report-1." January 21, 2020. www.who.int/docs/default-source/coronaviruse/situation-reports/20200121-sitrep-1-2019-ncov.pdf?sfvrsn=20a99c10_4.

"World Health Organization Novel Coronavirus (2019-nCoV) Situation Report-3." January 23, 2020. www.who.int/docs/default-source/coronaviruse/situation-reports/20200123-sitrep-3-2019-ncov.pdf?sfvrsn=d6d23643_8.

20

HIGH RISK OR LOW WORTH?

A few practical and philosophical COVID-19 issues surrounding the isolation of high-risk senior women

Lynnette Porter

Family folklore, backed by research, suggests that seniors who have retired and have nothing to look forward to, interest them daily, or connect them with a social network fade away as they become isolated from the people and activities important to them. Seniors who live alone may feel lonely, ignored, or unimportant in their isolation. Over time, they may become "invisible" because they are not actively part of others' daily lives. "Old age," for many seniors, implies social isolation and loneliness, likely leading to an earlier death.

The US stay-at-home or quarantine orders to prevent the spread of COVID-19 not only exacerbated concerns for isolated seniors but made longer-term self-quarantine likely for the many vulnerable-to-coronavirus older adults who could or should not join younger, healthier Americans in "reopening" the country once the official quarantine ended. Although *quarantine* is typically defined as enforced isolation from everyone else, usually to prevent the spread of disease, the quarantine as a result of state stay-at-home orders offered a few loopholes against total isolation indoors. Employees who were needed to provide "essential services," as defined by each state, could go to work. Everyone could leave home to buy groceries, fill prescriptions, or get medical assistance, for example. High-risk individuals, in particular, were highly recommended to stay indoors at all times, have food or medicine delivered, and have no contact with delivery or service persons. Everyone was reminded to sanitize any package coming into the home's "safe space" and immediately to use hand sanitizer or wash hands thoroughly after touching a potentially contaminated surface. Going outdoors for exercise was allowed if individuals wore masks and, preferably, came in contact with no one but the people with whom they live. High-risk seniors living in care facilities were locked down inside; no visitors were permitted, and residents could not leave their rooms. Even when stay-at-home orders officially expired, many high-risk seniors in care facilities remained in lockdown, and even those living at home often continued to self-quarantine under the same restrictive conditions. In a politicized society seeking to return to "normal" as quickly as possible, seniors inadvertently instigated questions about the value of human life and the "worth" of individuals during a pandemic.

Within my small circle of close family members and friends, seven women and I either fit the Centers for Disease Control's (CDC's) March 2020 definition of "high-risk" or "vulnerable" people most likely to have debilitating or deadly complications from COVID-19 or are current or future caregivers of someone who does. Specifically, a high-risk/vulnerable person is 65 years old or older, someone living in a long-term care facility, or anyone with an underlying medical condition. The long list of underlying medical conditions includes lung diseases (e.g., asthma, chronic obstructive pulmonary disease [COPD], lung cancer), serious heart conditions, compromised immune system, severe obesity, diabetes, liver disease, and chronic kidney disease (requiring dialysis) (CDC 2020). In this chapter, "high-risk" refers to seniors in general or specifically the women in my group who are at high risk of suffering complications or dying from COVID-19 because of age and underlying medical condition. Tables 20.1 and 20.2 introduce the women whose quarantine stories are included in this chapter.

As these women's COVID-19 quarantine stories explain, even people who live and safely interact with others every day may keenly feel the physical or emotional effects of being separated from loved ones not in quarantine with them. Although this is a very small group, their comments provide unique perspectives on social isolation even among privileged (e.g., White, middle-class) women. As both a participant in this group's COVID-19 discussions and chapter author, I recognize my bias. Nonetheless, I am in a unique position of reporting the group's anecdotal information in light of previous research about social isolation among seniors. Their comments provide interesting insights into individual experiences within the much larger US pandemic experience.

TABLE 20.1 Individuals in My "Study Group" Defined as "High Risk" for Complications or Death from COVID-19

Name	Age	US State of Residence	Underlying Chronic Medical Condition	Description of Residence
Janet	67	Texas	High blood pressure	Lives with spouse in a single-family house
Joanne	69	Florida	Cancer (survivor)	Lives alone in a house
Lynnette	63	Florida	Cancer	Lives alone in an apartment
Lynn	73	Florida	COPD	Lives with five family members in a single-family house but has her own suite
Marian	92	North Dakota	High blood pressure	Lives in a single-occupant room in an adult care facility

TABLE 20.2 Current or Future Caregivers of High-Risk Individuals in My "Study Group"

Name	US State of Residence	Relationship with High-Risk Individual
Donna	Florida	With Marian: Daughter, legally designated as one to make decisions regarding future care
Jen	Florida	With Lynn: Daughter, likely to be a future caregiver With Lynnette: Friend, legally designated as one to make decisions regarding future care
Sandy	Florida	With Joanne: Daughter, likely to be a future caregiver

Anecdotal information comes from conversations with each woman between March and June 2020, during a state's mandatory stay-at-home order and gradual reopening. These women's comments reflect concerns about quarantine and answers to these four questions: How can social isolation affect high-risk seniors? What is the relationship between social isolation and loneliness? What may be done to mitigate high-risk seniors' feelings of isolation and/or loneliness? How are high-risk seniors perceived by the rest of society during a pandemic? Because research about social isolation includes too many studies to be discussed in this chapter, only a few representative ones highlight the relationships among social isolation, loneliness, and health.

How can social isolation affect high-risk seniors?

A 2012 *Journal of Primary Prevention* article explains the prevalence of mental and physical health problems when, in particular, homebound seniors lack accessible social networks. More than a decade before the COVID-19 pandemic, up to 43% of community-dwelling seniors experienced social isolation, defined as occurring when an individual "lacks a sense of belonging socially, lacks engagement with others, [and] has a minimal number of [fulfilling, high-quality] social contacts" (Nicholson 2012, 137). Some possible physical effects of isolation include a greater possibility of heart disease or stroke and an increase in cognitive decline (152). The percentage of seniors experiencing social isolation in 2020 likely is far higher than that cited in this study. Even within my group, because of quarantine, all high-risk women were physically cut off from important people in our social network.

Sandy felt "happy" about the stay-at-home order as a way to protect her mother (Joanne) from exposure to COVID-19, even though staying at home kept Joanne from a social network of retirees. Sandy explained,

> I don't believe our citizens or our government took [COVID-19] seriously enough. I was able to convince my mom to stay home before the

stay-at-home order officially began, but she was also getting pressure from some of her friends in a retirees group to still go out to their monthly dinners. So, the stay-at-home orders not only validated my concern, but gave me (false) hope that we, as a nation, could effectively flatten the curve.

Although Joanne was physically isolated, she (as well as all high-risk women in my group) maintained virtual contact with those dearest to them.

Although Lynnette talked or texted with loved ones during the quarantine, she mourned her loss of physical freedom. Prior to the pandemic, she frequently visited close friends or went to theme parks, restaurants, theatres, and beaches with them. During the stay-at-home order, Lynnette lost these opportunities for in-person social activities. Yet, once the stay-at-home order was lifted, Lynnette, unlike the majority of her friends/family, was encouraged to stay home to stay safe – and even others' careful return to public spaces posed a higher risk of transmitting the virus to her. Whereas many people mentally "survive" quarantine by reminding themselves that it is temporary and looking forward to next year – or whenever they believe COVID-19 will be under control – Lynnette, in the final stage of terminal cancer, is not expected to enjoy a post-pandemic world. Losing the ability to spend time in person with loved ones is, therefore, even more devastating than might be expected.

Despite Lynn living with family members during quarantine, she still felt socially isolated from children and grandchildren who do not live in her household. She also questioned her role within the household because she no longer grocery shops for the family, a primary way she felt useful to her family and connected with the community. Additionally, shopping several times a week was a form of exercise no longer open to her during quarantine; walking around the house is not as stimulating as seeing different places and casually talking with strangers. Although she stays engaged with her family, she often feels "irrelevant" because of social separation and what she sees as a diminution of her role. In addition, she sometimes feels socially isolated because she, daughter Jen, and grandchildren have different interests and needs, often because of generation gaps in shared knowledge or experience. Although Lynn loves her family and feels loved by them, she may still feel lonely or socially isolated during quarantine.

Similarly, Janet felt socially isolated when she was "stuck indoors" for weeks. Even though she was quarantined with her husband, she missed teaching piano lessons in her home and frequently visiting her children and grandchildren. A typical pre-COVID-19 week involved going out to eat and heading to the cinema. Without these activities, she had "nothing to look forward to." When the stay-at-home order was lifted, some high-risk people, such as Janet, thus decided to take what they perceive as a manageable risk to go for a drive, pick up a carryout meal, or enjoy a family reunion in a public park – while staying the recommended six feet apart or wearing a mask.

Although it is too early to identify new long-term health problems as a result of the stay-at-home order or ongoing self-quarantine, short-term depression or heightened emotions reported by Lynnette, Janet, and Lynn indicate that an extended quarantine without ways to help alleviate persistent negative thoughts/feelings may be cause for concern about longer-term mental and physical health.

What is the relationship between social isolation and loneliness?

Loneliness and social isolation cannot be conflated, although high-risk seniors may experience both. Whereas *social isolation* includes a lack of social connections and activities, *loneliness* has been defined as "the perception or feeling that one is without meaningful social connections" (Taylor 2020, 141). Harry Owen Taylor's study of the effects of social isolation from "adult children, other family members, friends, living alone, being unmarried, and not participating in social activities" used data from a 2014 Wave of the Health and Retirement Study (141). In this study, "older adults" were defined as being 50 years or older. Taylor concluded that the greater the amount of social isolation/higher number of combined factors leads to greater loneliness. Taylor did not measure the quality of relationships and noted that social isolation from adult children was not a key factor when older adults have strained or negative relationships with their children (146). Positive, supportive relationships between older adults and their children may change the degree of loneliness and social isolation when mutually loving parents and children are physically separated. As Taylor (and other researchers) noted, loneliness and social isolation are associated with increased likelihood of mortality, health morbidities, and poorer self-rated mental or physical health (141).

In my group, all high-risk senior women who have adult children and the three women who now or in the future will care for a high-risk mother have positive, emotionally enriching parent-child relationships. Loneliness was described by Donna, Marian, Lynn, Jen, and Janet as being related to specific family members, rather than a general feeling of loneliness as a result of social isolation. Donna and Marian, for example, both expressed loneliness because of their separation, even though they talk on the phone to each other and have social interactions with others daily.

When that loved one is a very young child, the lost bonding time is difficult or impossible to make up. Watching a video of a toddler playing is very different from playing with the child. Jen, who is not at high risk, nonetheless expressed frustration and loneliness in being unable to visit her sister and one-year-old and five-year-old nephews, with whom she is very close and previously visited at least once a week for several hours. Lynn also commented sadly that she missed being with her grandchildren. Janet felt lonely when separated from a young grandchild who frequently had stayed overnight or with whom she shared "play dates." Because very young children may not remember the relatives they have not seen for months, their uncertainty or shyness about reuniting with "strangers" can be a devastating loss for the adults who love them.

As Kelly Rhea MacArthur (2021, this volume) notes,

> Scholars across academic disciplines agree that social relationships are at the center of what defines humanity, as well as what presents the biggest threat to well-being. Distancing during the coronavirus pandemic presents an even larger threat to public health if it creates patterns of social interaction that constrain relationships indefinitely.

Until a vaccine and/or other preventive or treatment measures prove efficacious in stopping the spread of COVID-19, older family members, in particular, are likely to face those indefinite constraints in their interactions with loved ones. Extended quarantines or social distancing may lead to longer-term health concerns in my study group, as well as in the larger senior population.

What may be done to mitigate high-risk seniors' feelings of isolation and/or loneliness?

Pragmatic strategies for making high-risk seniors feel not only remembered but also valued and for encouraging high-focus activities to even temporarily take their mind off COVID-19 can involve individual or group activities. Technology offers a range of communication experiences but, more importantly, helps connect high-risk seniors with the "outside" world. Other, longer-term strategies for helping high-risk seniors to control more aspects of their life may become more important during self-quarantine as states reopen.

Mitigating social isolation with technology

During states' stay-at-home orders resulting in a national quarantine for all but those deemed essential workers, television commercials and public service announcements began promoting the idea that families and friends separated during the quarantine can stay social through technology. Ads showed people laughing together as they video chatted. Social media touted Zoom movie nights or cocktail parties that brought people together virtually. Special events, such as the Together At Home concert spearheaded by Lady Gaga, brought together musicians and singers broadcasting from their homes (Watercutter 2020). In short, technology – whether permitting interactive participation or passive viewing – put the "together" in "we're all in this together." Whereas technology has been promoted as a way to minimize, if not eliminate, loneliness or social isolation during the pandemic, its benefits greatly vary among individuals who may be limited in their choice or use of technology; as well, not everybody may want to participate in online or multimedia communication.

A Pew study reported 42% of seniors have smartphones and 67% have Internet access (which may give them the opportunity to video chat, text, and post messages or media to social media accounts, as well as phone others). Yet, the possibilities for smartphone communication during quarantine were quickly put into perspective: Only about 25% of seniors feel "confident about using electronics to go online" (Poon and Holder 2020). Whereas some high-risk seniors learned how to work with new-to-them devices or software during the pandemic, others, of course, lacked access to technology or someone who can show them how to use it effectively. Some technologies also are not well suited to seniors with poor hearing or eyesight, arthritis, or other mobility problems (Poon and Holder 2020). These issues are commonly reported during "normal" times, but COVID-19 underscored the problems that many high-risk seniors face when confronted with an immediate need to use technology as a lifeline to reach the people they need in an emergency, especially doctors, delivery persons, and family members, or to ease loneliness and feelings of isolation.

Lack of digital communication was not an overwhelming concern for the women in my group. Almost everyone embraced at least some online or multi-media communication, as might be expected of people in their socioeconomic class. As well, Jen, Donna, Sandy, and Lynnette are university professors with more online experience because of their teaching or administrative roles. Janet's children own a computer support business and help companies manage their hardware and software needs. As a result, these high-risk women felt extremely comfortable using technology, possibly because they, unlike most COVID-vulnerable seniors, had readily available resource experts who encourage them to use a variety of technologies.

Only Marian chose not to connect by computer and turned down Donna's offer of setting her up with a laptop. Marian confided that she did not have any desire to go online. Instead, she prefers daily voice-only conversations with her sister and daughter. The every-afternoon phone call between Marian and Donna was established years before COVID-19. Marian explained, "we've done it so many years I take it for granted" but added "I'd like to see her." Prior to the pandemic, Donna flew to North Dakota to visit her mother for weeks in the summer and days during holiday breaks. They spent as much time together as possible, whether in Marian's room or during meals in a communal dining room. When the quarantined care center prohibited visitors and confined seniors to their room, Donna worried that her mother would indefinitely feel as if she were "in prison." Phone calls help maintain their connection but cannot replace in-person visits, which continue to be in limbo until COVID-19 is controlled.

The care center also helps mitigate seniors' loneliness, albeit in a limited way. Staff members bring meals and check on Marian a few times a day, but those kinds of encounters are superficial enough to be classified as casual social encounters – which can help alleviate social isolation more than loneliness. However, Marian considers the activities coordinator to be a friend; they had shared personal conversations prior to the lockdown and enjoy each other's company. About once a day, the activities coordinator stops by to chat a few minutes with Marian. The hardest part of dealing with COVID-19 is the "uncertainty of it all," and Marian wonders how long the pandemic will last. A personalized daily visit even lasting just a few minutes can help alleviate Marian's loneliness until she can connect with family members by phone.

Other individuals in my group tend to use some devices or services more often or for specific purposes. They prefer to rapidly text messages about everyday topics (e.g., how they are feeling, what they watched on Netflix, what is on the news); phone important or time-sensitive information; make Facebook posts (mostly photos, reposts of others' memes or texts, or status changes) to keep family and friends up to date, entertained, or enlightened; and set up less frequent Zoom meetings for adding a more personal touch to conversations or holding family reunions with three or more participants. Nevertheless, as Virginia Satir, one of the founding mothers of family therapy, emphasized, it takes 12 hugs a day for people to thrive, and nonsexual human touch can provide mental health benefits (Hartwell-Walker 2020). After being home alone for two months, Lynnette wondered if she would ever be hugged again, and Lynn and Janet especially missed hugging their grandchildren. Touching a screen or waving at an image is not the same as hugging a loved one.

High-focus activities

Without ways to break up prolonged social isolation, high-risk individuals may suffer more severe health effects. Researcher Nicholas Nicholson noted that seniors with poor social connections might resort to heavy drinking, poor eating habits, smoking, and a sedentary lifestyle (140). To maintain seniors' mental and physical health, Nicholson cautioned healthcare professionals to look for signs of isolation among seniors, especially those confined to home or a facility for long periods of time.

However, during the COVID-19 pandemic, healthcare professionals already are often overwhelmed by the health crisis or underemployed because medical facilities (at least temporarily) stopped elective procedures and regular appointments. During this pandemic, healthcare professionals may be unavailable to monitor high risk seniors' feelings of isolation and resulting detrimental changes to behavior or health. As a result, family and friends – even those not designated specifically as caregivers – may find themselves taking on that role more often during a pandemic. One way to engage high-risk seniors during the pandemic is to suggest events or provide activities they can look forward to or that help them focus on something other than COVID-19.

Most women in my group led more sedentary lives during the pandemic because they were limited to their homes, yards, or nearby vacant public spaces. During the stay-at-home orders, Sandy, Donna, and Jen shifted from working on campus to working at home. In addition, Jen had to monitor and assist three children with their online schoolwork. Thus, these women's high-focus activities most often involved computer work. Joanne, Janet, Lynn, and Marian are retired; Lynnette was on an academic sabbatical in spring 2020. These women needed something to help them pass the time safely and productively. Janet completed word puzzles and took up a new pastime – painting pictures. As soon as Lynn completed one jigsaw puzzle, she began another one. She equated completing puzzles as being her "job" during the pandemic, albeit one she enjoys. Joanne sewed masks as a useful pastime. Lynnette read one book after another, going through her library of books to read "someday" when she had more time. She also took advantage of free streaming entertainment, such as a weekly play made available on YouTube by the UK's National Theatre Live or a monthly art documentary that Exhibition on Screen showed on Facebook. (Unfortunately, these streamed events took place only during the national quarantine in the UK or US.) Janet, Lynn, and Lynnette often commented that they spent hours at a time focusing on their chosen "project," which made days seem to pass more quickly.

Stay-at-home orders permitted outdoor exercise, as long as social distance was maintained. The women in my group felt more positive and healthier when they could walk or garden outdoors. On sunny days, Lynnette walked a mile or more on sidewalks, through parking lots, or on paved paths to get out of the house but avoid people. She sometimes photographed flowers along the way as a way to focus only on that task and forget about everything else. Janet also enjoyed walking outdoors; the closest nature reserve was a mere 10-minute drive from home and provided solitary trails where she could enjoy nature. However, bad weather or malaise made staying indoors more desirable, and sometimes going for a walk just seemed too much trouble.

Despite attempting to maintain a daily routine, Janet, Lynnette, and Jen admitted to bingeing on something when they were bored in isolation or just needed a distraction from feeling overwhelmed. Jen spent a day catching up on episodes of a television serial, Janet sometimes turned to chocolate, and Lynnette enjoyed more wine than usual. Bingeing as a temporary high-focus activity became more common – even if what was binge-worthy was only a temporary focus. However, bingeing as a sedentary activity theoretically could become a problem if quarantine continues and no other activities seem available or desirable as a replacement.

Special events also give at-risk seniors something positive to anticipate and remind them that they have not been forgotten. During the state-mandated quarantine, media reported people drawing pictures or holding signs that could be seen through nursing home windows; neighbors sang or talked from a distance to seniors quarantined alone at home. Some musicians, storytellers, or artists continued to share their work with seniors remaining in quarantine after states began to reopen. As only one example, jazz musician Ethan Kogan and his friends formed M.A.S.Q. (Musicians Aiding Seniors in Quarantine) to play "free gigs in parking lots or outdoor spaces of nursing homes" in Chicago (Stevens 2020).

At times, special events fell into the "good intentions" category. Marian chuckled as she recalled a horse parade to entertain the seniors living in the care center.

Although she has never particularly been one to enjoy parades, she was persuaded to stand at the window to see the horse parade. As the appointed time came and went, Marian waited to see what would happen. Finally, the procession arrived – one horse, a Shetland pony, and a little girl walking with them. In hindsight, the horse parade was memorable primarily for what it was not. Nevertheless, it offered something different, if not necessarily special, for Marian to do one afternoon, and Donna shared a laugh when her mother told her the story.

Greater autonomy even when continued self-quarantine is recommended

A practical solution that gives high-risk persons more autonomy during the pandemic requires them to decide how much risk they are willing or have to assume in order to break the monotony of quarantine and if that level of risk may negatively affect others. Lynn or Lynnette, for example, must determine whether they should participate in family activities after the official stay-at-home order expired. As Jen explained, she cannot take responsibility for her mother's or friend's decisions regarding activities in which she, her children, or her husband are involved; it is important for both high-risk women to retain control over their life, even when family members/close friends may prefer them to stay safely at home. Undoubtedly, Lynn and/or Lynnette may decide it is not wise to venture to theme parks or theatres when everyone else can go. Jen recognizes that they may feel left out when they do not feel comfortable assuming risks that others can more easily accept. However, she noted that either or both of these high-risk individuals can participate in lower-risk activities with her family, such as a backyard barbecue with few people who have been self-quarantining at home or a trip to the beach where social distancing from "outsiders" can be maintained.

Jen, Jen's family, and Sandy self-quarantine for several days after leaving home for activities like shopping, doctor or dental appointments, or recreation in public spaces. Sandy diligently stays at home for 14 days before she visits her mother, whereas Jen, whose outside activities increased when children's or her appointments had to be made up after stay-at-home orders ended, separates higher-risk activities with two or more days at home. Everyone consistently wears masks in public and uses hand sanitizer frequently to help minimize the risk of coming in contact with the virus. Despite these measures, high-risk individuals could decide to stay away from loved ones until they feel the risk of meeting in person is low enough or is outweighed by the emotional need to see them masked face to masked face. Negotiating risk and sharing information about activities away from home can help high-risk individuals make informed choices about the level of risk they are willing to assume.

Of course, such autonomy is not possible in places like senior care centers, hospitals, or nursing homes, which remained locked down from visitation long after stay-at-home orders ended. Although many immunocompromised individuals have been restricted in their social activities and thousands of seniors resided in nursing homes or managed care facilities long before COVID-19, the number of high-risk individuals needing to stay at home/within a facility increased considerably during the pandemic. Social isolation as a result of COVID-19 may extend far beyond the phased reopening of states and include a larger permanent or long-term population of quarantined seniors. Finding ways to engage high-risk seniors is an ongoing task.

How are high-risk seniors perceived by the rest of society during a pandemic?

Yet another factor may play a uniquely important role in socially isolating seniors in general, but especially those who are at higher risk of COVID-19. Philosophical/ethical issues merged with political concerns during the US stay-at-home orders, and many of these issues involved high-risk seniors. More Americans publicly questioned who should live – and who should die – when the amount of medical equipment, number of hospital beds, number of vaccines, etc., is limited and not everyone can be assisted at the same time in the same geographic area. No matter how valuable individual seniors are valued by their loved ones, how seniors as a generation are perceived in the US may determine their public "worth" or "value."

Veteran newsman Ted Koppel (2020), age 80 when he interviewed doctors and bioethicists during the first surge of COVID-19 in hot spot New York City, confronted this ethical dilemma during a *CBS Sunday Morning* segment. Koppel described a horrific scenario to his interviewees: Koppel and a 25-year-old both have COVID-19 in the same hospital, both are healthy for their respective ages, both require a ventilator to live, but there is only one available ventilator. Who gets it? Predictably, the medical experts refused to say outright what Koppel concluded for his audience. Unless the 25-year-old had other health problems, age would be the deciding factor. Of course, not every medical decision is limited to a dichotomous choice. Nonetheless, questions like this can add to high-risk seniors' anxiety about what would happen should they contract the virus and require extreme life-saving measures.

In response to media reports that state officials were meeting to decide how to distribute health care, Peter Breen (vice president and counsel to the Thomas More Society) said that the "horrific idea of withholding care from someone because they are elderly or disabled is untenable and represents a giant step in the devaluation of each and every human life." Furthermore, as a published legal memorandum pointed out, rationing health care based on age or disability goes against federal law (Barnes 2020). Nonetheless, such public discussion about seniors' right to health care is a troubling trend.

Additionally, some politicians' and protesters' rhetoric about reopening the US economy focused on sacrificing the elderly, in particular, to speed up the recovery process. If COVID-19 could not be contained quickly enough, the argument went, and more people would become exposed to the virus when states reopened, undoubtedly the virus would be more easily transmitted to the most vulnerable. More seniors, many who suffer from chronic illnesses, would inevitably come into contact with virus carriers and die from COVID-19. Some people protesting a lengthy stay-at-home order carried signs indicating that seniors should be sacrificed so that more people could return to work and help improve the stalled economy. During a live broadcast of a protest in Nashville, for example, a woman standing behind the newscaster carried a sign proclaiming "Sacrifice the Weak" and "Re-open TN" (Evon 2020). Online debate ensued whether the protester, who was not identified or interviewed, was being sarcastic or serious. A California city board member was quoted as saying that if COVID-19 was allowed to run its course unchecked,

> We would have significant loss of life, we would lose many elderly, that would reduce burdens in our defunct Social Security System, health care cost . . . once the wave subsided – [a greater number of deaths would] make jobs available for others and it would also free up housing.
>
> *(Dillon 2020)*

Some politicians in more prominent positions also claimed that the oldest generation would (or should) be willing to sacrifice themselves so that their children and grandchildren could enjoy a faster economic recovery. Texas Lt. Governor Dan Patrick prominently voiced a "hypothetical deal . . . [that] would involve restarting the economy while possibly sacrificing those most vulnerable to covid-19, including older Americans." During a discussion with Fox News' Tucker Carlson, Patrick considered the pertinent question, "As a senior citizen, are you willing take a chance on your survival in exchange for keeping the America that all America loves for your children and grandchildren?" He replied, "And if that's the exchange, I'm all in" (Coughlin and Yoquinto 2020). Social Darwinism was posited as a way to protect the economic future of the fittest. In a political cost/benefit analysis, high-risk people, including but not limited to seniors, seemed to cost too much.

Not only the fact that these sentiments were prominently covered in national news but that they even existed could make vulnerable seniors worry about their safety. In addition, these sentiments further emotionally and socially isolate seniors from at least a percentage of Americans who really considered whether the oldest citizens were worth saving during extreme medical and economic crises.

Joanne's approach toward COVID-19 as Florida reopened perhaps provides the best advice for high-risk individuals who can choose if or how they can leave the relative safety of quarantine: "[C]ontinuing to stay home as much as possible is very important for my protection against COVID-19. . . . [I]t is very important to continue wearing a mask whenever it is necessary for me to venture out." She reiterates that everyone must remember that "all of the people who are going out without masks are not helping to stop the spread of the virus. They are certainly not thinking about their own health or the health of their community." Instead of believing in the previous mantra of national quarantine, "we're all in this together," high-risk seniors, their loved ones, and their caregivers more realistically understand that they have to look out for themselves, not only to avoid contracting COVID-19 but also from the deleterious effects of longer-term quarantine.

This stance seems not only appropriate but also increasingly necessary as parts of the US attempt to recreate a "normal" pre-COVID-19 environment during the pandemic. As numbers of new COVID-19 cases rose in Florida in mid-June 2020, Governor Rick DeSantis reiterated, "We're not shutting down, we're gonna go forward, we're gonna continue to protect the most vulnerable" (Kennedy and Anderson 2020). That statement, in reality, becomes a directive to the vulnerable and those who care about and for them to bear the responsibility for isolating high-risk seniors against COVID-19. The rhetoric surrounding COVID-19 in the US provides a worrisome social barometer regarding the current and future status of seniors. Although individual high-risk seniors, especially in my group, are highly valued by their friends and family and deemed of high worth simply for who they are, seniors vulnerable to COVID-19 might worry that the public only sees them as high risk and, therefore, worth only a low investment of very limited resources.

References

Barnes, Patricia. 2020. "Groups Warn Against Basing Life and Death Decisions in COVID-19 Pandemic on Age or Disability." *Forbes*, March 24. Accessed May 29, 2020. www.forbes.com/sites/patriciagbarnes/2020/03/24/groups-warn-against-basing-life-and-death-decisions-in-the-covid-19-pandemic-on-age-and-disability/#31381a2a6576.

Centers for Disease Control. 2020. "People Who Are at Higher Risk for Severe Illness." Accessed May 20, 2020. www.cdc.gov/coronavirus/2019-ncov/need-extra-precautions/people-at-higher-risk.html.

Coughlin, Joseph, and Luke Bryant Yoquinto. 2020. "Many Parts of America Have Already Decided to Sacrifice the Elderly." *Washington Post*, April 13. Accessed May 1, 2020. www.washingtonpost.com/outlook/2020/04/13/many-parts-america-have-already-decided-sacrifice-elderly/.

Dillon, Nancy. 2020. "California Official Removed from Board After Saying COVID-19 Should Be Allowed to 'Fix' Society by Culling Elderly, Weak, and Homeless." *New York Daily News*, May 1. Accessed May 1, 2020. www.nydailynews.com/coronavirus/ny-calif-official-who-said-coronavirus-could-fix-society-may-lose-job-20200501-crcpsikwejbnvpahwo5racbdgm-story.html.

Donna. Conversation with author, May 21, 2020.

Evon, Dan. 2020. "Was a 'Sacrifice the Weak' Sign Shown at a COVID-19 'ReOpen Tennessee' Rally?" *Snopes*, April 24. Accessed June 1, 2020. www.snopes.com/fact-check/sacrifice-the-weak-sign-real/.

Hartwell-Walker, Elizabeth. 2020. "Social Distancing Doesn't Have to Keep You Socially Distanced." *PsychCentral*, March 21. Accessed June 15, 2020. https://psychcentral.com/blog/social-distancing-doesnt-have-to-keep-you-socially-distant/.

Janet. Conversation with author. June 7, 2020.

Jen. Conversation with author. June 3, 2020.

Joanne. Email to author. June 16, 2020.

Kennedy, John, and Zac Anderson. 2020. "Florida Gov. Ron DeSantis Pledges to Keep State Open, Downplays Rise in Coronavirus Cases." *USA Today*, 17 June. Accessed June 22. www.usatoday.com/story/news/nation/2020/06/17/florida-governor-ron-desantis-keeping-state-open-coronavirus-cases-rises/3210417001/.

Koppel, Ted. 2020. "Coronavirus: Who Lives? Who Dies?" *CBS Sunday Morning*. YouTube Video, 7:38, March 22. www.youtube.com/watch?v=bF_sEYafNnU.

Lynn. Conversation with author. June 5, 2020.

MacArthur, Kelly Rhea. 2021. "Treating Loneliness in the Aftermath of a Pandemic: Threat or Opportunity?" In *COVID-19: Global Pandemic, Societal Responses, Ideological Solutions*, edited by J. Michael Ryan, 197–208. London: Routledge.

Marian. Conversation with author. May 25, 2020.

Nicholson, Nicholas R. 2012. "A Review of Social Isolation: An Important but Underassessed Condition in Older Adults." *Journal of Primary Prevention* (33): 137–52. DOI: 10.1007/s10935-012-0271-2.

Poon, Linda, and Sarah Holder. 2020. "The 'New Normal' for Many Older Adults Is on the Internet." *Citylab*, May 6. Accessed June 9, 2020. www.citylab.com/life/2020/05/seniors-tech-online-resources-computer-video-coronavirus/610405/.

Sandy. Email to author. June 16, 2020.

Stevens, Heidi. 2020. "Column: 'Musicians Need Audiences, and People Need Music.' Jazz Drummer Creates Impromptu Band to Play Free Gigs in Senior Living Parking Lots." *Chicago Tribune*, June 12. Accessed June 21, 2020. www.chicagotribune.com/columns/heidi-stevens/ct-heidi-stevens-jazz-musicians-play-at-nursing-homes-covid-0611–20200612-k4exov4vnnghnafm7feenjtotq-story.html.

Taylor, Harry Owen. 2020. "Social Isolation's Influence on Loneliness Among Older Adults." *Clinical Social Work Journal* (48): 140–51. DOI: 10.1007/s10615-019-00737-9.

Watercutter, Angela. 2020. "Lady Gaga's *Together at Home* Raised $128 Million for COVID-19 Relief." *Wired*, April 20. Accessed April 22, 2020. www.wired.com/story/lady-gaga-covid-19-coronavirus-relief/.

INDEX

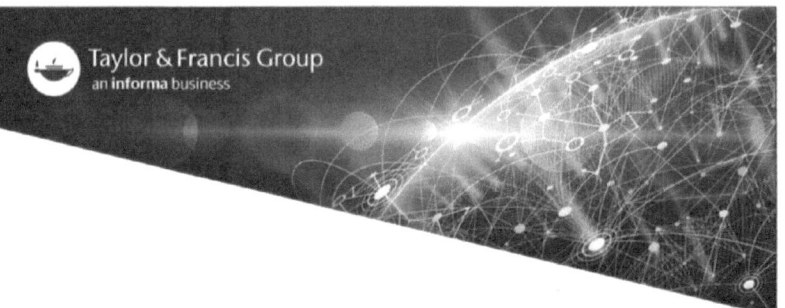
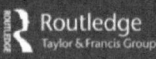
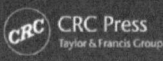